T0257464

Quality Control: Concepts and Applications

Quality Control: Concepts and Applications

Edited by **Theresa Heen**

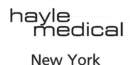

New York

Published by Hayle Medical,
30 West, 37th Street, Suite 612,
New York, NY 10018, USA
www.haylemedical.com

Quality Control: Concepts and Applications
Edited by Theresa Heen

International Standard Book Number: 978-1-63241-332-1 (Hardback)

Printed in the United States of America.

Contents

Preface

Quality control is a process that is used to ensure a certain level of quality in a product or service. Quality control is an important and growing aspect in every field of life. It might encompass whatever actions a business seems necessary to provide for the control and verification of certain characteristics of a product or service. With the improvement of technology, we come across new and complicated devices and methods in different fields. Quality control is necessary in all of those new techniques. Our objective was to gather information about quality control in various fields. This book aims at disseminating useful and practical knowledge about quality control in several fields such as quality control in radiology and clinical imaging, in energy, cosmetics, and in clinical laboratory medicine.

This book is a result of research of several months to collate the most relevant data in the field.

When I was approached with the idea of this book and the proposal to edit it, I was overwhelmed. It gave me an opportunity to reach out to all those who share a common interest with me in this field. I had 3 main parameters for editing this text:

1. Accuracy – The data and information provided in this book should be up-to-date and valuable to the readers.

2. Structure – The data must be presented in a structured format for easy understanding and better grasping of the readers.

3. Universal Approach – This book not only targets students but also experts and innovators in the field, thus my aim was to present topics which are of use to all.

Thus, it took me a couple of months to finish the editing of this book.

I would like to make a special mention of my publisher who considered me worthy of this opportunity and also supported me throughout the editing process. I would also like to thank the editing team at the back-end who extended their help whenever required.

Editor

Quality Control in Radiology and Clinical Imaging

Quality by Design and Risk Assessment for Radiopharmaceutical Manufacturing and Clinical Imaging

Kung-Tien Liu, Jian-Hua Zhao, Lee-Chung Men and Chien-Hsin Chen

Additional information is available at the end of the chapter

1. Introduction

Radiopharmaceuticals have been widely used in many clinical and nonclinical applications, such as *in vivo* and non-invasive diagnosis or treatment of human diseases. The quality of radiopharmaceuticals administered for a patient is primarily related for the radiation dose delivered to achieve optimizing diagnostic imaging or therapeutic efficacy. Radiopharmaceuticals with different half-lives (short, medium, and long), decay modes (alpha, beta, gamma, and electron capture), and biochemical properties (of ligands) can determine their utilities in medicine. Moreover, chemical and radiochemical impurities in a radiopharmaceutical can produce a serious trouble of diagnosis or treatment. Therefore, different requirements, regulations, and instrumentations for ensuring their high quality and high safety have been developed in many countries.

There are only few years for the progress of "Quality by Design (QbD)" in International Conference on Harmonisation (ICH) Guidelines, e.g. ICH Q8, ICH Q9, and ICH Q10 [1-3]. According to the requirement of ICH Q8, quality can not be tested into products; i.e., quality should be built in by design, i.e. QbD. Enhanced QbD approach to pharmaceutical development can improve the product and process knowledge.

In this chapter, we provide a harmonized framework of QbD for manufacturing and clinical applications of radiopharmaceuticals in accordance with the requirements and guidelines of U.S. Food and Drug Administration (FDA), International Atomic Energy Agency

(IAEA), World Health Organization (WHO) and European Association of Nuclear Medicine (EANM). The attributes of the components in the quality system (QA/QC), including organization, staffing and personnel, facilities, instrumentation and equipment, operation procedure, radiopharmaceuticals, protocol and conduct of a study or a treatment, records and reports, and audit framework were further characterized. Assessments and comparisons of critical quality attributes (CQAs) for assuring accurate radioactive dosimetry calculation in the efficiency tracing of absolute activity measurement and patient- and technologist-related risks for nuclear medicine imaging including Positron Emission Tomography (PET), Computed Tomography (CT), PET/CT, and Single Photon Emission Computed Tomography (SPECT) were identified.

2. Quality system design based on the Requirements and Guidelines

2.1. Quality policy and system

The quality system by design for radiopharmaceuticals and clinical imaging techniques is aimed to maintain and improve the qualified service for the patients, fulfill the regulatory requirements, optimize the safety and efficacy for patient care, demonstrate a proper equipment operating condition, and obtain a reliable quantitative performance in both diagnostic and therapeutic nuclear medicine procedures [4,5]. The pursuit of excellence in quality system is not a single action over a short period, instead, it is achieved through the whole life cycle of instruments, analytical methods or education for example, from planning and procurement to decommissioning based on advanced technology [6]. Continuous quality improvement implies a commitment to continuously struggle to advance based on state-of-the-art information and techniques developed by the nuclear medicine and metrology community at large [5].

Implementation of a quality system must be in accordance with the quality police, i.e. the overall quality intentions and direction of an organization, as formally expressed by top management. And quality system includes the structure, responsibilities, and procedures for implementing quality management. An integrated infrastructure of quality policy and system design is demonstrated as in Figure 1, which is mainly developed from the European Standard EN 28402 proposed by Bergmann et al. [7]. The attributes of the components in the quality sub-system (QA/QC), e.g. organization, personnel, facilities, instrumentation, operation procedures, preparation of radiopharmaceuticals, protocol and conduct, records and reports, and audit or inspection, were further integrated and classified in this article.

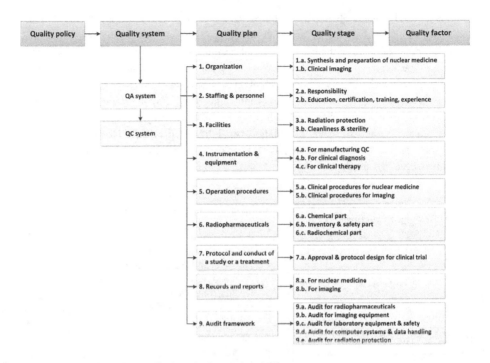

Figure 1. Quality policy and system for the radiopharmaceuticals [7].

2.2. Quality plan and key factors

2.2.1. Organization

The organization of quality system could be grouped into two categories: (a) synthesis and preparation of nuclear medicine and (b) clinical imaging as shown in Figure 2 [8-10]. For synthesis and preparation of nuclear medicine, three important guidelines were considered [11-13]. Basically, preparation of "classical" radiopharmaceuticals in "kit" procedures and in a "distinct chemical" procedures for PET radiopharmaceuticals are distinguished as two different parts [11].

For the clinical imaging, the major differences PET and SPECT in QbD are related to the properties and applications of a radiotracer. The most commonly used nuclides for PET imaging, such as carbon-11, oxygen-15, nitrogen-13, and fluorine-18, exhibit shorter half-life and more complicated labelling technology than that for SPECT imaging (Table 1)[14-31]. For example, the short half-lives of radionuclides used in PET modality allow for better detection sensitivity over a given period of time. This is because radiotracers with shorter half-lives can be injected in higher activities to the patient without posing any additional radiation damage to the patient (since overall accumulation over time remains the same) leading to the increased detectable radiation over a shorter time. Moreover, arguments that the natural occurrence of PET isotopes in biologically active molecules (as opposed to heavy isotopes used in SPECT) results in a less challenging task of synthesizing physiologically useful tracers in PET modality [32,33]. In general, PET generally has a higher resolution, higher sensitivity, and a better quantitation capability than SPECT. However, SPECT is more practical as a routine procedure [18] and is more cost-effective for the system setting or maintain than a PET facility [8].

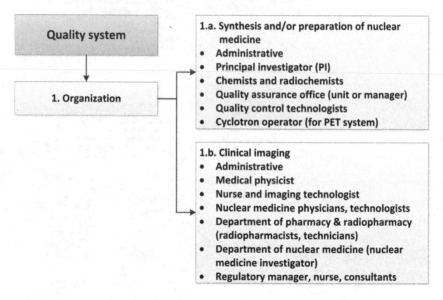

Figure 2. Quality system of organization [8-10].

Agents	Isotope	Half-life ($t_{1/2}$)	Radiopharmaceutical	Applications
PET imaging agents	C-11	20.4 min	C-11-raclopride	D2/D3 dopamine receptor
			C-11-MADAM	Serotonin transporter
	N-13	9.96 min	N-13-ammonia	Blood flow (ventricle)
	O-15	2.07 min	0-15 water	Myocardium perfusion, brain perfusion
	Ga-68	68 min	Ga-68-DOTA	Neuroendocrine tumours

F-18	109.8 min	F-18-fallypride	D2/D3 dopamine receptor
		F-18-FDG	Oncology imaging, metabolism of glucose in tumors, brain and myocardium
		F-18-NaF	Osseous metastasis
Cu-64	12.7 h	Cu-64-ATSM	Tumor hypoxia
I-124	4.12 d	I-124-FIAU	HSV1-tk expresssion
		I-124-HMFGI (IgG$_1$)	Breast ductal carcinoma
SPECT imaging Tc-99m agents	6 hr	Tc-99m-HMPAO	Brain perfusion
		Tc-99m-ECD	Brain perfusion
		Tc-99m-TRODAT-1	Dopamine transporter
		Tc-99m-Prostascint	Prostate cancer
		Tc-99m-CEA	Colon cancer
		Tc-99m-Depreotide	Lung cancer
		Tc-99m-Annexin-V	Acute myocardial infarction, chemotherapy response monitoring, apoptosis of lung tumors
		Tc-99m-sestabmbi	Myocardium perfusion
		Tc-99m-MAG3	Kidney perfusion
		Tc-99m-DTPA	Kidney perfusion
		Tc-99m-DMSA	Kidney perfusion
		Tc-99m pertechnetate	Thyroid
		Tc-99m sulfur colloid	Lymph nodes
SPECT imaging I-123 agents	13 hr	I-123-Iomazenil	Benzodiazepine (γ-aminobutyric acid) receptor
		I-123-IBZM	D2/D3 dopamine receptor
		I-123-iodobenzofuran	D2/D3 dopamine receptor
		I-123-epidepride	D2/D3 dopamine receptor
		I-123-FP-β-CIT	Dopamine-transporter
		I-123-ADAM	Serotonin transporter
		I-123-IMP	Brain perfusion
		I-123-NaI	Thyroid
In-111	2.8 d	In-111-Zevalin	Non-Hodgkin's lymphoma

		In-111-Octreotide	Somatostatin receptor (Neuroendocrine tumors)
	Tl-201	3.04 d	Tl-201	Myocardium perfusion
	Ga-67	3.3 d	Ga-67 citrate	Non-Hodgkin's lymphoma
Therapy agents	Sm-153	1.95 d	Sm-153 EDTMP	Metastatic bone pain palliation
	Sr-89	50.5 d	SrCl$_2$	Palliative treatment of bone cancers and for prostate cancer
	P-32	14.28 d	Orthophosphate	Metastatic bone pain palliation
	Re-186	3.78 d	Re-186-HEDP	Metastatic bone pain palliation
	Re-188	17 h	Re-188-bisphosphonate	Metastatic bone pain palliation
	Y-90	64.14 h	Y-90 Ibritumomab Tiuxetan	B-cell non-Hodgkin's lymphoma
	I-131	8 d	I-131 Tositumomab	B-cell non-Hodgkin's lymphoma
	Lu-177	6.7 d	Lu-177-DOTA-Tyr^3-Octreotate	Small cell lung cancer
	Ho-166	1.1 d	Ho-166-DOTMP	Multiple myeloma
	Sn-117m	13.6 d	Sn-117m-DTPA	Metastatic bone pain palliation
	At-211	7.2 h	At-211-81C6	Glioblastoma multiforme tumors

Table 1. Some examples of radiopharmaceutical classification and applications [14-31]. ADAM: 2-((2-((dimethylamino)-methyl) phenyl)thio)-5- iodophenylamine; DTPA: diethylenetriaminepentaacetic acid; ECD: ethyl cysteinate dimer; FDG: fluoro-deoxy-glucose; FIAU: 1-(2-fluoro-2-deoxy-ß-D-arabinofuranosyl)-5-[I-124]iodouracil; FP-ß-CIT: N-propyl-2-beta-carboxy-methoxy-3-beta(4-iodophenyl)-nortropane; HMPAO: hexamethyl propylene amine oxime; IBZM: iodobenzamide.

2.2.2. Staffing and personnel

Facilities should have written staff and personnel responsibilities and requirements. Two types of staff in the requirements for synthesis and preparation of nuclear medicine and clinical imaging are necessary [4]:

a. Personnel for synthesis and preparation of nuclear medicine may include such as facility management, administrative staff, study director (SD), principal investigator (PI), production chemists, QA manager or quality assurance unit (QAU), radiochemists, QC chemists, cyclotron operators, and technologists.

b. Personnel for PET and SPECT imaging examination may include such as facility management, administrative staff, medical physicists, nurses, referring physicians, nuclear medicine physicians, radiopharmacist, radiochemists, radiation protection® officer, engineers, QA manager or QAU, and technologists.

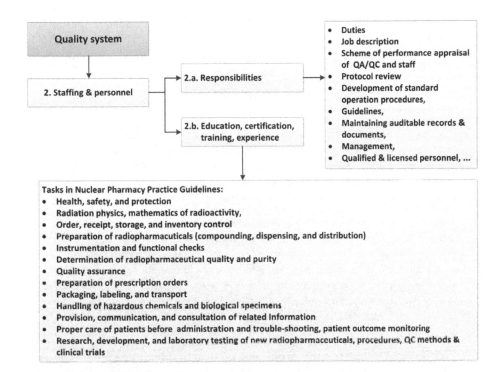

Figure 3. Quality system of staffing and personnel [9,34,35]

The responsibilities for staffing and personnel in a quality system are classified in Figure 3 [9,34,35] and briefly introduced below [4,6,7,36-38]:

a. Facility management: ensure the requirements, guidelines, and practices are complied within facility, sufficient qualified personnel, appropriate facilities, equipment, and materials are available, ensure that personnel clearly understand the functions they are to perform and appropriate and technically valid Standard Operating Procedures (SOPs) are established and followed, ensure that there is a QA manager or QAU with designated personnel and their responsibility is being performed, ensure that for each study an individual with the appropriate qualifications, training, and experience is designated by the management as the SD and PI, ensure that an individual is identified as responsible for the management of the archive.

b. Administrative staff: represent the first encounter a patient has with the centre. They receive the patients according to the established protocols. In collaboration with the medical and technical staff, they are responsible of the application of the procedures for scheduling studies.

c. SD and PI: they are responsible for approving, conducting, documenting, recording and archiving the overall of the study and for its final report.

d. Nuclear medicine physicians: responsible for quality encompasses the general services of the centre. In particular, supervises all patient care and management procedures and all clinical protocols. In addition, he/she supports and enforces the QA/QC of equipment, establish clinical review and auditing.

e. QA manager or QAU: all those planned and systematic actions necessary to provide adequate confidence that a product or service will satisfy given requirements for quality, express the closeness with which the outcome of a given procedure approaches some ideal, free from all errors and artefacts. Quality assurance embraces all efforts made to this end.

f. Radiopharmacist and Radiochemists (Nuclear pharmacy): they are responsible for compounding, dispensing, quality assessment, patient monitoring, drug use review, new drug development and evaluation, product selection and performance evaluation, pharmacokinetic modeling, drug information and educational services. They are also responsible for the performance of acceptance testing and organization/supervision of routine calibration and QC of all radiopharmacy equipment; QC of chemicals, enriched materials, precursors, and kits; QC of radiopharmaceuticals products and batch release.

g. Cyclotron operators: they are in charge of the daily operations, take part in the acceptance test of the cyclotron and related equipment, and are responsible for calibration and QC procedures for equipment.

h. Production chemists: synthesis and preparation of nuclear medicine.

i. QC chemists: the restriction of QC persons is independent of the production operations or must have independent oversight of these duties. The operational techniques and activities that are used to fulfill requirements for quality and are used in reference to the specific measures taken to ensure that one particular aspect of the procedure is satisfactory.

j. Medical physicists: specialized in nuclear medicine and responsible for the performance of acceptance testing and organization/supervision of routine calibration and QC of imaging and radiation measurement equipment, including radiation protection instrumentation.

k. Radiation protection officer: ensure the radiation safety for patient, staffing, and environmental.

l. Engineers and Technologists: contribute to the preparation of clinical examination protocols and the performance of patient examinations according to the established protocols, involved in the performance of routine calibration and QC of scanners.

m. Nurses: manage and care of the patient, collaborate in preparing protocols of patient management and information material as well as in checking the operation of other institutional services.

In IAEA, quality manager is responsible for the entire quality management system supervision, the authority to enforce it and act on its findings, and should be involved in the evaluation and periodic review of the results [5,6]. But, in EANM, the responsibility for overseeing the preparation operations of a qualified radiopharmaceutical is called QAU [11,12].

2.2.3. Facility

In a PET facility, it should include the facility for (a) PET/CT scanner, (b) cyclotron, and (c) radiopharmacy. The location of the facility is a very important issue for the flow of patients, materials, and radiation protection. According to the risk of radiation exposure, two areas are planned [4]:

a. low risk area, cold area or uncontrolled area is the area of offices, reception, waiting room, consulting room, cleaning utilities room or store, and

b. high risk area, hot area or controlled area is the area of hot laboratory, preparation, injection and uptake room, toilet, control and scanning room, post-examination waiting room, reporting room, and waste disposal room.

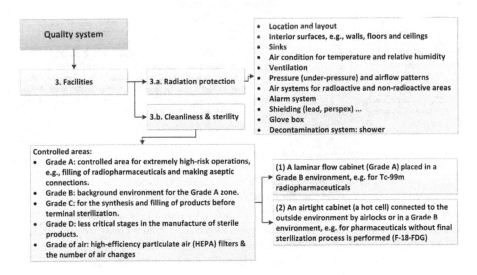

Figure 4. Quality system of facilities [34].

More considerations for the requirements of radiation protection and cleanliness are summarized in Figure 4 [34].

2.2.4. *Instrumentation and equipment*

The instrumentation and equipment in the quality system are summarized in Figure 5 [34,38]. Apparatus and equipment for the purposes of manufacturing QC, diagnosis, and therapy, including validated computerized systems, used for the generation, storage and re-trieval of data, and for controlling environmental factors relevant to the study should be suitably located and of appropriate design and adequate capacity. Apparatus used in a study should be periodically inspected, cleaned, maintained, and calibrated according to SOPs. Records of these activities should be maintained. Calibration should be traceable to national or international standards of measurement [39].

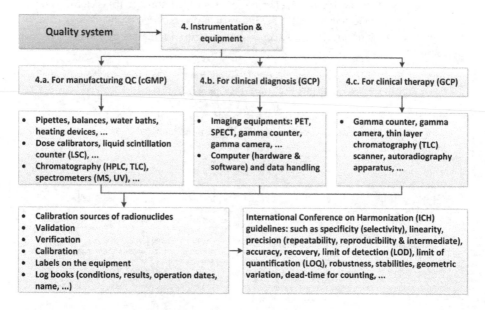

Figure 5. Quality system of instrumentation and equipment [34,38].

Performance tests and operation verification for the nuclear medicine units are achieved dai-ly, weekly, monthly, quarterly, or annually by a qualified medical physicist, a qualified nu-clear medicine technologist, or a medical physicist in training, with management by a qualified medical physicist. The tests results of intrinsic or system spatial resolution, uni-formity, center of rotation, sensitivity, energy resolution, counting rate parameters, multi-ple-window spatial registration, formatter and video display, linearity, leak test, overall system performance for imaging systems, interlocks, dose calibrators, thyroid uptake and counting systems must be reviewed and documented in an annual survey report in accord-ance with the ACR Technical Standard for Medical Nuclear Physics Performance Monitor-ing of Nuclear Medicine Imaging Equipment [37].

2.2.5. Operation procedures

A test facility should have written SOPs approved by facility management for ensuring the quality and integrity of the data generation. Deviations from SOPs related to the manufacturing, study, or treatment should be documented and should be acknowledged by the study director, the principal investigator, the medical physician, quality assurance personnel and/or radiopharmacist. The historical file of different version of all SOPs should be well recorded and stored. The requirements of SOPs for nuclear medicine manufacturing and imaging are summarized in Figures 6 and 7 [11,12,40-44].

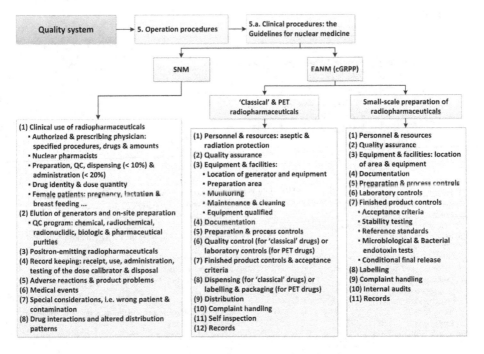

Figure 6. Quality system of clinical operation procedures for nuclear medicine [11,12,40].

2.2.6. Radiopharmaceuticals

(a) Manufacturing of radiopharmaceuticals

Manufacturing and quality control plans for radiopharmaceuticals are indicated in Figure 8 [34,40,45]. Radiopharmaceuticals might be manufactured or prepared in hospital radiopharmacies, centralized radiopharmacies, nuclear centers, institutes, industrial manufacturers, or PET centers in accordance with the requirements of good manufacturing practices (GMP) or Current Good Radiopharmacy Practice (cGRPP) [11-13,34].

Two categories of radiopharmaceuticals are classified in EANM Radiopharmacy Committee according to the significant difference of preparation procedures, i.e. "kit" and PET radiopharmaceuticals. Also, significant consideration in the "Guidelines on Current Good Radiopharmacy Practice (cGRPP) in the Preparation of Radiopharmaceuticals" is proposed by EANM Radiopharmacy Committee. Two types of preparation methods, i.e. in "classical" procedure and in "synthetical" procedure, have been distinguished in cGRPP [11]. According to WHO guideline, radiopharmaceuticals are divided into four categories including ready-to-use, radionuclide generators, "kits" for the labelled with a radioactive component, and precursors used for radiolabelling other substances before administration (e.g. samples from patients) [13].

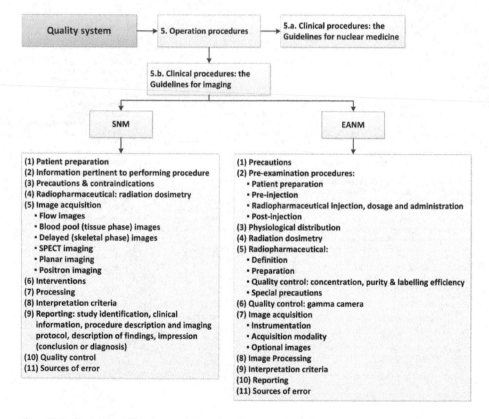

Figure 7. Quality system of clinical operation procedures for imaging [41-44].

Clinical investigations of radiopharmaceuticals can be approved by FDA as "legend drugs." The investigational radiopharmaceutical drug service (IRDS) is responsible for establishing study-specific procedures for radiopharmaceutical drug, including preparation, storage, dispensing and destruction of investigational drugs within the hospital [9]. Manufacturing or preparation of radiopharmaceuticals must follow the FDA 21CFR Part 212 "Current Good Manufacturing (cGMP) for PET drugs," USP Chapter <797> "Pharmaceutical Compounding-Sterile Preparations," USP Chapter <823> "Radiopharmaceuticals for Positron Emission Tomography - Compounding," and U.S. FDA Guidance: PET Drugs - Current Good Manufacturing Practice (CGMP) [10].

(b) Quality control of radiopharmaceuticals

Three essential parts i.e. chemical, inventory, and radiochemical QC diagrams for radiopharmaceuticals are also indicated in Figure 8 [30,50,45].

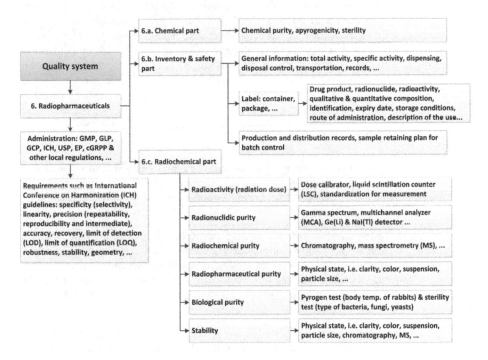

Figure 8. Quality system for radiopharmaceutical manufacturing and quality control [34,40,45].

Method developments for the chemical and radiochemical analysis of starting material, intermediates, precursor used for the radiolabelling, active pharmaceutical ingredient (APIs or drug substance), and finished product (drug product or finished dosage form) are essential requirements of Chemistry, and Manufacturing and Controls (CMC). In the applications of investigational new drug (IND), New Drug Application (NDA), and Abbreviated New Drug Application (ANDA), information on the CMC has to be filed as per 21 CFR 312.23(a) for a drug substance and drug product. The contents for the CMC sections of the

EU and U.S. are very much the same. However, the sequence and titles of the sections are quite different [46,47].

According to International Conference on Harmonization (ICH) guidelines, the parameters for the validation of analytical methods should basically include specificity (selectivity), linearity, precision (repeatability, reproducibility and intermediate), accuracy, recovery, limit of detection (LOD), limit of quantification (LOQ), robustness, and stability. However, instrument validation parameters for the radioactivity measurement or isotopic analysis, such as dose calibrator or liquid scintillation spectrometry, are partially different.

Radiopharmaceuticals are usually used before all quality control testing has been completed. The implementation of and compliance with the quality assurance program are therefore essential. Principal responsibilities of QA/QC are detailed by WHO and De vos et al., including preparation of detailed instructions for each test and analysis, ensuring the adequate identification, ensuring equipment and process validation, release or rejection of materials, evaluation of the quality and stability of the finished products, expiry dates, storage conditions, control procedures, specifications, and records keeping [13,34].

2.2.7. Protocol and conduct

Protocol for a medicine manufacturing study or imaging examination should be evaluated according to the purposes of a study, a treatment, or a clinical trial. Safety issue, such as algorithm proposed by ASNC for maximal benefit in patient radiation exposure must be included [33].

For each study and treatment, a written plan or protocol should exist prior to the initiation of the study. The protocol should be approved by dated signature of the study director, principal investigator or medical physician, facility management, sponsor and verified by quality assurance personnel and/or radiopharmacist. The study and treatment should be conducted in accordance with the study plan or protocol by using a unique identification to each study.

Clinical protocol should be evaluated based on the patient characteristics (e.g. patient history of disease or ability to complete the examination) and complexity of clinical situation in accordance with the current statements and guidelines [33]. For instance, advantages and disadvantages of assessing myocardial perfusion with PET, as compared to SPECT imaging, was reported and concluded that use of very short half-life tracers injected at very high activities, as well as the introduction of increasingly fast scintillators technology, which in turn has allowed reduction of random coincidences and introduced the possibility of time-of-flight (TOF) PET are expected to further contribute to high sensitivity imaging capabilities of PET [32].

An example for approving of protocol design for a clinical trial is shown in Figure. 9 [10,47]. Two pathways for the clinical studies of investigational radiopharmaceuticals are called Radioactive Drug Research Committee (RDRC) and IND. For an investigational medical product (IMP, investigation only), if there are adequate data from literature or original assessments that no pharmacologic effects are likely in humans, and the chosen radioactivity is small enough to result in the total radiation absorbed dose, clinical trial can be approved by National Competent Authority (NCA) and Ethical Committee (EC) in EU or approved by RDRC in U.S.. Otherwise, it is approved by EC in EU or approved by FDA in U.S., depending on the phase of drug development [47].

The FDA allows certain unique applications by the local RDRC, consisting of at least five individuals and three individual specialists in nuclear medicine, in formulate radioactive drugs, and in radiation safety, to approve and monitor for the use of radiopharmaceuticals in humans without IND approval. This is due to the low potential for toxicity of radiopharmaceuticals that are typically administered in tracer quantities. Requirements to establish a local RDRC at one's institution is outlined in regulation 21 CFR 361.1. And RDRC has to submit an annual report to the FDA as part of the procedures for maintaining an active and approved RDRC program [48].

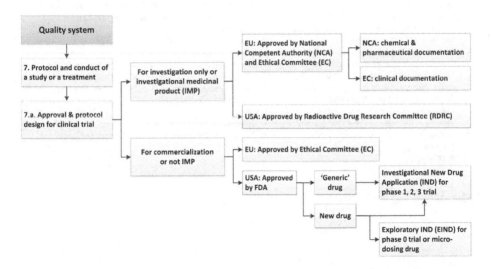

Figure 9. Quality system of protocol and conduct for a study or a treatment [10,47].

2.2.8. Records and reports

Records and reports for the manufacturing of radiopharmaceuticals and imaging trial or testing are summarized in Figure 10 [7,9,40-44]. All records and reports should be maintained at the radiopharmaceutical laboratory or another location that is accessible to responsible officials and to government employees designated to perform inspections [11,12]. Storage of records must ensure safekeeping for many years. Archive facilities of independent locations should be provided for the secure storage and retrieval of study plans, raw data, final reports, samples of test items and specimens. Archive conditions, e.g. fireproof, waterproof, and insect prevention are designed for protecting contents from untimely deterioration [38].

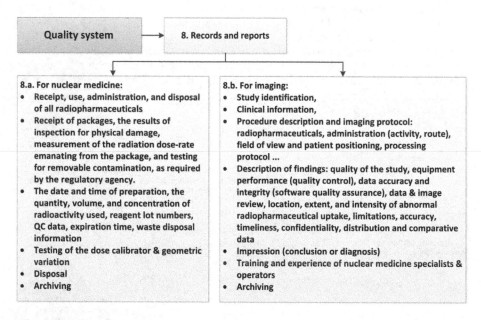

Figure 10. Quality system of records and reports [7,9,40-44].

2.2.9. Audit framework

Laboratory inspections and study audits should be established for periodical monitoring compliance with GLP, GCP, or GMP principles, study protocol, and SOPs [9,38]. Audits for radiopharmaceutical drug products typically begin by confirming the clinical site is appropriately licensed and authorized to receive, possess, store, handle, prepare and administer radiopharmaceuticals. The audit framework of quality system for radiopharmaceuticals, imaging equipment, laboratory equipment, safety, computer systems, data handling, and radiation protection are displayed in Figure 11 [9,39].

(a)

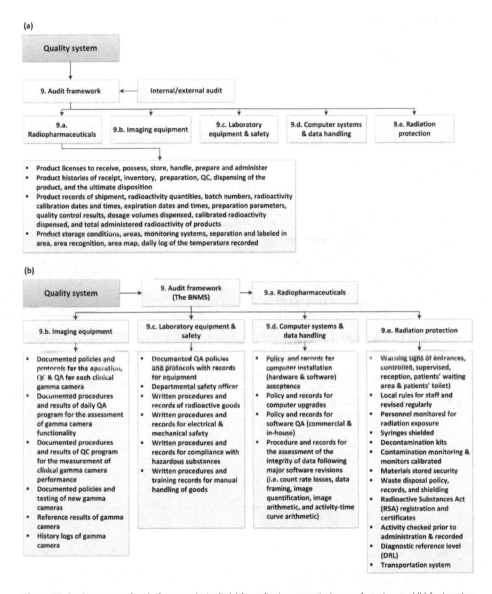

(b)

Figure 11. Quality system of audit framework. Audit (a) for radiopharmaceuticals manufacturing, and (b) for imaging equipment, laboratory equipment, safety, computer systems, data handling, and radiation protection. [9,39]

3. Quality evaluation and sources of uncertainty

3.1. Radiopharmaceuticals

3.1.1. Standardization: principle and applications

Quality control for the quantification of radiopharmaceutical activity is critical for accurate dosimetry calculations, from whole body to cell microscopy. Tumor uptake of radiopharmaceutical need to be correlated with tumor response and to be related to the tumor radiation absorbed dose. [14]

Isotope	Major decay modes	Method for standardization	Detection efficiency (ε)	Activity accuracy & uncertainty (U)	Ref.
-	β, γ, β-γ, EC, EC-γ, α, and mixed decay nuclides	LSC and C/N method	$\varepsilon_{pure\,\gamma}$: ~100% $\varepsilon_{pure\,EC}$: < 75% $\varepsilon_{EC-\gamma}$: ~100% ε_{α}: ~100%	U: 0.2-0.5% (pure β) U: 0.2-0.5% (β-γ)	51
Co-57	EC decay to Fe-57	4πβ-γ coincidence method	ε: ~75%	U: 2%	50
Ge-68/Ga-68 1. Ge-68 EC decay to Zn-68 2. Ga-68 β+, EC, γ decay to Zn-68		γ spectrometer x-ray spectrometer 4πβ-γ coincidence method LSC Calibrated IC	To ground state: β+ (87.85%), EC (8.92%) To 1077 keV: β+ (1.29%), EC (1.93%) Annihilation radiation: 178.29% γ-ray to 1077 keV: 3.22%	β+ U: 1%	52
Sn-117m-DTPA	Decay to Sn-117	4πβ LS and 4πγ methods		U_C: 0.60% (for DTPA by LS) U_C: 2.43% (for DTPA by NaI(T1))	17
Cs-131	EC decay to Xe-131	Coincidence methods: L Auger electrons plus L X-rays and K X-rays	-	U: 1%	53
Cs-134	β- and γ decay to Ba-134	LSC	ε: ~95%	3191 ± 8 kBq/g (0.54%)	54

		$4\pi\beta$-γ coincidence method	ε: 65-87%	3194 ± 12 kBq/g (0.88%)	
		$4\pi\gamma$ method	ε: ~83%	3174 ± 25 kBq/g (2.09%)	
		C/N method			
Tl-201	γ decays to Hg-201	High-pressure IC $4\pi\gamma$ coincidence method	γ ray (167.4 keV) probability: 0.1000 ± 0.0006	7.207 ± 0.033 (NIST) 7.197 ± 0.027 (NPL) 7.116 ± 0.050 (PTB)	55
Tl-204	β^- decay (97.4%) to Pb-204 and EC decay (2.6%) to Hg-204	Windowless 4π- CsI(Tl) -sandwich spectrometer, LSC, PPC			56
		$4\pi\beta$-γ coincidence method and Cs-134 tracer	ε_β: 71 - 91% ε_{EC} (~ ε_{AEs}): 50 - 100%	U_C: 0.76%	57
Pb-210	β decay to Bi-210 ($t_{1/2}$ 5.103 d), Po-210 ($t_{1/2}$ 138.4 d), and α decay to Pb-206	$4\pi\beta$-γ coincidence method Germanium γ spectrometry		U_C: 2.7%	58

Table 2. Some examples of absolute standardization of radiopharmaceuicals and related radioisotopes [17,50-58]

The theoretical counting efficiency, i.e. counts/disintegration or counts per minute/disintegration per minute (cpm/dpm), for a radionuclide can be used to examine the absolute activity, in disintegration or disintegration per minute (dpm) of the radionuclide. Different efficiency tracing methods has been developed for more than six decade by characterizing the effects of sample volume, medium composition (matrix), pulse discrimination conditions, photomultiplier voltage, amplifier gain, and luminophor concentration on counting efficiency of a radioactive species [49]. The use of $4\pi\beta$ scintillation counting and $4\pi\beta$-γ coincidence counting for the standardization of certain electron capture (EC) nuclides with simple decay schemes is established since 1952 [49] and 1957 [50].

Some examples of absolute standardization of radiopharmaceuicals and related radioisotopes are shown in Table 2 [17,50-58]. Below, we introduce different tracing methods, including (a) efficiency tracing (and extrapolation) method using a non-H-3 standard solution, (b) CIEMAT-NIST (C/N) efficiency tracing method, (c) non-extrapolation tracer method, (d) coincidence method by a $4\pi\beta$-γ system, (e) triple to double coincidence ratio (TDCR) method, and (f) $4\pi\gamma$ counting method.

(a) The efficiency tracing (and extrapolation) method using a non-H-3 standard solution

The efficiency tracer techniques, using Co-60, Cs-134, C-14, Cr-51, Mn-54 or Am-241 standard solution for the standardization of the β-γ nucides were developed. The 4π liquid scintillation (LS) consisted of the extrapolation of the 4π counting rate to the zero discrimination level for the standardization of the Tl-204 (97.6% β emission and 2.4% electron capture) solution was carried out for efficiency tracing using a Co-60 standard solution received in the framework of the 1997 BIPM comparison was carried out by Sahagia et al. [59]. A germanium spectrometer was calibrated for the standardization of Pb-210 using Am-241 as a normalizing agent has been proposed [58]. Instead, Dias et al. chose Cs-134 as an efficiency tracer to standardize Tl-204 as well as a 4πβ-γ coincidence system for the calibration [57]. This method can be also successfully used for the standardization of radionuclides such as Ir-192, Zn-65, Mn-54, with the detection of the β rays, Auger electrons, X rays, in the proportional counter (PC) [60]. Efficiency tracing with C-14 and zero detection threshold techniques with H-3 as tracers was applied for standardization of various β-emitting radionuclides, e.g. C-14, Cl-36, and Tl-204 using LS spectrometer [61].

Recently, different methodologies were proposed. Koskinas et al. developed a "dual-tracers", e.g. Cr-51 and Mn-54 procedure followed by the Laboratório de Metrologia Nuclear (LMN) for the standardization of EC nuclide, i.e. Fe-55. The efficiency was obtained by selecting a γ-ray window set at 320 keV (Cr-51) and at 834 keV (Mn-54) [62]. The activity of EC radionuclides is usually determined by 4π (proportional counter, PC)-γ coincidence counting and by an efficiency extrapolation method. However, an alternative method, called "wet extrapolation method", utilizes an absorption change during the drying of a water droplet added onto the source surface, variation of the PC detection efficiency can be achieved. Slopes of extrapolation curves and resulting activity values obtained are compared for several radionuclides (Mn-54, Ce-139, Y-88, and Co-57) [63].

(b) The CIEMAT-NIST (C/N) efficiency tracing method

CIEMAT/NIST (C/N) method, developed by Centro de Investigationes Energéticas, Medioambientales y Tecnologicas (CIEMAT), Spain and the National Institute of Standards and Technology (NIST), U.S. is used for standardization of radionuclides with Liquid Scintillation (LS) Spectrometry by calculating the counting efficiency of the radionuclide to be assayed and using H-3 as a tracer [61]. C/N program is suitable used for the calculation of the efficiency of nuclides decayed by β, β-γ, EC, EC-γ and nuclides with mixed decay [51]. The basic principle of C/N LS efficiency tracing method is a combination of a theoretical calculation of the counting efficiency and an experimental determination of correction factors in three steps [61,64]:

• Count rates (cpm) and the quench-indicating parameters (QIPs, i.e. tSIE) are determined for a set of samples of the nuclide to be measured, and for a set of H-3 standard samples, with a different quench. The tSIE values were calculated using the Ba-133 source inside of the instrument. By combining these data, a corresponding H-3 efficiency is obtained for each sample of the nuclide.

• The universal curve of Figure of Merit (FOM) as a function of tSIE was plotted. The efficiency of the nuclide is theoretically calculated as a function of the efficiency of the tracer nuclide H-3.

- This relation is used in conjunction with the measured data to calculate the efficiency for the nuclide and an activity value in dpm for each single measurement.

The parameters of emitters in different decay modes used for the C/N calculations are summarized as follows [51]:

- Pure β emitters (Sr-89, Sr-90, Y-90, and K-40): atomic number Z of the radionuclide, the mass number A, the endpoint energy EMax, and the shape parameters.

- Pure γ emitters (Nb-93m): the efficiency is nearly 100%.

- β+γ emitters, if the radionuclide has significant levels with half-lives in the order of the coincidence resolving time or the dead time of the equipment, a C/N calculation is not possible.

- Pure EC emitters: the input parameters are the capture probabilities, PK; PL; PM, and the atomic parameters for the rearrangement: the fluorescence yields ωK and ωL (averaged), the probabilities of the X-rays (PKL, PKX, and PLX) and their average energies (EKL, EKX, and ELX), the emission probabilities of the Auger electrons (PKLL, PKLX, PKXY, and PLXY) and their average energies (EKLL, EKLX, EKXY, and ELXY).

- EC+γ emitters (Co-57, Se-75, Sr-85, and Ba-133): the calculation method is the same as for β+γ nuclides.

- The efficiency of LSC systems with respect to alpha radiation is in each case very close to unity. A tracer method is not necessary.

(c) The non-extrapolation tracer method

An alternative called "non-extrapolation tracer method" was proposed by Steyn et al. in 1979, where Fe-55 was used as a tracer to establish the figure-of-merit (FOM) of the detection system for the calculation of counting efficiency [65]. The liquid scintillation method, for the determination of absolute activity of Mn-54 and Zn-65 from 4π(LS)e-γ data by direct calculation without efficiency extrapolation was performed. The non-extrapolation LS method relies on determining the probability of the γ-ray interacting with the scintillator solution, is described and validated by measurements made on Co-60 [66].

(d) The coincidence method by a 4πβ-γ system

Coincidence method comes from the additional coincidence channel, which records a disintegration event when it is detected in both β- and γ-channels. Typically, the system for absolute standardization is usually consisted of a gas-flow or pressurized proportional counter with 4π geometry as the α, β, electrons or X-ray detector and coupled to a pair of NaI(Tl) scintillation counters or a semiconductor detector, as γ detectors. The 4πβ-γ coincidence technique has been considered a primary standardization method due to its high accuracy and because it can obtain the radionuclide activity depending only on observables quantities [57,67].

Alternatively, solid or liquid scintillation counters (LSC) are used in place of gas-flow proportional counters. Advantages of using LSC counting in the 4π channel are that self-absorption does not occur, leading to Auger electrons being detected with relatively high efficiency; source preparation is easy; and the source geometry is highly reproducible. The latter leads to good reproducibility of the counting efficiency of the X-rays and Auger electrons, which in turn gives rise to consistent results amongst the counting sources. The efficiency data can generally be fitted with a linear function, particularly in the high-efficiency region, or by a low-order polynomial expression, giving rise to reliable extrapolated activity values [68].

Several examples for the applications of the coincidence method by a $4\pi\beta$-γ system are such as standardization of Ho-166m using the normal gas flow $4\pi\beta$-γ coincidence method [69], standardization of Tl-204 using Cs-134 as tracer and a $4\pi\beta$-γ coincidence system was used for the calibration [57], directly measured of radionuclides with EC decay schemes, e.g. I-125, Ir-192, Zn-65, and Ce-139 by a LS coincidence extrapolation technique [68], and standardization of Fe-55 using a "dual-tracers" method coupled with a $4\pi\beta$-γ coincidence calibration system [62].

(e) The triple to double coincidence ratio (TDCR) method

The TDCR method was first developed at the R.C., Poland and at the LNHB, France. The equipment consists in a detection unit, provided with three photomultipliers (PMs), acted by the light emitted in the vial containing the radioactive solution dissolved in a liquid scintillator, and the electronic unit [60]. TDCR, allowing the observation of three kind of double coincidences (2-photodetectors) and triple coincidence (3-photodetectors) method in LSC, is a fundamental measurement method suitable to the standardization of pure-beta emitters, i.e. H-3, C-14, P-32, Ni-63, Tc-99, Tl-204 and some low energy electron-capture emitters, i.e. Fe-55 [59,60,70,71]. Detection efficiency variation can be achieved using techniques of chemical quenching, coaxial grey filters and PM tubes defocusing. The two former processes reduce the mean quantity of light emitted and the later reduces the detection probability [71]. Basically, the specific experimental parameter (K) is equal to the ratio of the triple coincidences counting rate (N_T) to the sum of double coincidences counting rate (N_D). Determination of a counting efficiency (ε_D) for each counting point (N_D) leads to the activity of the source (N_0). The efficiency functions ε_T and ε_D are nonlinear functions for a particular emitter and counting system [70].

Two innovative TDCR instrumentations were developed:

- The TDCR method of LSC is well established for measuring the activity of pure beta emitting and electron capture radionuclides. Recently, a new TDCR counting system was designed by the National Physical Laboratory (NPL) for activity assays of low-energy, pure β-emitting radionuclides and EC nuclides. Three photomultiplier tubes (PMT) were arranged in the optical chamber as well as a NaI(Tl) detector was mounted below the optical chamber. The detector allows $4\pi\beta$-γ coincidence measurements to be performed in parallel [72].

- Radionuclides such as P-32, Sr-89, Y-90, Tl-204, and Rh-106 were successfully studied using an in-house built new TDCR-Čerenkov counter developed by Kossert. Since Čerenkov counting acts as natural discrimination for αemitters and low-energy β emitters, some potential radioactive impurities or progenies will not disturb the measurements. Two standard sources, e.g. Cl-36 and P-32 were used to determine the free parameter and to calculate the Čerenkov counting efficiencies. Since Čerenkov counting is more sensitive to changes in the computed β spectra, the method was extensively used to investigate β shape factor functions [73].

(f) The $4\pi\gamma$ counting method.

An ionization chamber system referring to a long living and stable standard source is very adequate for the comparison of γ-ray emitting radio-nuclides. In most cases Ra-226 sealed sources have been used as the reference because the Ra-226 sources were widely used in radiotherapy [69]. Zimmerman et al. standardized and compared solution of Sn-117m by $4\pi\beta$ liquid scintillation (LS) spectrometry and 4π γ-ray spectrometry (NaI(Tl) and high-purity germanium detectors). Massic activities were measured for determining the dose calibrator factor settings [17].

3.1.2. Uncertainty of measurement

Examples for the evaluation of detection efficiency (ε), activity accuracy, and measurement uncertainty (U) of absolute activity of radiopharmaceuicals and related radioisotopes are shown in Table 2. Components of combined uncertainty were further summarized in this section.

(a) Uncertainty for the efficiency tracing (and extrapolation) method using a non-H-3 standard solution

Components of combined uncertainty in the activity determination include counting statistics, background, dead time, weighing, decay scheme parameter, half life, and extrapolation of efficiency curve [57]. Source of uncertainty evaluated by Woods et al. in the absolute standardization of low energy β emitter, i.e. Pb-210 are counting, background, half life, β dead time, γ dead time, resolving times, choice of fit, count rate dependence, dead time formula, weighing, separation time, extrapolation range, contaminants, and reproducibility [58].

(b) Uncertainty for the C/N efficiency tracing method

Component of uncertainty in the standardization of Re-186 by the C/N method of LS efficiency tracing with H-3 include source preparation, scintillator stability, dead time, liquid-scintillation measurements, uncertainty due to H-3 reference standard, EC/β⁻ branching ratio, spectral distributions for EC and β⁻ branches. [74]

The contributions to the uncertainty of the value of the specific activity are volatility of H2 [GeCl6] during the preparation of solid sources for coincidence measurements, drop masses, counting statistics, background variation, accidental coincidences and dead time losses, Compton continuum of the 1077 keV peak included in the γ window around the 511 keV peak, decay scheme correct ion factor, correction factor for non-vanishing εEC, impurities and half-life uncertainty, and detection of 511 keV quanta in the β detector due to its γ sensitivity [52].

The components contributing to the uncertainty of $4\pi\beta$-γ coincidence method were estimated as follows: counting statistics and background variation, instrumental corrections, impurities, half-life uncertainty, decay scheme correction factor, and mass of droplet. Standard deviation of LSC composed of the following contributions: counting statistics, background variation, scintillator stability, comparison with H-3 tracer, instrumental corrections (dead time), dilution factor, droplet mass, radioactive impurities, half-life uncertainty, main decay data, uncertainty of the ε calculation due to the K-L model, capture probabilities P_K, P_L, fluorescence yields, ω_K, ω_L, spectral distribution of β particles, and average energy of weak Auger electrons [75].

Source of the uncertainty: counting statistics, mass, dead time, background, timing, chemical effects (adsorption, sample spread, impurities), input parameters and statistical model, quenching, kB influence, decay scheme parameters, and pulse shape discriminator setting. [76]

(c) Uncertainty for the non-extrapolation tracer method

The quoted total uncertainty (1σ) of 0.85% comprised mainly the components due to counting statistics (0.28%), afterpulsing (0.40%) and the evaluated decay-scheme data (0.63%). ε_M: double tube detection efficiency of Mn-54, $\varepsilon_M{}^*$: reduced Mn-54 efficiency due to quenching caused by the addition of the Fe-55 aliquot [65].

(d) Uncertainty for the coincidence method by a $4\pi\beta$-γ system

Uncertainty components assayed by Koskinas et al. for the standardization of Eu-152 were counting statistics, weighing, dead time, impurities, half life, extrapolation of efficiency curve [77].

(e) Uncertainty for the TDCR method

The main source of uncertainty of TDCR method comes from the model describing the nonlinearity of the scintillator due to the ionization quenching phenomenon [71]. Type A standard uncertainty, i.e. counting statistics and type B standard uncertainty, i.e. extrapolation (interception uncertainty), spurious pulses, nonuniformity of sources, tracer activity, E. C. correction, dead-time, background, half-life, weighing were evaluated by Sahagia et al. [59].

(f) Uncertainty for the $4\pi\gamma$ counting method.

Construction of an ionization chamber efficiency curve is not a straightforward process as the curve has to be extracted from experimental calibration points analytically. The efficiency curve is implicitly contained in individual radionuclide coefficients and these are obtained experimentally or by Monte Carlo modelling or calculated back from the efficiency curve. Due to this variety, the interpretation and intercomparison of different efficiency curves is often hard and transferring individual radionuclide calibration coefficients between ionization chambers of different constructions is not a simple process [78].

3.1.3. International measurement program

One of the most important components in the quality system of radiopharmaceuticals is to establish the measurement traceability to international standards for ensuring the accurate and consistent of measurement results [5]. Traceability of activity measurements is the critical part in the production and use of unsealed radioactive sources in nuclear medicine. The U.S. Nuclear Regulatory Commission (NRC) defines a medical event as a patient receiving an injected activity greater than 20% different from the prescribed dosage. Tthe Society of Nuclear Medicine (SNM) guidelines also recommend that the measurement be with 10% of the prescribed dosage. Moreover, the instruments being used are capable of accurate measurements to within 5% [79]. Therefore, programs for the establishment and dissemination of activity measurement standards in nuclear medicine are held in many countries.

International comparison of standard sources and solutions, such as P-32, Mn-54, Zn-65, Ir-192, Tl-204, and Am-241, which is organized by the International Committee of Weights and Measures (CIPM), the EUROMET system, the former COMECOM, and bilateral comparisons, has been held since 1962 [60].

South Africa's national radioactivity measurement standard is maintained by the National Metrology Laboratory (NML) of the Council for Scientific and Industrial Research (CSIR). Standardizations are undertaken by a number of direct methods utilizing liquid scintillation counting (LSC) [80].

Comparisons of activity measurements for I-131, Tl-201 and Tc-99m with radionuclide calibrators were organized in Cuba since 2002. During 2002, the Radionuclide Metrology Department of the Isotope Center (CENTIS-DMR) has organized several comparisons with various radionuclides in order to obtain information on the quality of the activity measurements during production and administration of radiopharmaceuticals in Cuba [81].

The Australian Radiation Protection and Nuclear Safety Agency (ARPANSA) conducts a series of Radiopharmaceutical Quality Assurance Test Program under a Memorandum of Understanding (MOU) between ARPANSA and the Therapeutic Goods Administration (TGA). For example, in 2005, 46 batches of 24 different types of radiopharmaceuticals, e.g., ready to use radiopharmaceuticals and kits for the preparation of Tc-99m were tested. Two percent in 46 batches of radiopharmaceuticals tested was failure to meet full specifications [82].

International comparison program of national metrological institutes for the standardization of Fe-55, which is a suitable radionuclide standard for X-ray spectrometers, was held by the Comité Consultative pour les Etalons de Mesures des Rayonnements Ionisants (CCEMRI) of the Bureau International des Poids et Mesures (BIPM) [62]. National Metrology Institute of Japan - Advanced Industrial Science and Technology (NMIJ/AIST, Japan) and National Institute of Ionizing Radiation Metrology (ENEA-INMRI, Italy) have been involved in recent years, particularly those relevant in the frame of the international cooperation coordinated by the BIPM and the International Committee for Radionuclide Metrology (ICRM). Particular research activities are devoted on the field of the nuclear safety, nuclear medicine and environmental radionuclide measurements. [83]. International comparisons held by BIPM also can be traced by laboratories such as National Institute for Physics and Nuclear Engineering (Romania) [59], Laboratorio de Metrologia Nuclear (Brazil) in collaboration with the Laboratório Nacional de Metrologia das Radiações Ionizantes, from Rio de Janeiro [57], Radiation Safety Systems Division, Bhabha Atomic Research Centre (India) [61], and Electrotechnical Laboratory (ETL) (Japan) [69].

The Ce-139 measurements formed part of a regional comparison organized by the Asia Pacific Metrology Programme (APMP) [68].

The National Institute of Standards and Technology (NIST) maintains a program for the establishment and dissemination of activity measurement standards in nuclear medicine, i.e. Ga-67, Y-90, Tc-99m, Mo-99, In-111, I-125, I-131, and Tl-201 for more than ten years. These standards are disseminated through Standard Reference Materials (SRMs), Calibration Services, radionuclide calibrator settings, and the NIST Radioactivity Measurement Assurance Program (NRMAP, formerly the NEI/NIST MAP). For over 3600 comparisons, 96% of the participants' results differed from that of NIST by less than 10%, with 98% being less than 20%. The percentage of participants results within 10% of NIST ranges from 88% to 98% [79].

Measurements from a variety of types of detectors including, ionization chambers, radionuclide calibrators, solid state detectors, Ge detectors, NaI(Tl) detectors, liquid scintillation counters (LSC), Cherenkov counting, and proportional counter are reported [79].

3.2. Nuclear medicine imaging

3.2.1. PET, CT, PET/CT, and SPECT imaging

PET, CT, PET/CT, and SPECT are non-invasive imaging tools and applied for creating two dimensional (2D) cross section images of three dimensional (3D) objects. PET and SPECT can potentially provide functional or biochemical information by measuring distribution and kinetics of radiolabelled molecules, whereas CT visualizes X-ray density in tissues in the body. The PET imaging in oncology has been migrating from the use of dedicated PET scanners to the use of PET/CT tomographs. This is due to the advantages that PET/CT offers over dedicated PET. One of these advantages is that the integration of PET and CT imaging into a single scanning session allows excellent fusion of the acquired data. Although these nuclear medicine imaging tools provide many advantages and applications in diagnosing diseases clinically, they also poses some challenges and induce artifacts and quantitative errors that can affect the image quality.

3.2.2. Risks of artifact in PET, CT, and SPECT imaging

Artifacts and pitfalls can arise at any stage in the process of nuclear medicine imaging and can be grouped into issues related to the (i) patient, (ii) the equipment, or the technologist.

(a) Patient-related risks:

In PET/CT, the patient-related artifacts commonly found are due to metallic implants, truncation, and respiratory motion (or patient motion). These artifacts occur because the CT scan is used to replace a PET transmission scan for the purpose of attenuation correction of the PET data.

Metallic implants, such as dental fillings, hip prosthetics, or chemotherapy ports, cause high CT numbers and generate streaking artifacts on CT images due to their high photon absorption [85,86]. This increase CT numbers causes correspondingly high PET attenuation coefficients, resulting in an overestimation of the PET activity and thereby to a false-positive PET finding.

In PET/CT, truncation artifacts occur due to the difference in size of the field of view between the CT (50 cm) and PET (70 cm) tomographs [87,88] and frequently seen in large patients or patients scanned with arms down, such as in the case of melanoma and head and neck indications. When a patient extends beyond the CT field of view, the extended part of the anatomy is truncated and consequently is not represented in the reconstructed CT image. Truncation also causes streaking artifacts at the edge of the CT image, leading to an overestimation of the attenuation coefficients used to correct the PET data. This increase in attenuation coefficients creates a rim of high activity at the truncation edge, resulting in the misinterpretation of the PET scan.

The most prevalent artifact in PET/CT imaging is respiratory motion during scanning. The artifact is due to the discrepancy between the chest position on the CT image and the chest position on the PET image. PET images are acquired over time periods (time frames) that can vary from a few seconds to tens of minutes. Therefore, during such time periods various motions may have significant effects on the PET images. Both respiratory and contraction induced heart motions have major effect (source of error) on PET imaging of cardiac and thoracic regions. Some equipment, e.g., dose calibrators for the measurements of quantitative measurements is calibrated against or traceable to a reference source of whole body tomographs [89]. Because of the long acquisition time of a PET scan, it is acquired while the patient is freely breathing. The final image is hence an average of many breathing cycles. On the other hand, a CT scan is usually acquired during a specific stage of the breathing cycle. This difference in respiratory motion between PET scans and CT scans results in breathing artifacts on PET/CT images. Several literatures have described this problem [90-91]. The artifacts resulted from respiratory motion or patient motion is also commonly found in myocardial perfusion SPECT. This is because that SPECT requires that the object of interest remains constant for the duration of the acquisition [92-93]. Visually detectable patient motion has been reported in 36% of clinical studies in one study [94] and 43% in another [95].

Source of clinical problems of the patients were also indicated by Hladik III, including (i) special patient populations, e.g., pregnant or breast-feeding women, pediatric and geriatric patients, patients requiring dialysis, incontinent, catheterized or miscellaneous patients, (ii) insufficient patient care, education, and preparation, e.g. insufficient patient instruction, shielding or protection in exposure and contamination problems, pregnancy testing, withholding xanthine-containing foods and drug-drug interaction prior to imaging, delay in the administration or imaging, metal implants of patient, (iii) improper behavior of patient, e.g., excessive movement, contamination from incontinence, attenuation from jewelry, prostheses, or implants, etc., and (iv) unexpected altered biodistributions may be undetectable, adverse reactions or untoward effects, [96]

(b) Equipment- or technologist-related risks:

There are several patient-related artifacts and interpretation pitfalls that can potentially compromise nuclear medicine imaging, as discussed above. In order to minimize or identify these artifacts, technologists play an important role in recognizing and correcting them. For example, technologists should ask patients to remove all metallic objects before imaging and should document the location of non-removable metallic objects to minimize or identify the

artifacts from metallic implants. In PET/CT imaging, it is crucial for technologists to carefully position patients at the center of the field of view and with arms above head to reduce
truncation artifacts. Moreover, in order to minimize the artifacts from respiratory motion
and produce accurately quantifiable images, it is also essential that technologists instruct patients about breath-hold techniques before the scanning session.

Moreover, sources of clinical problems of error medication also include fail of (i) patient
identification, (ii) dosage prescription and administration, (iii) radionuclide administration,
(iv) radiopharmaceutical prescription and administration in kinetics or finished product purity testing, (v) interventional medications, (vi) injection technique, (vii) radiopharmaceutical labelled, (viii) preparation or execution of diagnostic or therapeutic procedure, and (ix)
radiation protection [7,96].

QC performed on nuclear medicine cameras provides the confidence to technologists and
physicians that a scan supplies an accurate representation of the radioisotope distribution in
the patient. The instrumentation for nuclear medicine imaging is more complex than that
used for whole-body and planar imaging, and requires careful quality control to ensure optimum performance. According to the standards, the main performance parameters are divided into two groups. The first group includes basic intrinsic measurements: spatial
resolution in axial and transaxial directions, sensitivity, count rate capabilities by measuring
the system dead time and the generation of random events at different radioactivity levels,
and scatter fraction of γ rays emitted by the annihilation of positron. The second group includes measurements of the accuracy of corrections for physical effects, specifically: uniformity correction, scatter correction, attenuation correction, and count rate linearity
correction. Other possible tests to be added to the list of acceptance or performance tests
such as: noise equivalent count rate, partial volume and spillover, motion artefacts, image
quality test, and PET/CT image co-registration [89].

Nuclear medicine imaging increases the accuracy of diagnosis by combining anatomic information with functional imaging. It is highly dependent on a host of technical considerations.
Knowledgeable technologists can minimize or reduce artifacts and other potential problems
with image acquisition and, in that way, produce better-quality images.

4. Conclusion

Implement of ICH QbD for the radiopharmaceutical manufacturing and imaging technology
can be harmonized to a globalized framework in accordance with the regulations and requirements of U.S. FDA, IAEA, WHO and EANM. The attributes of the components in the
quality unit (QA/QC), including the aspects of organization, staffing and personnel, facilities, instrumentation and equipment, operation procedure, radiopharmaceuticals, protocol
and conduct of a study or a treatment, records and reports, and audit were reviewed and
indentified. Critical quality attributes (CQAs) for assuring accurate radioactive dosimetry
calculation in the efficiency tracing of absolute activity measurement and in the patient- and
technologist-related risks for nuclear medicine imaging (PET, CT, and SPECT), i.e. potential

sources of error or uncertainty, were elucidated. Although there still have many hard-to-controlled quantitative errors and artifacts that can eventually affect the quality of imaging, therapeutic efficacy, or safety, it is important for the facility staffs to be aware and continual improvement of these quality factors. By reducing uncertainty and risk or increasing process knowledge and product understanding resulting from QbD can significantly improve the efficiency of manufacturing processes.

5. Abbreviations

API Active pharmaceutical ingredient

ARPANSA Australian Radiation Protection and Nuclear Safety Agency

BNMS British Nuclear Medicine Society

BIPM Bureau International des Poids et Mesures (France)

CT Computed Tomography

CFR Code of Federal Regulations (U.S.)

CMC Chemistry, and manufacturing and controls

CQAs Critical quality attributes

CSIR Council for Scientific and Industrial Research

CGMP Current Good Manufacturing Practice

CGRPP Current Good Radiopharmacy Practice (EU)

EC Ethical Committee (EU)

EANM European Association of Nuclear Medicine (EU)

EDQM European Directorate for the Quality of Medicines & HealthCare

EIND Exploratory IND (FDA, U.S.)

FDA U.S. Food and Drug Administration

HPLC High-performance liquid chromatography

ICH International Conference on Harmonisation

IMP Investigational Medicinal Product (for drugs used in clinical trials of EU)

IND Investigational new drug

IAEA International Atomic Energy Agency

IRDS Investigational Radiopharmaceutical Drug Service

LSC Liquid scintillation counting

MA Marketing authorization (EU)

MS Mass spectrometry

MOU Memorandum of Understanding

NRC Nuclear Regulatory Commission

NCA National Competent Authority (EU)

PET Positron emission tomography

QA Quality assurance

QC Quality control

QP Qualified persons who are professional responsible for the release of a drug in Europe

QbD Qulaity by design

RPR Responsible person for the small-scale preparation of radiopharmaceuticals

RDRC Radioactive Drug Research Committee (FDA, U.S.)

SPECT Single photon emission computed tomography

SSRP Small-scale "in-house" radiopharmaceutical

SOP Standard operating procedure

TGA Therapeutic Goods Administration

TLC Thin layer chromatography

USP United States Pharmacopeia

WHO World Health Organization

Author details

Kung-Tien Liu[1*], Jian-Hua Zhao[2], Lee-Chung Men[2] and Chien-Hsin Chen[1]

*Address all correspondence to: ktliu@ecic.com.tw

1 Everlight Chemical Industrial Corporation,, Taiwan

2 Chemistry Division, Institute of Nuclear Energy Research,, Taiwan

References

[1] International Conference on Harmonisation. (2009). *ICH Harmonised Tripartite Guideline, Pharmaceutical Development, Q8 (R2).,* http://www.ich.org/fileadmin/

Public_Web_Site/ICH_Products/Guidelines/Quality/Q8_R1/Step4/Q8_R2_Guideline.pdf.

[2] International Conference on Harmonisation. (2005). *ICH Harmonised Tripartite Guideline, Quality Risk Management, Q9.*, http://www.ich.org/fileadmin/Public_Web_Site/ICH_Products/Guidelines/Quality/Q9/Step4/Q9_Guideline.pdf.

[3] International Conference on Harmonisation. (2008). *ICH Harmonised Tripartite Guideline, Pharmaceutical Quality System, Q10.*, http://www.ich.org/fileadmin/Public_Web_Site/ICH_Products/Guidelines/Quality/Q10/Step4/Q10_Guideline.pdf.

[4] International Atomic Energy Association. (2010). Planning a Clinical PET Centre. http://www-pub.iaea.org/MTCD/publications/PDF/Pub1457_web.pdf.

[5] Zimmerman, B. E., Herbst, C., Norenberg, J. P., & Woods, M. J. (2006). International Guidance on the Establishment of Quality Assurance Programmes for Radioactivity Measurement in Nuclear Medicine. *Applied radiation and isotopes*, 64(10), 1142-1146.

[6] International Atomic Energy Association. (2009). Quality Assurance for SPECT systems. http://www-pub.iaea.org/MTCD/publications/PDF/Pub1394_web.pdf.

[7] Bergmann, H., Busemann-Sokole, E., & Horton, P. W. (1995). Quality Assurance and Harmonisation of Nuclear Medicine Investigations in Europe. *European Journal of Nuclear Medicine and Molecular Imaging*, 22(5), 477-480.

[8] Chuck, A., Jacobs, P., Logus, J. W., St, Hilaire. D., Chmielowiec, C., & Mc Ewan, A. J. B. (2005). Marginal Cost of Operating a Positron Emission Tomography Center in a Regulatory Environment International. *Journal of Technology Assessment in Health Care*, 21(4), 442-451.

[9] Norenberg, J. P., Petry, N. A., & Schwarz, S. (2010). Operation of a Radiopharmacy for a Clinical Trial. *Seminars in Nuclear Medicine*, 40, 347-356.

[10] Decristoforo, C., & Schwarz, S. W. (2011). Radiopharmacy: Regulations and Legislations in Relation to Human Applications. *Drug Discovery Today: Technologies*, 8(2-4), e71-77.

[11] European Association of Nuclear Medicine. (2007). *Guidelines on current good Radiopharmacy Practice (cGRPP) in the Preparation of Radiopharmaceuticals, Version 2.*, http://www.eanm.org/publications/guidelines/gl_radioph_cgrpp.pdf.

[12] Elsinga, P., Todde, S., Penuelas, I., Meyer, G., Farstad, B., Faivre-Chauvet, A., et al. (2010). Guidance on Current Good Radiopharmacy Practice (CGRPP) for the Small-Scale Preparation of Radiopharmaceuticals. *European Journal of Nuclear Medicine and Molecular Imaging.*, 37(5), 1049-1062.

[13] World Health Organization. (2003). *WHO Expert Committee on Specifications for Pharmaceutical Preparations- WHO Technical Report Series, 908-Thirtyseventh Report.*, http://whqlibdoc.who.int/trs/who_trs_908.pdf.

[14] Barbet, J., Kraeber-Bodéré, F., & Chatal, J. F. (2008). Review: What Can Be Expected from Nuclear Medicine Tomorrow? *Cancer biotherapy and radiopharmaceuticals*, 23(4), 483-504.

[15] International Atomic Energy Agency. (2001, 18-22 January 1999). Paper presented at Therapeutic Applications of Radiopharmaceuticals, Proceedings of an International Seminar, Held in Hyderabad,, India. http://www-pub.iaea.org/MTCD/ publications/PDF/te_1228_prn.pdf.

[16] Atkinson, B. J., & Tu, S. M. (2011). Radiopharmaceuticals: Present and Future. *Journal of Supportive Oncology*, 9(6), 206-207.

[17] Zimmerman, B. E., Cessna, J. T., & Schima, F. J. (1998). The Standardization of the Potential Bone Palliation Radiopharmaceutical 117mSn (+ 4) Dtpa. *Applied radiation and isotopes.*, 49(4), 317-328.

[18] Kung, H. F., Kung, M. P., & Choi, S. R. (2003). Radiopharmaceuticals for Single-Photon Emission Computed Tomography Brain Imaging. *Seminars in Nuclear Medicine*, 33(1), 2-13.

[19] Imam, S. K. (2005). Molecular Nuclear Imaging: The Radiopharmaceuticals (Review). *Cancer biotherapy and radiopharmaceuticals*, 20(2), 163-172.

[20] Wong, F. C., & Kim, E. E. (2009). A Review of Molecular Imaging Studies Reaching the Clinical Stage. *European Journal of Radiology*, 70(2), 205-211.

[21] Glaser, M., Luthra, S. K., & Brady, F. (2003). Applications of Positron-Emitting Halogens in Pet Oncology (Review). *International Journal of Oncology*, 22(2), 253-268.

[22] Elsinga, P. H. (2002). Radiopharmaceutical Chemistry for Positron Emission Tomography. *Methods*, 27(3), 208-217.

[23] Srivastava, S., & Dadachova, E. (2001). Recent Advances in Radionuclide Therapy. *Seminars in Nuclear Medicine*, 31, 330-341.

[24] Jastrzebski, J. (2012). Radioactive Nuclei for Medical Applications. *Acta Physica Polonica B*, 43(3), 49-70.

[25] Miederer, M., Scheinberg, D. A., & Mc Devitt, M. R. (2008). Realizing the Potential of the Actinium-225 Radionuclide Generator in Targeted Alpha Particle Therapy Applications. *Advanced drug delivery reviews*, 60(12), 1371-1382.

[26] International Atomic Energy Agency. (2009). *Therapeutic Radionuclide Generators: Sr-90/Y-90 and W-188/Re-188 Generators..*, http://www-pub.iaea.org/MTCD/publications/PDF/trs470_web.pdf.

[27] Al-Nahhas, A., Win, Z., Szyszko, T., Singh, A., Nanni, C., Fanti, S., et al. (2007). Gallium-68 PET: A New Frontier in Receptor Cancer Imaging. *Anticancer research*, 27(6B), 4087-4094.

[28] Anderson, C. J., & Ferdani, R. (2009). Copper-64 Radiopharmaceuticals for PET Imaging of Cancer: Advances in Preclinical and Clinical Research. *Cancer Biotherapy and Radiopharmaceuticals.*, 24(4), 379-393.

[29] Farncombe, T. H., Gifford, H. C., Narayanan, M. V., Pretorius, P. H., Frey, E. C., & King, M. A. (2004). Assessment of Scatter Compensation Strategies for 67Ga SPECT Using Numerical Observers and Human Lroc Studies. *Journal of Nuclear Medicine,* 45(5), 802-812.

[30] Rajendran, J. G., Eary, J. F., Bensinger, W., Durack, L. D., Vernon, C., & Fritzberg, A. (2002). High-Dose 166Ho-Dotmp in Myeloablative Treatment of Multiple Myeloma: Pharmacokinetics, Biodistribution, and Absorbed Dose Estimation. *Journal of Nuclear Medicine.*, 43(10), 1383-1390.

[31] Schmitt, A., Bernhardt, P., Nilsson, O., Ahlman, H., Kölby, L., Maecke, H. R., et al. (2004). Radiation Therapy of Small Cell Lung Cancer with 177Lu-Dota-Tyr3-Octreotate in an Animal Model. Journal of Nuclear Medicine.; , 45(9), 1542-1548.

[32] Rahmim, A., & Zaidi, H. (2008). Pet Versus Spect: Strengths, Limitations and Challenges. *Nuclear Medicine Communications,* 193-207.

[33] Bateman, T. M. (2012). Advantages and Disadvantages of PET and SPECT in a Busy Clinical Practice. *Journal of Nuclear Cardiology,* 19, S3-S11.

[34] De Decker, M., & Dierckx, R. A. (2005). The Good Laboratory Practice and Good Clinical Practice Requirements for the Production of Radiopharmaceuticals in Clinical Research. *Nuclear Medicine Communications,* 575-579.

[35] Patidar, A. K., Patidar, P., Tandel, T. S., Mobiya, A. K., Selvam, G., & Jeyakandan, M. (2010). Current Trends in Nuclear Pharmacy Practice. *International Journal of Pharmaceutical Sciences Review and Research,* 5(2), 145-150.

[36] Laven, D. L., & Martin, W. R. (1989). Justification for Hospital-Based Nuclear Pharmacy Services. *Journal of Pharmacy Practice,* 2(3), 152-161.

[37] Mac, Farlane. C. R. (2006). Acr Accreditation of Nuclear Medicine and PET Imaging Departments. *Journal of Nuclear Medicine Technology,* 34(1), 18-24.

[38] Jarritt, P. H., Perkins, A. C., & Woods, S. D. (2004). Audit of Nuclear Medicine Scientific and Technical Standards. *Nuclear Medicine Communications,* 77-75.

[39] Organisation for Economic Co-operation and Development. (1998). OECD Series on Principles of Good Laboratory Practice and Compliance Monitoring. , OECD Principles on Good Laboratory Practice , 1

[40] Callahan, R. J., Chilton, H. M., Ponto, J. A., Swanson, D. P., Royal, H. D., & Bruce, A. D. (2007). Procedure Guideline for the Use of Radiopharmaceuticals 4.0. *Journal of Nuclear Medicine Technology,* 35(4), 272-275.

[41] Bombardieri, E., Aktolun, C., Baum, R. P., Bishof-Delaloye, A., Buscombe, J., Chatal, J. F., et al. (2003). Bone Scintigraphy: Procedure Guidelines for Tumour Imaging. *European Journal of Nuclear Medicine and Molecular Imaging*, 30(12), 99-106.

[42] Donohoe, K. J., Brown, M. L., & Collier, B. D. ((2003).). Society of Nuclear Medicine Procedure Guideline for Bone Scintigraphy. Bone Scintigraphy , 205-209.

[43] Delbeke, D., Coleman, R. E., Guiberteau, M. J., Brown, M. L., Royal, H. D., Siegel, B. A., et al. (2006). Procedure Guideline for SPECT/CT Imaging 1.0. *Journal of Nuclear Medicine*, 47(7), 1227-1234.

[44] Strauss, H. W., Miller, D. D., Wittry, M. D., Cerqueira, M. D., Garcia, E. V., Iskandrian, A. S., et al. (2008). Procedure Guideline for Myocardial Perfusion Imaging 3.3. *Journal of Nuclear Medicine Technology*, 36(3), 155-161.

[45] Stelmach, H., & Quinn, J. L. (1974). Radiopharmaceutical Quality Control. *Seminars in Nuclear Medicine*, 4, 295-303.

[46] Ahuja, S., & Scypinski, S. (2001). Handbook of Modern Pharmaceutical Analysis. Academic Press.

[47] Harapanhalli, R. S. (2010). Food and Drug Administration Requirements for Testing and Approval of New Radiopharmaceuticals. *Seminars in Nuclear Medicine*, 40, 364-384.

[48] Hoffman, J. M., Gambhir, S. S., & Kelloff, G. J. (2007). Regulatory and Reimbursement Challenges for Molecular Imaging1. *Radiology.*, 245(3), 645-660.

[49] Belcher, E. H. (1953). Scintillation Counters Using Liquid Luminescent Media for Absolute Standardization and Radioactive Assay. *Journal of Scientific Instruments*, 30, 286-289.

[50] Troughton, M. E. C. (1966). The Absolute Standardization of Cobalt-57. *The International Journal of Applied Radiation and Isotopes*, 17(3), 145-150.

[51] Günther, E. (2002). What Can We Expect from the Ciemat/Nist Method? *Applied Radiation and Isotopes*, 56(1-2), 357-360.

[52] Schönfeld, E., Schötzig, U., Günther, E., & Schrader, H. (1994). Standardization and Decay Data of 68ge/68ga. *Applied Radiation and Isotopes*, 45(9), 955-961.

[53] Plch, J., Zderadicka, J., & Kokta, L. (1974). Coincidence Methods of Standardization for 131cs and Measurement of Decay Parameters. *The International Journal of Applied Radiation and Isotopes.*, 25(10), 433-444.

[54] Barquero, L., & Roteta, M. (2002). Standardization of 134cs by Three Methods. *Applied Radiation and Isotopes.*, 56(1-2), 211-214.

[55] Funck, E., Debertin, K., & Walz, K. F. (1983). Standardization and Decay Data of 201tl. *International Journal of Nuclear Medicine and Biology*, 137-140.

[56] Hult, M., Altzitzoglou, T., Denecke, B., Persson, L., Sibbens, G., & Reher, D. F. G. (2000). Standardisation of 204tl at Irmm. *Applied Radiation and Isotopes*, 52(3), 493-498.

[57] Dias, M. S., & Koskinas, M. F. (2003). Standardization of a 204tl Radioactive Solution. *Applied Radiation and Isotopes*, 58(2), 235-238.

[58] Woods, D. H., Bowles, N. E., Jerome, S. M., de Lavison, P., Lineham, S., Makepeace, J. L., et al. (2000). Standardisation of 210pb. *Applied Radiation and Isotopes*, 52(3), 381-385.

[59] Sahagia, M., Razdolescu, A., Grigorescu, E. L., Luca, A., & Ivan, C. (2000). The Standardization of a 204tl Solution. *Applied Radiation and Isotopes*, 52(3), 487-491.

[60] Sahagia, M., Razdolescu, A. C., Grigorescu, E. L., Luca, A., & Ivan, C. (2006). Results Obtained by the Radionuclide Metrology Laboratory of IFIN-HH, in the International Comparisons of Standard Solutions, During 2002-2004. *Romanian Journal of Physics*, 51, 21-26.

[61] Kulkarni, D. B., Reddy, P. J., Bhade, S. P. D., Narayan, K. K., Narayanan, A., Krishnamachari, G., et al. (2006). Comparison of Efficiency Tracing and Zero Detection Threshold Techniques with Ciemat/Nist Standardization Method under Different Quench Conditions with Liquid Scintillation Spectrometer. *Current science*, 90(1), 83-87.

[62] Koskinas, M. F., Pires, C. A., Yamazaki, I. M., et al. (2008). Standardization of 55Fe by Tracing Method. Kidlington, Royaume Uni: Elsevier.

[63] Sochorová, J., Auerbach, P., & Havelka, M. (2008). Application Of "Wet" Extrapolation Method for Activity Standardisation of Electron Capture Radionuclides. *Applied Radiation and Isotopes.*, 66(6), 919-924.

[64] Gunther, E. W. (1994). Standardization of 59Fe and 131I by Liquid Scintillation Counting. *Nuclear Instruments and Methods in Physics Research Section A: Accelerators, Spectrometers, Detectors and Associated Equipment*, 339(1-2), 402-407.

[65] Simpson, B. R. S., & Meyer, B. R. (1998). Activity Measurement of 55Fe by an Efficiency Calculation Method. *Applied Radiation and Isotopes*, 1073-1076.

[66] Simpson, B. R. S., & Morris, W. M. (2004). Direct Activity Determination of 54Mn and 65Zn by a Non-Extrapolation Liquid Scintillation Method. *Applied Radiation and Isotopes*, 60(2), 475-479.

[67] Dias, M. S., Silva, F. F. V., & Koskinas, M. F. (2010). Standardization and Measurement of Gamma-Ray Probability Per Decay of 177Lu. *Applied Radiation and Isotopes*, 1349 -1353 .

[68] Van Wyngaardt, W. M., & Simpson, B. R. (2006). Absolute Activity Measurement of the Electron-Capture-Based Radionuclides 139Ce, 125I, 192Ir and 65Zn by Liquid Scintillation Coincidence Counting. *Applied radiation and isotopes: including data, in-*

strumentation and methods for use in agriculture, industry and medicine, 64(10-11), 1454 -1458.

[69] Hino, Y., Matui, S., Yamada, T., Takeuchi, N., Onoma, K., Iwamoto, S., et al. (2000). Absolute Measurement of 166mHo Radioactivity and Development of Sealed Sources for Standardization of γ-Ray Emitting Nuclides. *Applied Radiation and Isotopes,* 52(3), 545-549.

[70] Broda, R., Péron, M. N., Cassette, P., Terlikowska, T., & Hainos, D. (1998). Standardization of 139Ce by the Liquid Scintillation Counting Using the Triple to Double Coincidence Ratio Method. *Applied Radiation and Isotopes,* 1035-1040.

[71] Cassette, P., Broda, R., Hainos, D., & Terlikowska, T. (2000). Analysis of Detection-Efficiency Variation Techniques for the Implementation of the TDCR Method in Liquid Scintillation Counting. *Applied Radiation and Isotopes,* 52(3), 643-648.

[72] Johansson, L. C., & Sephton, J. P. (2010). Validation of a New TDCR System at NPL. *Applied radiation and isotopes,* 1537 -1539 .

[73] Kossert, K. (2010). Activity Standardization by Means of a New Tdcr-Cerenkov Counting Technique. *Applied radiation and isotopes,* 68(6), 1116-1120.

[74] Coursey, B. M., Cessna, J., Garcia-Torano, E., Golas, D. B., Grau, Malonda. A., Gray, D. H., et al. (1991). The Standardization and Decay Scheme of Rhenium-186. *International Journal of Radiation Applications and Instrumentation Part A Applied Radiation and Isotopes.,* 42(9), 865-869.

[75] Schönfeld, E., Janssen, H., Schotzig, U., Gunther, E., & Schrader, H. (1994). Standardization and Decay Data of 186Re. *Nuclear Instruments and Methods in Physics Research Section A: Accelerators, Spectrometers, Detectors and Associated Equipment,* 339(1-2), 174-179.

[76] Günther, E. (2000). Standardization of 237np by the Ciemat/Nist Lsc Tracer Method. *Applied Radiation and Isotopes.,* 52(3), 471-474.

[77] Koskinas, M. F., Fonseca, K. A., & Dias, M. S. (2002). Disintegration Rate Measurement of a 152Eu Solution. *Applied Radiation and Isotopes,* 56, 1-2, 441-445.

[78] Švec, A. (2009). Interpretation of Ionization Chamber Efficiency Curves. *Metrologia,* 43-46.

[79] Cessna, J. T., & Golas, D. B. (2012). The Nist Radioactivity Measurement Assurance Program for the Radiopharmaceutical Industry. *Applied radiation and isotopes.*

[80] Simpson, B.R.S. (2002). Radioactivity Standardization in South Africa. *Applied Radiation and Isotopes,* 56(1-2), 301-305.

[81] Oropesa, P., Hernández, A. T., Serra, R., Martinez, E., & Varela, C. (2003). Comparisons of Activity Measurements with Radionuclide Calibrators. *Applied Radiation and Isotopes,* 59(5-6), 383-387.

[82] Ivanov, Z. (2006). Results of the Quality Assurance Testing Program for Radiopharmaceuticals (2005), Version 3. *Australian: Australian Radiation Protection and Nuclear Safety Agency*, http://www.arpansa.gov.au/pubs/technicalreports/tr144.pdf.

[83] Capogni, M., De Felice, Y., Saito, N., & De Felice, P. (2011). *Ionising Radiation Metrology in the Field of Nuclear and Life Science Applications*, http://www.enea.it/it/internazionali/eventi-internazionali/enea-in-japan-2011/radiation-metrology/capogni.pdf.

[84] Hino, Y., & Ohgaki, H. (1998). Absolute Measurement of 192Ir. *Applied Radiation and Isotopes*, 1179-1183.

[85] Goerres, G. W., Hany, T. F., Kamel, E., von Schulthess, G. K., & Buck, A. (2002). Head and Neck Imaging with PET and PET/CT: Artefacts from Dental Metallic Implants. *European journal of nuclear medicine*, 29(3), 367-370.

[86] Kamel, E. M., Burger, C., Buck, A., von Schulthess., G. K., & Goerres, G. W. (2003). Impact of Metallic Dental Implants on CT-Based Attenuation Correction in a Combined PET/CT Scanner. *European radiology*, 13(4), 724-728.

[87] Carney, J., Townsend, D. W., Kinahan, P. E., Beyer, T., Kachelriess, M., Kalender, W. A., et al. (2001). CT-Based Attenuation Correction: The Effects of Imaging with the Arms in the Field of View. *Journal of Nuclear Medicine (suppl)* , 42, 56P-57P.

[88] Mawlawi, O., Pan, T., & Cody, D. D. (2004). Evaluation of a New CT Truncation Correction Algorithm for Accurate Quantification of PET/CT Images. *Journal of Nuclear Medicine (suppl)*: , 45, 413P.

[89] Teräs, M. (2008). Performance and Methodological Aspects in Positron Emission Tomography. Finland, University of Turku.

[90] Osman, M. M., Cohade, C., Nakamoto, Y., & Wahl, R. L. (2003). Respiratory Motion Artifacts on PET Emission Images Obtained Using CT Attenuation Correction on PET-CT. *European journal of Nuclear Medicine and Molecular Imaging*, 30(4), 603-606.

[91] Cohade, C., Osman, M., Marshall, L. T., & Wahl, R. L. (2003). PET-CT: Accuracy of PET and CT Spatial Registration of Lung Lesions. *European Journal of Nuclear Medicine and Molecular Imaging*, 30(5), 721-726.

[92] Botvinick, E.H., Zhu, Y.Y., O'Connell, W. J., & Dae, M. W. (1993). A Quantitative Assessment of Patient Motion and Its Effect on Myocardial Perfusion SPECT Images. *Journal of Nuclear Medicine*, 34(2), 303-310.

[93] Cooper, J. A., Neumann, P. H., & Mc Candless, B. K. (1992). Effect of Patient Motion on Tomographic Myocardial Perfusion Imaging. *Journal of Nuclear Medicine*, 33(8), 1566-1571.

[94] Wheat, J. M., Currie, G. M., & Ramsay, B. (2006). Visual Quality Control of Gated Myocardial Perfusion SPECT. *The Internet Journal of Cardiology*, 4(1).

[95] Wheat, J. M., & Currie, G. M. (2004). Incidence and Characterization of Patient Motion in Myocardial Perfusion SPECT: Part 1. *Journal of Nuclear Medicine Technology*, 32(2), 60-65.

[96] Hladik, W. B., & Norenberg, J. P. (1996). Problems Associated with the Clinical Use of Radiopharmaceuticals: A Proposed Classification System and Troubleshooting Guide. *European Journal of Nuclear Medicine and Molecular Imaging*, 23(8), 997-1002.

Chapter 2

Quality Assurance in Diagnostic Medical Exposures in Ghana - A Medical Physicist's Perspective

Stephen Inkoom

Additional information is available at the end of the chapter

1. Introduction

It is well known that medical expsoure procedures such as diagnostic radiology, nuclear medicine and radiotherapy remains the largest source of man made exposure to ionising radiation and continues to grow substantially. This makes the role of quality assurance (QA), an important tool in medical exposure procedures. This paper reviews the future of quality assurance in diagnostic medical exposures in Ghana from the perspective of a Medical Physicist, since a viable QA programme must be developed under the guidance and supervision of a medical physicist who is qualified in this area of expertise by education, training and experience. The Medical Physicist is expected to give guidance and supervision to the Technologists and other staff to execute the programme but should be prepared to perform higher level QA procedures as required. The focus of this review is on diagnostic radiology since it is the dominant mode of medical exposure as compared to nuclear medicine and radiotherapy procedures in Ghana as per the database of the Regulatory Authority Information System "(RAIS)" of the Radiation Protection Institute. It is also worth noting that most of the issues under consideration for discussion mirrors similar conditions in many developing countries. The main goal of a diagnostic quality assurance programme is to make sure that radiation doses to patients, staff and public are as low as reasonable achievable (ALARA) consistent with high quality diagnostic images of patients. An adequate diagnostic QA program involves periodic checks of all major components in the respective diagnostic imaging modalities. On the other hand, an optimum QA programme for any individual diagnostic facility will depend on some items such as the type of procedures performed, type of equipment utilized, patient workload, etc. The current scope of diagnostic imaging procedures in Ghana covers conventional, fluoroscopy, dental, computed tomography, interventional procedures and nuclear medicine scans. Interventional radiology procedures performed are quite few but the future looks promising in this field. The performance of QA practices are done on three fronts; namely at the hospital, equipment engineers and the Regulatory Authority (RA). The hospital based QA are done mainly by the Radiographic Technologist through their routine equipment warm ups and minor quality checks. Equipment Engineers perform engineer related QA checks through installation and acceptance testing, performance tests and periodic preventative maintenance procedures. On the other hand, the RA is largely in charge of major QA procedures through it's on site safety assessment inspections by assessing the compliance of the equipment within regulatory requirements. This is largely so because the RA has the technical expertise and equipment. Due to the expansion of diagnostic imaging procedures in medicine coupled with rapid technological advances, the availability of qualified and trained personnel is crucial if the desired quality is to be achieved. Some measures have been put in place for human resource development, but there is room for improvement. On the way forward, there is a strong need for the establishment of National Quality Control Centre for Diagnostic Radiology. This body must be equipped with the requisite state of the art equipment, highly qualified and trained personnel in order to coordinate all QA activities in the country. Such a body can initiate some guidelines on the minimum instrumentation requirements for all imaging modalities. Nevertheless, a good QA programmme is not a guarantee for the assurance of the radiation safety of patients, staff and public. What is also needed is a separate radiation safety programme, which is very essential in every diagnostic imaging facility and must also be under the direction of a qualified expert in radiation protection.

2. Overview of quality assurance

The 2008 United Nations Scientific Committee on the Effects of Atomic Radiation (UNSCEAR) report on medical exposures from the assessment of the global population dose from medical exposures for the period 1997-2007 indicates that medical exposure remains the largest source of man made exposure to ionizing radiation and continues to grow substantially. (UNSCEAR, 2008). A summary of the annual per caput effective dose to the global population due to all sources of ionizing radiation is illustrated in Table 1.

It is evident that diagnostic examinations result in a per caput effective dose of 0.66 mSv, while medical exposures now contribute around 20% of the average annual per caput dose to the global population. Medical exposures are defined as; (i) exposure of patients as part of their medical diagnosis or treatment; (ii) exposure of individuals as part of health screening programmes; and (iii) exposure of healthy individuals or patients voluntarily participating in medical, biomedical, diagnostic or therapeutic research programmes. These exposures include diagnostic radiology, nuclear medicine and radiation therapy (Fig. 1), out of which diagnostic radiology accounts for the largest contribution. Diagnostic radiology generally refers to the analysis of images obtained using x-rays. In nuclear medicine, a radiopharmaceutical is administered to the patient and concentrates primarily in a specific region of the body which allows: (i) external imaging of the body to evaluate structure and/or function, and (ii) or delivery of a large radiation dose to control a specific disease. Radiation therapy involves the use of intense radiation beams and high-activity sources for the treatment of many types of cancer.

Source	Annual per caput effective dose (mSv)	Contribution (%)
Natural background	2.4	79
Diagnostic medical radiology	0.62	20
Diagnostic dental radiology	0.0018	<0.1
Nuclear medicine	0.031	1.1
Fallout	0.005	<0.2
Total	3.1	100

Source: UNSCEAR 2008 report on medical radiation exposures. (UNSCEAR, 2008).

Table 1. Sources of ionizing radiation and the annual per caput effective dose to the global population.

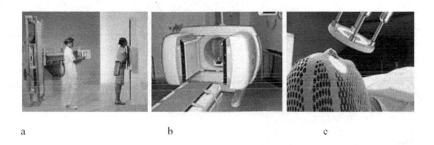

a   b   c

Figure 1. An illustration of (a) diagnostic radiology, (b) nuclear medicine and (c) radiation therapy procedures.

This makes the role of (QA), an important tool in medical exposure procedures. Quality assurance procedures must aim at to produce images of optimal diagnostic quality while ensuring that the radiation exposures to patients, staff and the public are kept as low as practicable. In achieving this goal, QA procedures if well implemented would ensure that any problem in the imaging chain will be dealt without a compromise in the diagnostic quality of the images. The World Health Organization (WHO), (WHO, 1982), indicates that achieving adequate diagnostic information and least possible exposure of the patient to radiation should be done at the lowest possible cost. An adequate diagnostic QA program involves periodic checks of all major components in the respective diagnostic imaging modalities. On the other hand, an optimum QA programme for any individual diagnostic facility will depend on some items such as the type of procedures performed, type of equipment utilized, patient workload, etc. Any QA procedure must be in agreement with the relevant national and international legislation or regulations on the protection and safe uses of ionising radiation. Another form of QA is to establish clinical audit, which is an essential tool for quality improvement in any diagnostic centre. For instance, the European Council directive (Commission of the European Communities. 1997) defines clinical audit as: "a systematic examination or review of medical radiological procedures which seeks to improve the quality and the outcome of patient care, through structured review whereby radiological practices, procedures, and results are examined against agreed standards for good medical radiological procedures, with modifications of the practices where indicated and the application of new standards if necessary."

This paper reviews the future of quality assurance in diagnostic medical exposures in Ghana from the perspective of a Medical Physicist, since a viable QA programme must be developed under the guidance and supervision of a medical physicist who is qualified in this area of expertise by education, training and experience. The Medical Physicist is expected to give guidance and supervision to the Technologists and other staff to executive the programme but should be prepared to perform higher level QA procedures as required.

3. Current status of quality assurance in diagnostic medical exposures

The types of diagnostic medical exposure procedures in Ghana are;

• Plain radiography

• Mammography

• Fluoroscopy

• Computed Tomography

• Dental

In addition to the above procedures for diagnosis, some hospitals perform interventional or invasive procedures on a limited scale. On the other hand, the types of medical exposure in nuclear medicine procedures are the use of gamma camera and single photon emission computed tomography (SPECT/CT) for imaging various organs. Plain radiography (screen-film and digital systems) is the dominant mode of all the diagnostic medical procedures, accounting for more than 80% of the total contribution of all the imaging modalities. (RAIS, 2011).

The performance of QA practices are done on three fronts; namely at the hospital, equipment/service engineers and the (RA). The hospital based QA are done mainly by the Radiographers/Radiologic Technologist through their routine equipment warm ups and minor quality checks. In this scenario, a qualified Medical Physicist with the requisite expertise must supervise such QA procedures. Unfortunately, there are not many Medical Physicists in diagnostic departments as compared to radiation therapy centres. Equipment/service engineers perform engineer related QA checks through installation and acceptance testing, performance tests and periodic preventative maintenance procedures as well as when there is equipment down time. On the other hand, the RA is largely in charge of major QA procedures through it's on site safety assessment inspections by assessing the compliance of the equipment within regulatory requirements. This is largely so because the RA has the requisite technical expertise and equipment.

In Ghana, Medical Physicists are engaged in service, teaching, research and administration activities. They perform some of the tasks outlined by the International Organisation for Medical Physics (IOMP) in its definition of who a Medical Physicist is and the roles and responsibilities (International Organisation for Medical Physics, 2010) such as:

- teaching principles of medical physics to physicians, residents, graduate students, medical students, technologists, and other health care professionals by means of lectures, problem solving, and laboratory sessions.

- conducting research into various human disorders, illnesses and disabilities, develop instrumentation, mathematical analysis and applications of computers in medicine; investigating biophysical techniques associated with any branch of medicine. Research is very important for advancement of medical physics as a profession and science.

- responsible for ensuring the quality, safety testing and correct maintenance of all radiation emitting devices in order to get an accurate diagnosis of illnesses. Medical Physicists also involved in the formulation of radiation protection guides and procedures specific to clinical environment and producing protocols to minimize radiation exposure of patients, staff and the general public.

- in administration, they supervise and manage radiation workers and other health professional workers.

- participating in and contributing to the development and implementation of national and

- prepares guidance on education and training drawing-up standards and guidance relating to medical devices.

- preparing, publishing and presenting scientific papers and reports

Ghana is involved in several International Atomic Energy Agency (IAEA) Technical and Research Projects. Some of the Projects in which Medical Physicists are involved are:

- RAF/9/033 - Strengthening Radiological Protection of Patients and Medical Exposure Control.

- RAF/9/034 - Establishment of National Capabilities for Response to a Radiological and Nuclear Emergency.

- RAF/9/035 - Education and Training in Support of Radiation Protection Infrastructure.

- RAF/9/032 - Development of Technical Capabilities for the Protection of Health and Safety of Workers Exposed to Ionizing Radiation.

- RAF/9/027 - National Regulatory Control and Occupational Radiation Protection Programmes.

- RAF/9/031 - Strengthening National Regulatory Infrastructure for the Control of Radiation Sources.

- GHA/6/015 - Upgrading and Expansion of Radiotherapy and Nuclear Medicine Services

- INT/6/054 - Strengthening Medical Physics in Radiation Medicine

- RAF/2/008 - Strengthening and Expanding Radiopharmacy Services in Africa (AFRA)

- RAF/6/032 - Promoting Regional and National Quality Assurance Programmes for Medical Physics in Nuclear Medicine (AFRA II-7)

- RAF/6/041 - Supporting the Development of Comprehensive National Cancer Control Programmes

- RAF/6/044 - Medical Physics in Support of Cancer Management (AFRA II-8)

- RAF/6/045 - Enhancing Accessibility and Quality in the Care of Cancer Patients (AFRA II-10)

The main objectives of some of the projects are discussed. For instance in RAF/9/033, the objectives are to upgrade / strengthen radiological protection of the patient in medical exposures due to:

i.   Diagnostic Radiology and Interventional Radiological procedures

ii.   Nuclear Medicine procedures

iii.   Radiotherapy practice

The objectives of other projects are as follows:

- GHA/6/015 - To consolidate existing radiotherapy and nuclear medicine facilities at two leading Teaching Hospitals located in the southern part of the country, and establish a third one in the northern part to cater for the diagnosis, curative and palliative treatment of cancer patients and the efficient diagnosis and management of other diseases.

- INT/6/054 - To promote the recognition of medical physics in radiation medicine and to harmonize educational material in order to ensure safe and effective diagnosis and treatment of patients.

- RAF/2/008 - To strengthen radiopharmacy in support of in vivo and in vitro nuclear medicine in Africa.

- RAF/6/032 - To improve the effectiveness and safety of nuclear medicine procedures by providing support for design and implementation of quality assurance (QA) programmes and by establishing training and education programmes in medical radiation physics, focusing on aspects related to the application of nuclear medicine techniques.

- RAF/6/041 - To assist Member States in performing comprehensive cancer capacity need assessments and national cancer strategic planning via collaboration with IAEA, WHO, and other partners under the Programme of Action for Cancer Therapy (PACT) umbrella.

- RAF/6/044 - To strengthen national and regional medical physics capabilities to ensure efficient support of cancer management in AFRA Member States and to sustain quality assurance/quality control (QA/QC) programmes, including the promotion of safety culture and innovative practices in dosimetry.

- RAF/6/045 - To establish national and regional networks in clinical radiation oncology. To interact with National Organizations with the aim to promote the comprehensive management of commonest cancers. Support academic education, training and accreditation, patients and personnel safety in radiotherapy improvement of documentation of clinical outcomes through regular patient assessment.

4. Regulatory guidelines for quality assurance procedures

The National Competent/Regulatory Authority in Ghana charged with the responsibility for authorization and inspection of practices using ionizing radiation sources and radioactive materials is the Radiation Protection Board (RPB) (Radiation Protection Instrument LI 1559, 1993). However, the operational functions of the RPB are carried out by RPI, which was established in 2000 to provide scientific and technical support for the enforcement of the provisions in LI 1559. Details about how the RA was established and the main activities have been described elsewhere (Inkoom et al, 2011). There are plans to establish a new Regulatory Body to regulate the peaceful uses of nuclear energy and technology which will be independent of any governmental agency. Currently, the RA is answerable to the Ghana Atomic Energy Commission (GAEC) which is a promoter for the peaceful uses of nuclear energy and technology and also plays the role of a regulator. However, the new RA is expected to be only a regulator and not a promoter of the application of nuclear technology.

5. Human resource development

The categories of Radiographic Staff available in Ghana are Radiologists, Medical Physicists, Biomedical Engineers and Radiographers/X-ray Technicians. Most of our Radiologists were trained overseas until the last few years when local training of Radiologists started and the accreditation is given by either the Ghana College of Surgeons or the West African College of Physicians and Surgeons. Similarly, the other professionals were also trained overseas. Currently, the School of Allied Health Sciences (SAHS), College of Health Sciences (CHS) of the University of Ghana (UG) is responsible for churning out medical and dental technical graduates in physiotherapy, medical laboratory science and radiography. There are plans to establish another Allied Health University and some private institutions are also running some of the programmes. A Post-Graduate School of Nuclear and Allied Sciences which was established jointly by the GAEC and UG, in co-operation with the IAEA is training the Medical Physicists, Radiation Protection Professionals, Nuclear Engineers, etc. at the National and Sub-Regional levels.

6. Recent trends in quality assurance

The increasing expansion of diagnostic imaging procedures in medicine coupled with rapid technological advances makes the availability of qualified and trained personnel to be very crucial if the desired quality is to be achieved. This come with a lot challenges to the medical imaging community. This offers practitioners the opportunity to continually undergo retraining and other continuous professional development programmes in their respective fields. Also with the emergence of picture archiving and communication system (PACS) in many hospitals, there is the need for the development of appropriate on line QA procedures and in corporating them into hospital PACS systems. Special attention must also be given to the emergence of digital technology over the last decade as one of the greatest technological advances in medical imaging. This new technolgy poses a great challenge in medical imaging, requiring re-training of staff on the safe use of equipment and radiation protection issues. In Ghana for instance, the RPI of GAEC, in collaboration with the IAEA, has in the previous years developed a lot of expertise in the training of occupationally exposed workers in Ghana and the rest of Africa, spanning a period of almost two decades (Boadu et al. 2011). This local expertise in training can be tapped. In this regard, a critical review of all QA procedures that were developed for screen-film systems needs special attention.

7. The way forward

Various practitioners in the medical imaging community must brace themselves in order to face challenges of technological developments. With the advent of digital radiography: advances in computed radiography, direct digital radiography, digital subtraction angiography, new digital receivers, image processing techniques, computer applications in radiology and PACS offers enormous challenges. The advantages of digital technology:post-processing capabilities, decreased costs, multiple viewing options, electronic transfer, possibilities of archiving, wide dynamic range of flat panel detectors and increased detection quantum efficiency has led to a high demand of this technology by the medical imaging community. Therefore, the development of the requisite human resource must be continued and sustained in order to deal with the challenges.

There is a strong need for the establishment of National Quality Control Centre for Diagnostic Radiology. This body must be equipped with the requisite state of the art equipment, highly qualified and trained personnel in order to coordinate all QA activities in the country. Such a body can initiate some guidelines on the minimum instrumentation requirements for all imaging modalities. With the training of more Medical Physicists sand Radiation Protection Professionals, it is expected that they would take up positions in all major hospitals which have a myriad of imaging modalities. The Ghana Society of Medical Physics, RA, Ministry of Health and other stakeholders must initiate procedures for the establishment of Medical Physics Departments in such hospitals. This would give the necessary recognition to the profession of Medical Physics in Ghana, which has been given recognition by the International Labour Organization (ILO) in its International Standard Classification of Occupations (ISCO) (ILO, 2008). With this recognition, Medical Physics has been accepted as modern applied branch of physics. Clinical audit should also be incorporated in the overall QA procedures in the country.

As the uses of ionizing radiation continue to increase in medicine, it is also expected that the services of Medical Physicist would increase. As such, more physicists would be required to be trained in subsequent years. Appropriate accreditation bodies charged with issuing accreditation certificates, for a period of years must be put in place to regulate the profession of Medical Physics and maintain international standards of practice.

8. Conclusion

The role of an effective QA programme in any diagnostic department cannot be overemphasized especially if the desired quality of producing good diagnostic images and the least radiation exposure are to be achieved. Nevertheless, a good QA programmme is not a guarantee for the assurance of the radiation safety of patients, staff and public. What is also needed is a separate radiation safety programme, which is very essential in every diagnostic imaging facility and must also be under the direction of a qualified expert in radiation protection or a Medical Physicist expert. With significant contributions in clinical service, education, and research, Medical Physics continues to grow in importance both as a profession and as science, driven by the technological developments of societies in general and medicine in particular.

Acknowledgements

The support received from the Radiation Protection Institute of Ghana Atomic Energy Commission is appreciated.

Author details

Stephen Inkoom

Radiation Protection Institute, Ghana Atomic Energy Commission, Legon, Accra, Ghana

References

[1] Boadu, M., Schandorf, C., Emi-Reynolds, G., Faanu, A., Inkoom, S., Kwabena, Gye-kye. P., & Kaikor, M.C. (2011). Systematic approach to training of occupationally exposed workers in Ghana andthe rest of Africa. *Health Phys*, 101(2: S116YS120).

[2] Commission of the European Communities. (1997). Council Directive 97/43/ Euratom of 30 Juneon health protection of individuals against the dangers of ionizing radiation in relation to medical exposure, and repealing Directive 84/466 Euratom. *Off. J. Eur. Commun. Rep. L.*, 180(1997), 22-27.

[3] International Labour Organization (ILO). *International Standard Classification of Occupations (ISCO), Geneva, Switzerland, (ISCO-08), 2008.*

[4] International Organisation for Medical Physics (IOMP). (2010). IOMP Policy Statement No.1. *The Medical Physicist: Role and Responsibilities, IOMP Working Group on Policy Statement* [1].

[5] Radiation Protection Instrument LI 1559. (1993). *Provisional National Defence Council Law 308, Accra, Ghana. Date of Gazette Notification: 2nd April, 1993.*

[6] Regulatory Authority Information System [RAIS]. (2011). *Radiation Protection Institute, Ghana Atomic Energy Commission, Accra, Ghana.*

[7] Inkoom, S., Schandorf, C., Reynolds, G. E., & Fletcher, J. J. (2011). Quality Assurance and Quality Control of Equipment in Diagnostic Radiology Practice-The Ghanaian Experience. *Wide Spectra of Quality Control, Isin Akyar (Ed.)*, 291-308, 978-9-53307-683-6, InTech, http://www.intechopen.com/articles/show/title/quality-assurance-and-quality-control-of-equipment-in-diagnostic-radiology-practice-the-ghanaian-exp.

[8] United Nations Scientific Committee on the Effects of Atomic Radiation. (2008). *Sources and effects of ionizing radiation. Report to the General Assembly with scientific annexes (UNSCEAR).*

[9] World Health Organization (1982). Quality Assurance in Diagnostic Radiology, Macmillan Procrom,9-24154-164-4

Chapter 3

Unified Procedures for Quality Controls in Analogue and Digital Mammography

Barbara Testagrossa, Giuseppe Acri, Federica Causa,
Raffaele Novario, Maria Giulia Tripepi and
Giuseppe Vermiglio

Additional information is available at the end of the chapter

1. Introduction

Breast cancer is the most commonly diagnosed cancer in women [1]. Current attempts to control breast cancer concentrate on early detection by means of massive screening campaign, via periodic mammography and physical examination, because ample evidence in dicates that such screening indeed can be effective in lowering the death rate [2]. Early diagnosis of breast cancer plays a leading role in reducing the mortality and improving the prognosis of this disease [3].

Mammography consists in imaging the female breast using X-rays with low contrast (to keep the delivered dose low), but at the same time high resolution (especially used for early detection).

The goal of mammography is to achieve the image quality required for a given detection task, while ensuring that the patient-absorbed dose is kept as low as reasonably achievable [4]. As practised now, it normally requires a dedicated X-ray tube with special anode materials such as molybdenum or rhodium, small focal spots, operating at a tube voltage around 25 to 32 kV, and carefully chosen films and screens in dedicated cassettes. Stationary or moving grids are used as in other branches of plain film radiography. Present-day mammography can be described as a low-dose procedure [5]. In recent years, advances in screen-film technology and film-processing techniques have contributed to major improvements in the quality of mammographic images. At present, two distinct mammographic techniques exist:

- Analogue mammography in which the image is recorded on a film.

- Digital mammography in which the image is digitalised.

The production of analogue or digital mammography images is based on two distinct concepts of image formation [6].

The analogue image is a continuous representation of spatial and intensity variations of the X-ray pattern transmitted by the tissue under analysis. Traditionally, the mammographic image is analogue, obtained using conventional screen-film image receptors as the standard detector [7]. The advantages of screen-film mammography are: high spatial resolution and low contrast sensitivity achieved through improvements in X-ray tube design, screen-film combinations, grids, and film processing [8]. Thus, analogue mammography permits high image quality, low patient dose, and most importantly, the ability to detect small, nonpalpable breast cancers.

In digital systems, image acquisition and display are two independent processes [4]. In such systems images are captured as a digital signal, making electronic transfer and storage of images possible. Digital systems offer a large dynamic range of operation, improving visualization of all areas of the breast and increasing exposure latitude. Also, the digital format allows grayscale adjustment to optimize contrast for any imaging task.

In addition, with the digitalization of the diagnostic image, new medical applications have now emerged, such as Computer-Aided Diagnosis (CAD), stereo mammography, tomosynthesis, contrast medium imaging and dual energy imaging [7].

For a successful screening function the mammograms should contain sufficient diagnostic information to be able to detect breast cancer, using a radiation dose as low as reasonably achievable (ALARA principle). In this context, it is necessary to establish and actively maintain regular and adequate Quality Assurance (QA) procedures that take into account medical, organisational and technical aspects. The QA procedure should include periodic tests to ensure accurate target and critical structure localization. Such tests are referred to as Quality Controls (QC). They are fundamental for the QA procedure because they help ascertain that the equipment performs consistently at a high quality level.

However, whilst the requirement for standardisation is impelling, the Italian legislation (D.L.vo 187/00) is not keeping pace with the advances in mammographic technology. Indeed, at present both analogue and digital formats are used in an un-regulated way, without introducing a proper regulation especially for digital mammography. As a consequence, the QA protocols have been adapted ad hoc to the new digital technology, thus resulting in multiple protocols, some of which valid only for specific machines, resulting in high costs of operation.

On the other hand, at the European level, QA procedures for both analogue and digital mammography systems have been properly addressed and defined, [European guidelines for quality assurance in mammography screening – 4th Edition, Section 2]. In both cases, in fact, the QC of the physical and technical aspects must guarantee the best possible diagnostic information obtainable and image quality stability, within the limits imposed by the ALARA principle.

However, for the case of digital systems the imaging chain can be divided into three independent parts, as cited in [9]:

a.   Image acquisition, including X-ray generation system, image receptor and (in some systems) image receptor corrections;

b.   Image processing software;

c.   Image presentation, including monitor, imaging presentation software, printer and viewing box.

To produce images with adequate quality, each part of the imaging chain must function within the limits dictated by the standards of screen-film mammography [9], although the definition of such limits for digital systems is still in progress.

In the EUREF protocol it is assumed that digital mammography should perform at least as screen-film mammography.

In this context, a unified protocol is proposed here that can be used with either analogue or digital mammography systems, with the view of reducing the volume of verification procedures to test the operation of such equipment. The advantage of the proposed protocol is that it can be applied as is to both analogue and digital mammography. The results obtained from the application of this protocol to analogue and digital mammography are presented in Section 3, with particular emphasis on image quality. The remaining part of this Section is dedicated to a review of mammographic techniques.

1.1. Screen-film mammography

In screen-film mammography, the film is used as the medium for both image acquisition and display. However, whilst providing excellent spatial resolution in high contrast structures, screen-film mammography has limited detection capability for low-contrast lesions in dense breasts [10]. On phantoms, the highest spatial resolution can be as high as 15–20 lp/mm but with a very low associated contrast. In addition, noise can limit the reliability of detection, especially for the small or subtle structures [11]. Although considerable advances in film-screen mammography have occurred over the past 20 years, some inherent limitations to further technical improvement exist [12]. One such limitation results from the trade - off between dynamic range (latitude) and contrast resolution (gradient) [13]. The relationship between X-ray exposure, image density, and contrast is illustrated by the Hurter and Driffield (H&D) sigmoid curve (Fig. 1) which uniquely characterises a given type of screen-film system under specific conditions [14].

Because of the sigmoid shape of the characteristic curve, the range of X-ray exposures over which the film display gradient is significant, i.e., the image latitude, is limited. The parts of the H&D curve where the slope is flat indicate poor contrast (i.e. over- or under-exposed images) [12, 16].

In screen-film mammography, the automatic exposure control (AEC) has the critical role of ensuring that the appropriate amount of radiation reaches the image receptor to produce a target optical density on the processed film [16]. In AEC systems, an ion chamber or other radiation detector is placed beneath the film cassette and connected electrically to the exposure time control circuit. When a pre-set amount of radiation has been detected, the exposure is automatically terminated. Other limitations of film-screen mammography include (a) noise caused by the random fluctuation of X-ray quantum absorption by the fluorescent screen and the film emulsion, which can limit the detection of subtle structures, (b) the trade-off between spatial resolution and detection efficiency of the film and screen, and (c) the inefficiency of rejection of scatter radiation by the mammographic grid [12].

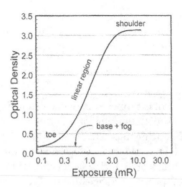

Figure 1. The Hurted & Driffield (H&D) curve describes optical density (OD) vs. the logarithm (base 10) of exposure [15].

1.2. Digital mammography

Digital mammography is an emerging technology, first approved in January 2000 [17], in which the image acquisition, display and storage functions can be performed independently, allowing for optimisation of each function. It offers several potential advantages including wider dynamic range, improved contrast, increased signal to noise ratio for overcoming the limitations of the film–screen combination (limited latitude, limited display contrast, low detection efficiency and noise), and therefore, increasing the sensitivity and specificity of breast cancer detection [18, 19]. Moreover, digital images offer a variety of new and improved applications. The digital image will provide image archiving and retrieval advantages over film, and will facilitate the use of computer-aided diagnosis [11, 20]. Other advanced applications made possible through digital imaging, such as dual energy and 3D tomosynthesis are expected to further improve diagnostic sensitivity and specificity.

In particular, Full Field Digital Mammography (FFDM) offers the promise of revolutionizing the practice of mammography through its superior dose and contrast performance [20]. In FFDM the screen-film is substituted by a fixed or removable digital detector. The digital image is obtained by sampling the X-ray pattern at discrete increments of spatial position and image signal intensity. Any digital image is a 2-dimensional grid of picture elements (pixels), which is defined by its size and bit depth. The size of an image is given by the length by width (in pixels) product. The bit depth is the number of shades of gray that can be displayed [1].

In a digital imager a detector absorbs the X-rays and produces an electronic signal at each pixel. The signal is then translated into a digital value by an analog-to-digital converter

(ADC). Once the digital image is stored in the computer memory it can be displayed with contrast independent of the detector properties [12].

Digital mammography systems, unlike screen-film mammography systems, allow manipulation of fine differences in image contrast by means of image processing algorithms [10]. The physical properties of the digital image (contrast, resolution and noise) can vary noticeably according to the detection technology used. There are two methods of image capture used in digital mammography that represent different generations of technology: indirect conversion and direct conversion [20].

Indirect conversion digital detectors uses a two step process for X-rays detection, similar to screen-film [1].

Direct conversion should not be confused with "direct readout", which is a capability of all electronic detectors.

Fully digital mammography (FDM) detectors are the final class of detectors. These detectors are sealed units that are permanently mounted to a mammography system. FDM detectors are electronic devices that directly capture X-ray images. In general, such devices require that a new mammography system be installed [8].

1.2.1. Photostimulable phosphors (Computed Radiography systems)

Computed Radiography (CR) is at this moment the most common digital radiography modality in radiology departments, in place of conventional screen film systems [21].

CR for mammography system employ as the X-ray absorber a storage photostimulable phosphor imaging plate (typically $BaFBr:Eu^{+2}$, where the atomic energy levels of the europium activator determine the characteristics of light emission), that replaces the traditional screen-film combination [22]. In this case, the removable detector or the Imaging Plate (IP) is inserted as a cassette in a conventional mammography unit. So, the IP can be used in a standard mammography machine without modification [7].

X-ray absorption mechanisms are identical to those of conventional phosphors. The peculiarity here is that the useful optical signal is not derived from the light that is emitted in prompt response to the incident radiation, but rather from the subsequent emission.

CR digital phosphor plates have shown promise in mammographic imaging because of the wide exposure latitude and linear response [23].

The potential advantages of this technology are the small detector-element size, the fact that the plates can be used also in conventional mammography units, the ease of having multiple plate sizes, and the relatively low cost. In addition the plates are reusable since they can be readily erased optically [8].

However scattering of the light within the phosphor causes the release of traps over a greater area of the image than the size of the incident laser beam. This results in loss of spatial resolution [24].

1.2.2. Optical detector

The detector consists of a phosphor screen, a charged coupled device (CCD) camera, and a fiberoptic taper to couple the light from the screen to the camera. It now represents the most widely used digital mammography technique for cassette-free imaging [8].

The imaging performance of these systems depends on a number of factors, including the characteristics of the phosphor screen, the choice of CCD and the method used to optically couple the phosphor to the CCD.

A CCD is an integrated circuit formed by depositing a series of electrodes, called 'gates' on a semiconductor substrate to form an array of metal-oxide-semiconductor (MOS) capacitors [22].

CCDs are particularly well suited to digital radiography because of their high spatial resolution capability, wide dynamic range and high degree of linearity with incident signal.

1.2.3. Flat panel

The active matrix flat panel technology is the most promising digital radiographic technique [25, 26].

The active matrix detector is based on large glass substrates on which imaging pixels are deposited.

This flat panel plate consists of a matrix of approximately 5 million photodiodes that form the readout for each image. The charge produced on the diode in response to light emitted from the phosphor surface is collected and digitized [1].

2. Quality Control (QC)

QCs are fundamental to guarantee that the radiological equipment performs consistently, with standard and constant physical and technical operational parameters.

The technological advances of the past ten years have revolutionised imaging techniques for diagnostics. As a consequence, QC procedures need to be updated to suit the new technologies and related protocols. This is particularly true for mammographic equipment, for which the physical parameters to be monitored to guarantee high-quality imaging are identified in specific documents.

The European Protocol for "Quality Control of the Physical and Technical Aspects of Mammography Screening" [9] gives guidance on physical, technical and dose measurements, and the periodicity of the corresponding tests to be performed as part of mammography screening programmes.

On the other hand, in the case of the Italian regulation, the relevant legislation (D.L.vo 187/00) was approved before the commercialisation of CR and digital mammography. Therefore, guidelines and procedures for CR and digital mammography are missing.

This shortcoming is particularly relevant in the case of mammography because it is well known that both image quality and breast dose depend on the equipment used and the radiographic technique employed.

For a complete and accurate estimate of image quality and delivered dose, the following components and system parameters should be monitored [9]:

• X-ray generation and exposure control system

• Bucky and image receptor

• Film processing (for screen-film systems)

• Image processing (for digital systems)

• System properties (including dose)

• Monitors and printers (for digital systems)

• Viewing conditions

		Screen-film mammography	Digital mammography
X-ray generation	X-ray source	Focal spot size	
		Source-to-image distance	
		Alignment of X-ray field/Image receptor	
		Film/bucky edge	
		Radiation leakage	
		Output	
	Tube voltage	Reproducibility	
		Accuracy	
		HVL	
	AEC	Central opt. dens. control settings	Exposure control steps: central value
		Opt. dens. control step	Exposure control steps: difference per step
		Target opt. dens. control settings	------
		Short-term reproducibility	Short-term reproducibility
		Long-term reproducibility	Long-term reproducibility / Variation in SNR
			Variation in dose

		Screen-film mammography	Digital mammography
		Object thickness and tube voltage compensation	Object thickness and tube voltage compensation / CNR per PMMA thickness
		Adjustable range	-----
		Spectra	-----
		Correspondence between AEC sensors	------
		Back-up timer and security cut-off	
Compression		Compression force	
		Maintain force for 1 minute	
		Compression force indicator	
		Compression plate alignment, symmetric	
Bucky and image receptor	Anti scatter grid	Grid system factor	
	Screen-film	Inter cassette sensitivity variation (mAs)	-----
		Inter cassette sensitivity variation (OD range)	-----
		Screen-film contact	-----
	Response function	-----	Linearity
		-----	Noise evaluation
	Missed tissue at chest wall side detector homogeneity	-----	Variation in mean pixel value (on image)
		-----	Variation in SNR (on image)
		-----	Variation in mean SNR (between images)
		-----	Variation in dose (between images)
	Detector element failure	-----	Number of defective dels
		-----	Position of defective dels
	Uncorrected dels	-----	Number of uncorrected defective dels
		-----	Position of uncorrected defective dels

	Screen-film mammography	Digital mammography
Inter plate sensitivity variations	-----	Variation in SNR
	-----	Variation in dose
Dosimetry	Glandular dose per PMMA thickness	
Image quality	Threshold contrast visibility	
	Exposure time	
	Spatial resolution	MTF and NPS
	-----	Scanning time
	-----	Geometric distortion
	-----	Artifact evaluation
	-----	Ghost image factor

Table 1. Operational parameters relevant to analogue and digital mammographs [9].

Some of the above components are suitable only for analogue systems, others only for digital ones, and some are common to both systems although requiring dedicated QC procedures.

With reference to QCs for mammography, the EU legislation is subdivided in two parts: Section 2a for screen-film mammography, Section 2b for digital mammography. In both cases, several measurements should be undertaken by medical physicists. The components that are common to both analogue and digital mammographic systems are listed in Table 1 with corresponding operational parameters specific for the two cases. As expected, the methodology to be used for QC in the two different cases are substantially different particularly with respect to image quality monitoring.

For example, in the case of traditional, analogue mammography, spatial resolution and threshold contrast visibility can be used to uniquely characterise the image quality. On the other hand, in digital mammography image quality is assessed by monitoring the Modulation Transfer Function (MTF), Noise Power Spectrum (NPS) and Nyquist frequency. MTF represents the efficiency or fan imaging system in reproducing subject contrast at various spatial frequencies [7, 20, 27]. The Nyquist frequency, instead, indicates the maximum spatial resolution that can be visualized in an image. NPS provides information on noise at different spatial frequencies. In digital mammography, in fact, spatial resolution is obtained from MTF and Nyquist frequency.

The combination of MTF and NPS gives the Detective Quantum Efficiency (DQE), regarded as the best overall indicator of the image quality of digital radiographic systems. DQE is the efficiency with which a detector uses the incident photons to form an image [28]. Systems with higher DQE can produce higher quality images, at the same dose. Further, there are also other parameters that need to be monitored in digital techniques to defined the image quality. These are listed in Table 2.

Metric	Performance attribute
MTF	Resolution properties of the image/detector/system
NPS	Noise properties of the image/detector/system
DQE	SNR transfer properties of the detector
eDQE	SNR transfer properties of the system
Dark noise	Noise in the absence of signal
Uniformity	Signal uniformity in the absence of an object
Exposure Indicator	Accuracy of exposure indication by the system
Linearity	Exposure response behavior of the system
High-contrast resolution	Ability of the system to represent high-contrast patterns
Low-contrast resolution	Ability of the system to represent low-contrast patterns
Distortion	Geometrical accuracy of images
Artifact	Non-uniform artifactual features in the images
Ghosting	Appearance of shadows of prior images on subsequent images
Throughput	Speed by which a system can sequentially capture images
Normal exposure	Target exposure values for clinical use reflecting system speed

Table 2. List of parameters for digital image quality control [27].

The problem is to define a unified protocol that can be applied to any (analogue, CR, digital) type of mammographic system.

On the basis of procedures developed previously [29, 30], and to minimise problems arising from the use of different QC procedure to monitor different physical parameters for analogue and digital mammographs it is proposed here to monitor only parameters related to the beam at the output of the RX tube. The resulting QC procedure is then flexible and applicable universally to any type of mammograph.

The only additional pieces of equipment needed to execute the proposed QC is a phantom coupled to a solid-state exposure meter (PHAN-EX).

The phantom is a 4.5 cm thick block of PMMA, simulating a standard breast, including details simulating those of clinical interest (micro-calcification, tumoral mass, fibrous structures). This is coupled to an RX exposure meter composed of a photodiode and a digital counter, thus capable of measuring the exposure and the quality of the mammographic image [31]. The proposed protocol was tested on different (analogue and digital) mammographs, to assess its versatility and accuracy, independent of the physical characteristics of the mammographic system. Results on AEC tests obtained from the implementation of the proposed protocol implemented on analogue and digital mammographs, are presented and discussed in Section 3.

Acoustic and light signaling	Acceptance test, status test and constancy test. The acoustic and light signals should function properly. Operating procedure: The test of acoustic and light signalling will be performed with the exposure. Frequency: Daily
Security cut-off	Acceptance test, status test and constancy test. The security cut-off should function properly. Operating procedure: To verify the correct functioning of the security cut-off produce an exposure with a high mAs value and report the measured dose. Then, produce a second exposure releasing the switch before the set time and report the new measured dose. This value had to be considerably smaller than the previous one. Frequency: Daily
Source-to-image distance	Acceptance test. Manufacturers specification, typical ≥ 600 mm. Operating procedure: if the focal spot is indicated, measure the distance between the focal spot indication mark on the tube housing and the top surface of the bucky. Add the distance between bucky surface and the top of the image receptor to the resulting value. Alternatively, calculate the source-to-image distance by the magnification of an object of known dimension.
Long-term reproducibility	Constancy test. Deviations from the reference value of exposures ≤ ± 2%. Operating procedure: the long term reproducibility of the AEC system is calculated by determining the deviation of the exposures obtained from the phan-ex and from the reference value (45 mm PMMA test block), with the exposure meter accurately placed on the plate holder. The measured counts per second (cps) should be recorded. Frequency: Yearly
Short term reproducibility	Acceptance test, status test and constancy test. Deviations from the mean value of exposures < ± 5%. Operating procedure: the short term reproducibility of the AEC system is calculated by the deviation of the 3 routine exposures (45 mm PMMA test block) of the phan-ex, with the exposure meter accurately placed on the plate holder. The measured counts per second (cps) should be recorded. Frequency: Yearly
Object thickness compensation	Acceptance test, status test and constancy test. Deviations from the reference value of exposures (45 mm PMMA test block) ≤ ± 15%. Operating procedure: the object thickness compensation of the AEC is calculated by determining the deviation of exposures of the phan-ex detector, accurately placed on PMMA plates of 30, 45 and 60 mm thickness, from the reference value (45 mm PMMA) at 28 kV. The measured counts per second (cps) should be recorded. Frequency: Yearly
Tube voltage compensation	Acceptance test, status test and constancy test. Deviations from the reference value of exposures (45 mm PMMA test block, imaged at 28 kV) ≤ ± 15%.

Operating procedure: the tube voltage compensation of the AEC is calculated by imaging the 45 mm PMMA test block, setting the tube voltage at 26 kV, 28 kV and 30 kV, with the exposure meter of the phan-ex accurately placed on the test block. The measured counts per second (cps) should be recorded.

Frequency: Yearly

Difference per step	Acceptance test, status test and constancy test.
	All the deviation in the measured exposures between successive steps: 0.1 - 0.2 per step.
	Operating procedure: The optical density control step can be determined by placing the phan-ex on a 45 mm PMMA plate and taking an exposure at all possible steps, setting the operating voltage at 28 kV. The measured counts per second (cps) should be recorded.
	Frequency: Yearly
Uniformity	Acceptance test, quality control.
	Parallel to the axis tube, the exposure value should decrease by 30-35 % at a height of 12 cm from the chest wall. Perpendicularly to the axis tube, a typical value of exposure decrease is < 7% from the centre of the X-ray field to 10 cm, for each side.
	Operating procedure: Beam uniformity can be determined by positioning the exposure meter on a 45 mm PMMA plate, first at the centre of the PMMA plate and, successively, at the top, right, bottom and left of the test block. Image the plate and report the measured counts per second (cps).
	Frequency: Yearly
Spatial resolution (at high frequency)	Acceptance test, status test and constancy test.
	Spatial resolution should be ≥ 12 line pairs per mm (lp/mm)
	Operating procedure: It can be estimated by imaging two resolution lead bar patterns, up to 20 line pairs per mm (lp/mm) each, placed on a 45 mm-thick PMMA plate. Image the patterns using a Mo/Mo target-filter combination at 28 kV.
	Frequency: Yearly
Threshold contrast visibility	Acceptance test, status test and constancy test.
	Minimum detectable contrast for a 5-6 mm detail < 1.3%.
	Operating procedure: It can be estimated by imaging a suitable phantom containing 5-6 mm circular details. The phantom is accurately placed on a 45 mm PMMA plate. Image the phantom using a Mo/Mo target-filter combination at 28 kV.
	Frequency: Yearly
Alignment of X-ray field/image receptor	Acceptance test, status test and constancy test.
	X-rays must cover the film by no more than 5 mm outside the film parallel to the axis tube, laterally X-rays must totally cover the film.
	Operating procedure: The alignment of the X-ray field and image receptor at the chest wall side can be determined by using two loaded cassettes and two X-ray absorbers. Produce an exposure
	Frequency: Every three months
Tube Voltage Accuracy	Acceptance test, status test.
	Accuracy for the range of clinically used tube voltages (25 –31 kV): < ± 1 kV.
	Operating procedure: The equipment should be tested over the range of clinically used settings (typically 25 – 31 kV) at intervals of 1 kV. To determine the tube voltage accuracy, the kV-meter

should be accurately placed. The resulting measured kV should be recorded. After having assessed that the differences between measured and nominal tube voltage values are within 1 kV, the exposures can be repeated at 1 kV intervals, after positioning the exposure meter, by recording the resulting counts per second (cps).

Constancy test.

Accuracy for the range of clinically used tube voltages (25 –31 kV): measured mGy vs nominal kV curve should be within the error bar.

Operating procedure: Adequately position the exposure meter and report the counts per second (cps) measured at intervals of 1 kV.

Frequency: Yearly

Tube Voltage Reproducibility	Acceptance test, status test and constancy test. Reproducibility (at 28 kV): < ± 0.5 kV. Operating procedure: To determine tube voltage reproducibility, accurately position the kV-meter and make at least three exposures at a fixed tube voltage that is normally used clinically (e.g. 28 kV). When the deviation from the mean value is < ± 0.5 kV and repeat the exposures, after positioning the exposure meter, and record the resulting counts per second (cps). Constancy test. Reproducibility (at 28 kV): < ± 2 %. Operating procedure: Adequately position the exposure meter. Make at least three exposure at a fixed tube voltage that is normally used clinically (e.g. 28 kV) and report the measured counts per second (cps). Frequency: Yearly
Exposure time	Acceptance test, status test and constancy test. Exposure time needed to image a 45 mm PMMA phantom: < 2 sec. Operating procedure: After accurately positioning the PMMA phantom and the sensor, the time for a routine exposure is measured. Frequency: Yearly
Reference dose	Acceptance test, status test and constancy test. Entrance dose: ≤10 mGy (40 mm PMMA test block); ≤ 12 mGy (45 mm PMMA test block); ≤ 20 mGy (50 mm PMMA test block). Operating procedure: Accurately position the exposure meter on the PMMA test block of known thickness. Report the counts per second (cps) measured at the entrance. Frequency: Yearly
Output rate	Acceptance test, status test and constancy test. Output rate must be < / 7.5 mGy/s (at the focus-to-film distance). Operating procedure: The output rate should be measured using a Mo/Mo target-filter combination at 28 kV, in the absence of scatter material and attenuation, and reporting the counts per second (cps). After calculating the exposure value, calculate the output rate at a distance equal to the focus-to-film distance (FFD). Frequency: Yearly
Average glandular dose (AGD)	Acceptance test, quality control. AGD (45 mm PMMA): < 2 mGy.

Operating procedure: After determining the tube load (mAs) necessary to image the phan-ex, accurately position the exposure meter on the 45 mm PMMA test block and report the measured counts per second (cps), without backscattering. After calculating the exposure value, calculate the output rate at a distance equal to the focus-to-film distance (FFD) and convert this value into the average glandular dose.

Frequency: Yearly

| Grid system factor | At acceptance and when dose or exposure time increases suddenly. |

Grid system factor must be ≤ 3.

Operating procedure: The grid system factor can be estimated by accurately positioning the phan-ex and measuring counts per second (at 28 kV), without compression, and with and without the grid system.

Grid imaging

Acceptance test, status test and constancy test.

No significant non uniformity

Operating procedure: image the bucky at the lowest position of the AEC-selector, without PMMA. Verify the image uniformity.

Frequency: Yearly

Back-up timer

Acceptance test, quality control.

The back-up timer should function properly.

Operating procedure: Make an exposure of a 1 mm lead sheet and verify if the AEC system terminates the exposure.

Frequency: Yearly

Half Value Layer (HVL)

Acceptance test, status test and constancy test.

For 28 kV Mo/Mo target-filter combination the HVL must be between 0.30 and 0.40 mm Al equivalent.

Operating procedure: Position the exposure detector at the reference ROI (since the HVL is position-dependent) on top of the bucky. Place the compression device halfway between focal spot and detector. Select a Mo/Mo target/filter combination, 28 kV tube voltage and an adequate tube loading (mAs-setting), and expose the detector directly. The filters can be placed on the compression device and must intercept the whole radiation field. Use the same tube load (mAs) setting and expose the detector through each filter.

Frequency: Yearly

Focal spot size

At acceptance and when resolution has changed, quality control.

For 28 kV Mo/Mo target-filter combination, focal spots size are reported in the following table.

Focal spot size	Reference values	
	Length (cm)	Width (cm)
1 × 1	0.1 ÷ 0.15	0.1 ÷ 0.15
2 × 2	0.2 ÷ 0.3	0.2 ÷ 0.3
3 × 3	0.45 ÷ 0.65	0.3 ÷ 0.45
4 × 4	0.6 ÷ 0.85	0.4 ÷ 0.6

Operating procedure: Produce a magnified image of the pinhole and measure, on the image, the length and the width, in cm. Repeat for all available focal spots.

Frequency: Yearly

Compression force

Acceptance test, status test and constancy test.

	Maximum automatically applied force: 130 - 200 N.
	Operating procedure: The compression force can be estimated using a compression force test device or a bathroom scale.
	Frequency: Yearly
Compression plate alignment	Acceptance test, status test and constancy test.
	The difference between the measured distances at the left and right side of the compression paddle should be ≤ 5 mm for symmetrical load.
	Operating procedure: The alignment of the compression device at maximum force can be visualized and measured when a piece of foam-rubber is compressed.
	Frequency: Yearly

Table 3. Proposed protocol for mammography QC and technical specification of the parameters to be monitored.

3. Results and discussion

The chosen protocol can be used equally for acceptance, status and constancy tests. It was successfully implemented for both analogue and digital mammographs.

In particular, it was implemented for constancy tests of all parameters relevant to the exposure, utilising the same phantom-exposure meter pair.

In addition to the protocol, Table 3, the QC report worksheet is proposed in which the raw results (counts per second, cps) can be reported, Fig. 2-3. The raw data is then elaborated to estimate the entrance dose.

The proposed protocol and QC report were tested on different (analogue and digital) mammographs, to assess their versatility and accuracy, independent of the physical characteristics of the mammograph.

As an example, the AEC test results obtained for a digital mammographic system are reported in Figs. 4-6 to show that the same protocol can also be used on digital instruments.

The results obtained from the object thickness compensation are represented in Fig. 4. In particular, in Fig. 4 (a), the value of the dose (mGy) normalised to the tube load value (mAs) for the reference PMMA test block thickness (45 mm), is constant and within the error bar (± 15 %). The dose as a function of the PMMA plate thickness is presented in Fig. 4 (b). This curve shows that, with increasing dose, the normalised dose is constant, indicating the correct operation of the AEC system.

The results obtained from the tube voltage compensation are presented in Fig. 5 (a). Differently from the previous test, where the tube voltage was kept constant (28 kVp) varying only the tube load, in this type of test two parameters are varied: tube voltage and tube load. Therefore, in this test the parameter chosen to assess the tube voltage compensation is the logarithm (base 10) of the dose. Also in this case the results show that the logarithm of the dose is within the limit values (± 15 % calculated for a reference tube voltage of 28 kVp and for a 45 mm PMMA test block).

TEST RESULTS

DATE __/__/__

QC REPORT

(A) ACCEPTANCE TEST ☐
(B) STATUS TEST ☐
(C) CONSTANCY TEST ☐

Monitored parameters

1) Acoustic and light signalling [(A), (B), (C)]

Acoustic signal functions property: yes ☐   no ☐
Light signal functions properly: yes ☐   no ☐

2) Security cut-off [(A), (B), (C)]

Exposure value   ____ cps;
Terminated exposure: ____ cps;

3) Source-to-image distance [(A), (B)]

Nominal value: manufacturers specification: ____ cm
Focus indication to Bucky: ____ cm
Bucky to cassette (or receiver image) ____ cm
Source-to-image distance: ____ cm

4) AEC-system [(A), (B), (C)]

• Long term reproducibility [(C)] and short term reproducibility [(A), (B), (C)]

Limit: ≤ ± 2% (long term reproducibility)
≤ ± 5 % (short term reproducibility)

• Difference per step [(A), (B), (C)]

Limit: 0.1 – 0.2 per step

PMMA test block: 45 mm   Tube voltage: 28 kVp;

Step	Tube load (mAs)	Counts per second (cps)
-2		
-1		
0		
+1		
+2		

5) Uniformity [(A), (B), (C)]

Limit: < 30-35 % (parallel to the axis tube)
< 7 % (perpendicular to the axis tube)

Exposure meter position	Counts per second (cps)
Centre	
Top	
Right	
Bottom	
Left	

6) Spatial resolution [(A), (B), (C)]

Limit: ≥ 12 lp/mm

Target-filter combination: Mo/Mo
Tube voltage: 28 kVp   Tube load: ____ mAs
Resolution: ____ lp/mm

PMMA test block: 45 mm;   Tube voltage: 28 kVp;

exposure	Tube load (mAs)	Counts per second (cps)
1		
2		
3		
4		
5		

• Object thickness compensation [(A), (B), (C)]

Limit: ≤ ± 15%

Tube voltage: 28 kVp;

PMMA test block (mm)	Tube load (mAs)	Counts per second (cps)
30		
45		
60		

• Tube voltage compensation [(A), (B), (C)]

Limit: ≤ ± 15%

PMMA test block: 45 mm;

Nominal tube voltage (kV)	Tube load (mAs)	Counts per second (cps)
26		
28		
30		

7) Threshold contrast visibility [(A), (B), (C)]

Limit: ≥ 1.3 %

Target-filter combination: Mo/Mo
Tube voltage: 28 kVp   Tube load: ____ mAs

Diameter disc: ____ mm   Contrast: ____ %
Diameter disc: ____ mm   Contrast: ____ %
Diameter disc: ____ mm   Contrast: ____ %
Diameter disc: ____ mm   Contrast: ____ %

8) Alignment of X-ray field/image receptor [(A), (B), (C)]

Limit: < 5 mm (chest)
totally cover the film (otherwise)

Left: ____ mm
Nipple: ____ mm
Right: ____ mm
Chest: ____ mm

9) Tube voltage [(A), (B), (C)]

• Accuracy [(A), (B), (C)]

Limit: ≤ ± 1 kVp [(A): (B)]
measured mGy vs nominal kV curve should be within the error bar [(C)]

Nominal tube voltage (kVp)	25	26	27	28	29	30	31
Measured tube voltage (kVp)							
Counts per second (cps)							
Tube load (mAs)							

• Precision [(A), (B), (C)]

Limit: ≤ ± 0.5 kVp [(A): (B)]
≤ ± 2.0 % [(C)]

Nominal tube voltage (kVp)	28		
Measured tube voltage (kVp)			
Counts per second (cps)			
Tube load (mAs)			

Figure 2. QC report worksheet for raw data recording (part 1)

10) **Exposure time [(A), (B), (C)]**

Limit: ≤ 2 second

PMMA test block: 45 mm
Tube voltage: 28 kVp;   AEC settings: _____

Exposure time: _____ sec

11) **Reference dose [(A), (B), (C)]**

Limit: ≤ 10 mGy (40 mm PMMA test block)
≤ 12 mGy (45 mm PMMA test block)
≤ 20 mGy (50 mm PMMA test block)

PMMA test block: _____ mm;
Tube voltage: _____ kVp   Tube load: _____ mAs
Counts per second: _____ cps

12) **Output rate [(A), (B), (C)]**

Limit: > 7.5 mGy/s (at the focus-to-film distance)

Tube voltage: 28 kVp;   Tube load: ____ mAs   Exposure time: ___ sec
FFD: _____ cm   Counts per second: _____ cps

13) **Average glandular dose [(A), (B), (C)]**

Limit: ≤ 2 mGy (45 mm PMMA test block)

Tube voltage: 28 kVp   Tube load: ____ mAs
FFD= _____ cm   Tube output = ____ cps/mAs

14) **Anti scatter grid [(A), (B), (C)]**

- **Grid system factor [(A)]**

Limit: ≤3

Grid	Counts per second (cps)	Tube load
Present		
Absent		

- **Grid imaging [(A), (B), (C)]**

Artefacts are present: yes ☐   no ☐
Description of artefacts: _____

15) **Back-up timer [(A), (B), (C)]**

Exposure terminates by exposure limit :

yes ☐   no☐

16) **Half-Value Layer (HVL) [(A), (B), (C)]**

Limit: 0.3 mm Al ≤ HVL ≤ 0.4 mmAl (Mo/Mo filter-tube combination).

Tube voltage: 28 KVp;   Tube load: ___mAs;

no filter	0 mm	cps = _____
filter 1	____ mm	cps = _____
filter 2	____ mm	cps = _____
filter 3	____ mm	cps = _____
filter 4	____ mm	cps = _____
filter 5	____ mm	cps = _____

17) **Focal spot size [(A), (B), (C)]**

Limits:

Nominal focal spot size (mm)	Length (cm)	Width (cm)
1 x 1	0.1 - 0.15	0.1 - 0.15
2 x 2	0.2 - 0.3	0.2 - 0.3
3 x 3	0.45 - 0.65	0.3 - 0.45
4 x 4	0.6 - 0.85	0.4 - 0.6

Nominal focal spot size (mm)	Measured Length (cm)	Measured Width (cm)
1 x 1		
2 x 2		
3 x 3		
4 x 4		

18) **Compression force [(A), (B), (C)]**

Limit: maximum automatically-applied force 130-200 N

Measured compression force: _____ N
Compression force after 1 min: _____ N

19) **Compression plate alignment [(A), (B), (C)]**

Limit: ≤ 5 mm

	Left (mm)	Right (mm)
Rear		
Front		

Figure 3. QC report worksheet for raw data recording (part 2).

The dose radiated by the AEC system as a function of the tube voltage is presented in Fig. 5 (b), as measured with the phan-ex. From the results of Fig 5 (b) it is noticed that as the tube voltage increases, the dose decreases, further confirming that the AEC system is functioning correctly.

Results from the test on the "difference per step" are reported in Fig. 6. Also in this case, the logarithm of the dose was calculated at each step. The obtained values are within the limit values (0.2 – 0.4 as the step difference was 2), Fig. 6 (a). The corresponding values of the dose per step are reported in Fig. 6 (b).

For the short-term reproducibility test, exposure values were measured, from which the average dose value was determined with respect to the tube load supplied by the AEC system (mGy/mAs), Fig. 7, to show the proposed unified protocol is equally applicable to analogue and digital mammographic system.

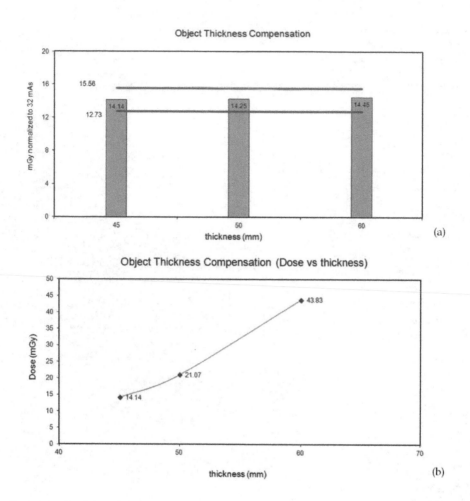

Figure 4. Results of object thickness compensation test: (a) the dose (mGy) normalised to the tube load value (mAs); (b) the dose (mGy) as a function of PMMA plate thickness.

The use of the phan-ex, coupled with the proposed protocol, is useful also to verify parameters related to the exposure such as tube voltage precision and accuracy, and exposure time.

Most importantly the proposed protocol permits the evaluation of the functional parameters of the instruments by utilising a single phantom, thus significantly reducing the number of additional dedicated equipment and simplifying the task of the Medical Physics Expert.

The results obtained from raw data analysis obtained following the proposed protocol were found to be consistent with those obtained from standard procedures [32-35], thus highlighting the usefulness and versatility of the proposed unified protocol to test all relevant parameters in analogue and (direct or indirect) digital instruments. The simplification is even more relevant in the latter type of mammographs for which the QC procedures currently used present considerable difficulties in the interpretation of the measurement protocols.

The applicability of the proposed phantom can be further extended to the measurement of parameters other than those relevant to the exposure even for the next generation of mammographs which are still under development. One such instrument is the SYRMEP, equipped with a Si-based microstrip detector and a synchrotron X-Ray source characterised by superior performance with respect to typical X-Ray tubes [36].

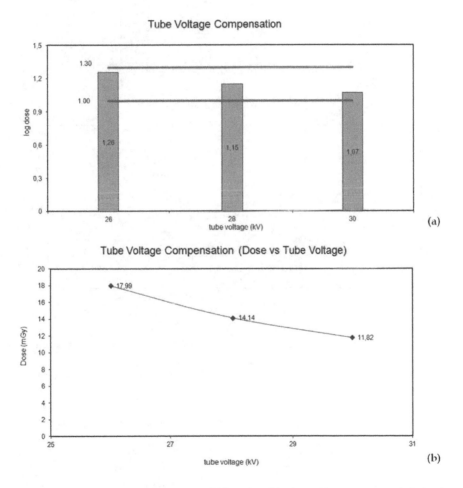

Figure 5. Results of tube voltage compensation test: (a) logarithm of the dose, red lines representing the limit values (± 15 %) with respect to 28 kVp reference tube voltage; (b) the dose (mGy) as a function of tube voltage (kVp).

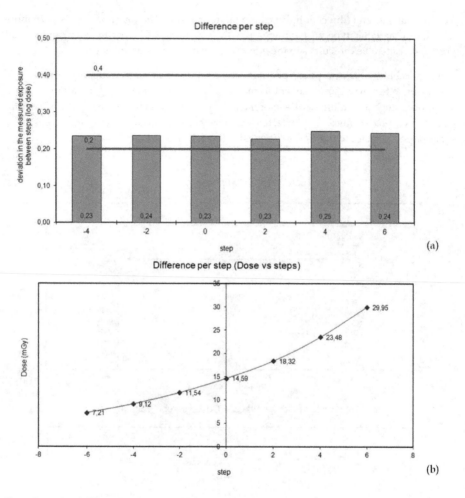

Figure 6. Results of difference per step test: (a) logarithm of the dose, red lines representing the limit values (0.2 – 0.4 per step); (b) the dose (mGy) per step.

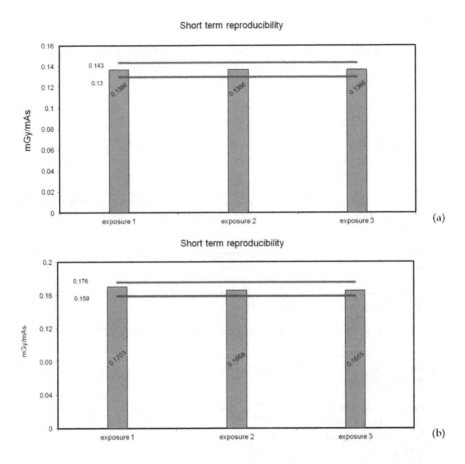

Figure 7. Results of short term reproducibility test, dose to tube load ratio (mGy/mAs) for three different exposures : (a) digital, (b) analogue mammograph;

Author details

Barbara Testagrossa[1], Giuseppe Acri[1], Federica Causa[1], Raffaele Novario[2], Maria Giulia Tripepi[1] and Giuseppe Vermiglio[1*]

*Address all correspondence to: vermigli@unime.it

1 Environmental, Healh, Social and Industrial Department - University of Messina, Italy

2 Department of Biotechnologies and Life Sciences– University of Insubria, Italy

References

[1] Shah, A. J., Wang, J., Yamada, T., & Fajardo, L. L. (2003). Digital Mammography: A Review of Technical Development and Clinical Applications. *Clinical Breast Cancer*, 4(1), 63-70.

[2] Feig, S. A. (1988). Decreased breast cancer mortality through mammographic screening: results of clinical trials. *Radiology*, 167, 659-665.

[3] Skaane, P., & Skjennald, A. (2004). Screen-film mammography versus full-filled digital mammography with soft-copy reading: screening program. *The Oslo II study. Radiology*, 232(1), 197-204.

[4] Huda, W., Sajewicz, A. M., & Ogden, K. M. (2003). Experimental investigation of the dose and image quality characteristics of a digital imaging system. *Medical Physics*, 30(3), 442-448.

[5] Law, J. (2006). The development of mammography. *Physics in Medicine and Biology*, R155-R167.

[6] Noel, A., & Thibauld, F. (2004). Digital detectors for mammography: the technical challenges. *European Radiology*, 14, 1990-1998.

[7] James, J. J. (2004). The current status of digital mammography. *Clinical Radiology*, 59, 1-10.

[8] Maidment, A. D. A. (2003). Digital mammography. *Seminars in Roentgenology*, 38(3), 216-230.

[9] Perry, N., Broeders, M., de Wolf, C., Törnberg, S., Holland, R., & von Karsa, L., Ed. (2006). *European guidelines for quality assurance in breast cancer screening and diagnosis* (4th Edition), Luxembourg, Office for Official Publications of the European Communities.

[10] Pisano, E. D., Cole, E. B., Hemminger, B. M., Yaffe, M. J., Aylward, S. R., Maidment, A. D. A., Johnston, E., Williams, M. B., Niklason, L. T., Conant, E. F., Fayardo, L. L., Kopans, D. B., Brown, M. E., & Pizer, S. M. (2000). Image processing algorithms for digital mammography: a pictorial essay. *Radio Graphics*, 20, 1479-1491.

[11] Muller, S. (1999). Full-field digital mammography designed as a complete system. *European Journal of Radiology*, 31, 25-34.

[12] Feig, S. A., & Yaffe, M. J. (1996). Current status of digital mammography. *Seminars in Ultrasound, CT, and MRI*, 17(5), 424-443.

[13] Cherie, M. Kuzmiak. (2012). *Digital Mammography, Imaging of the Breast- Technical Aspects and Clinical Implication, Laszlo Tabar (Ed.)*, 978-9-53510-284-7, InTech, Available from, http://www.intechopen.com/books/imaging-of-the-breast-technical-aspects-and-clinical-implication/digital-mammography-chapteraccessed 5 June 2012.

[14] Feig, S. A., & Yaffe, M. J. (1998). Digital mammography. *Radio Graphics*, 18, 893-901.

[15] Screen-Film Radiography II. (2012). http://myweb.dal.ca/halem/phyc2250/09_-_Screen-Film_Radiography_II.pdf, accessed 25 June 2012.

[16] Pisano, E. D., & Yaffe, M. J. (2005). State of the art: Digital Mammography. *Radiology*, 234(2), 353-362.

[17] Berns, E. A., Hendrick, R. E., Solari, M., Barke, L., Reddy, D., Wolfman, J., Segal, L., De Leon, P., Benjamin, S., & Willis, L. (2006). Digital and screen-film mammography: comparison of image acquisition and interpretation times. *American Journal of Roentgenology*, 187, 38-41.

[18] Yaffe, in., Haus, A., & Yaffe, M. J., Eds. (1992). *Syllabus of Categorial Course on Technical Aspects of Mammography*, Radiological Society of North America, Oak Book, IL.

[19] Säbel, M., & Aichinger, H. (1996). Recent development in breast imaging. *Physics in Medicine and Biology*, 41, 315-368.

[20] Smith, A. P. (2003). Fundamentals of Digital Mammography: Physics, Technology and Practical Consideration. *Radiology Management*, 25(5), 18-24, 26-31.

[21] Rampado, O., Isoardi, P., & Ropolo, R. (2006). Quantitative assessment of computed radiography quality control parameters. *Physics in Medicine and Biology*, 51, 1577-1593.

[22] Panagiotakis, G. (2012). Mammographic detectors. *PhD Thesis*, University of Patras, http://www.hep.upatras.gr/class/download/bio_sim_eik/mammographic detectors.pdf, accessed 5 June 2012.

[23] Kruger, D. G., Abreu, C. C., Hendee, E. G., Kocharian, A., Peppler, W. W., Mistretta, C. A., & Mac Donald, C. A. (1996). Imaging Characteristics of x-ray capillary optics in digital mammography. *Medical Physics*, 23(2), 187-196.

[24] Pisano, E. D., Yaffe, M. J., & Kuzmiak, C. M. (2004). *Digital mammography*, Lippencott, Williams & Wilkins, Philadelphia.

[25] Yaffe, M. J., & Rowlands, J. A. (1998). X-ray detectors for digital radiography. *Physics in Medicine and Biology*, 42, 1-39.

[26] Kasap, S. O., & Rowlands, J. A. (2000). X-ray photoconductors and stabilized a-Se for direct conversion digital flat-panel X-ray image detectors. *Journal of Materials Science: Materials in Electronics*, 11, 179-198.

[27] Samei, E., & Ravin, C. E. (2008, March 12-13, 2008). Washington DC, USA. *Assuring image quality for classification of digital chest radiographs: conference proceedings*, NIOSH Scientific Workshop.

[28] Ranger, N. T., Samei, E., Dobbins, J. T., I. I. I., & Ravin, C. E. (2007). Assessment of Detective Quantum Efficiency: intercomparison of a recently introduced international standard with prior methods. *Radiology*, 243(3), 785-795.

[29] Vermiglio, G., Tripepi, M. G., Mannino, G., Sansotta, C., & Testagrossa, B. (2005, 14-17 June 2005). Prove periodiche di funzionalità in mammografia mediante misure di esposizione. Verona, Italy. *In: Polimetrica S.a.s. (ed.) Proceedings of 4° Congresso Nazionale AIFM*, 672-675.

[30] Testagrossa, B., Sansotta, C., Acri, G., Tripepi, M. G., & Vermiglio, G. (2007, October 1-3 2007). Vasto Marina (CH), Paper presented at XXXIV Convegno AIRP "Sicurezza e qualità in radioprotezione". *Fantoccio multiuso per controlli di qualità in mammografia tradizionale e digitale: conference proceedings.*

[31] *Controllo di qualità in mammografia PHAN-EX*, Operating handbook.

[32] Italian Regulation 26 Maggio 2000, n. 187. Attuazione della direttiva 97/43/Euratom in materia di protezione sanitaria delle persone contro i pericoli delle radiazioni ionizzanti connesse ad esposizioni mediche. Gazzetta Ufficiale n. 157 del 7 luglio 2000. Suppl. Ordinario n. 105. http://www.camera.it/parlam/leggi/deleghe/00187dl.htm (accessed 25 June 2012).

[33] Linee Guida ANPEQ-ISPESL relative al controllo sugli impianti radiologici e accessori. (2004). http://www.anpeq.it/download/app_radiologiche.pdf, accessed 27 June 2012.

[34] Corrado, F., Gennaro, G., Golinelli, P., & Rossetti, V. (2004). Protocollo Italiano per il controllo di qualità degli aspetti fisici e tecnici in mammografia. *AIFM Report*, http://www.fisicamedica.it/aifm/report/2004_n1_ReportAIFM.pdf, accessed 27 June 2012.

[35] Norma CEI 62-27 ed.2 (CEI EN 60601-2-7). (1999). Apparecchi elettromedicali. *Parte 2: Norme particolari per la sicurezza di generatori ad alta tensione dei generatori radiologici per diagnostica.*

[36] Castelli, E. (2012). Un sistema di rivelazione per mammografia digitale con luce di sincrotrone. *PhD Thesis*, University of Trieste, http://www.infn.it/thesis/PDF/256-Bergamaschi-laurea.pdf, accessed 25 June 2012.

Quality Control in Energy

Chapter 4

The Quality Management of The R&D in High Energy Physics Detector

Xuemin Zhu and Sen Qian

Additional information is available at the end of the chapte

1. Introduction

Particle physics, also recognized as high energy physics, is a basic subject focusing on the research of the elementary elements of materials and their mutual actions. One distinguished characteristic of particle physics study is that the experimental equipments involved are always huge and special ones. Therefore, big science projects, including the R&D of large detectors, are usually required in high energy physics experiments. Those projects are complicated systematic engineering, involving many front and technology fields. It is impossible for a single institute to finish those large projects by its own. Cooperation among different institutes or organizations is necessary for big science projects in particle physics, especially international ones.

1. 1. The Institute of High Energy Physics [1]

The Institute of High Energy Physics (IHEP) is the biggest and comprehensive fundamental research center in Chinese Academy of Science. The major research fields of IHEP are particle physics, accelerator physics and technologies, radiation technologies and application, Particle physics experiments and Accelerator physics and technology are two of the leading research areas. The main research facilities at IHEP include Beijing Electron Positron Collider (BEPC) and Beijing Spectrometer (BES), DayaBay Neutrino Experiment, Chinese Spallation Neutron Source, etc. IHEP has extensive cooperation with all high energy physics laboratories and participates in many important particle physics experiments in the world.

1.2. The Beijing Electron Positron Collider [2] and the Beijing Spectrometer [3]

The Beijing Electron Positron Collider (BEPC) consists of the injector, the storage ring, the transportation line, the Beijing Spectrometer (BES), the Beijing Synchrotron Radiation Facility (BSRF) and the computer center. Beijing Spectrometer (BES) is a general purpose magnetic spectrometer in the South IP of the storage ring. The general layout of the BEPC is shown in Fig.1.

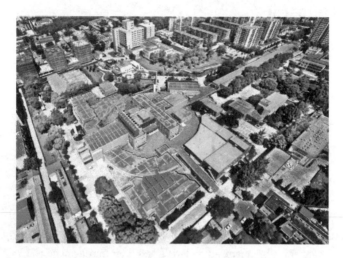

Figure 1. The airscape of the BEPC.

BEPC started construction in 1984 and the first electron-proton collider was produced in Oct. 1988. BEPCII was installed in 2003 and finished five years later in 2009. IHEP establishes comprehensive and long-term cooperation with high energy laboratories and universities all over the world, especially in USA, Japan and Europe. With the international cooperation, IHEP have gained huge success in 30 years. For example, IHEP took part in the research of CMS and ATLAS detectors of Large Hadron Collider (LHC), which is the world's largest, highest-energy particle accelerator and the collider at the beginning of 21 centuries, built by CERN [4]. BESIII is also organized by IHEP and participated by 51 institutions and universities around the world, 34 from Asian, 12 from Europe and 5 from USA.

1.3. The Daya Bay Neutrino Experiment [5]

The Daya Bay Neutrino Experiment is a neutrino-oscillation experiment designed to measure the mixing angle q13 using anti-neutrinos produced by the reactors of the Daya Bay Nuclear Power Plant (NPP) and the Ling Ao NPP.

The Daya Bay Neutrino Experiment is a major international joint research program, mainly organized by China working closely with researchers from other countries. In terms of both money and people, it is among the largest scientific collaborations between US and China. More than 200 scientists from China, include Hong Kong and Taiwan, the US, Russia, the Czech Republic are involved in the Daya Bay experiment. During the cooperation, China is in change of the laboratory construction, R&D of Anti-neutrino detector (AD), Gd-loaded

Liquid Scintillator, Muon Veto Detector, Readout Electronic and Data acquisition system (DAQ) etc. While America is in responsible of the construction of water Cherenkov detector and so on.

Scientists from the Chinese Academy of Sciences (CAS) and the U.S.-based Brookhaven National Laboratory and the Lawrence Berkeley National Laboratory will participate in the underground experiment. An international funding commission comes into existence in the funding agency to discuss fee issues and instruct the experiment process and fee management through experimental supervision organization. The project management of the Daya Bay Neutrino Experiment adopts the advanced and mature modern management idea used for managing large international joint project and big science experimental research project. An international cooperation group is built and management rules are made. Besides, a cooperation group commission is founded, during which executive board and spokesperson is elected for overall supervision of the whole project. The Daya Bay Neutrino Experiment is initiated in 2007 and finished in 2012.

1.4. Chinese Spallation Neutron Source [6]

Chinese Spallation Neutron Source (CSNS) is designed to build a device with the power of proton beam reaching up to 100 kW effective and the flux of pulsed neutrons coming out top in the world, along with other three spallation neutron sources built in America, Japan and British. CSNS is also a large cooperative project, supported by Chinese Academy of Sciences and Guangdong government. The normal operation for uses is foreseen in 2018. IHEP is the main construction institution in the project with the Institute of Physics Chinese Academy of Sciences as the co-operation unit. The construction team bring together three generations of outstanding scientific and technical researchers in China. An international CSNS neutron technology advisory committee is set up for reviewing the key experimental work. The experts of the advisory committee are from well-known laboratories in America, Japan, Germany, Australia and other countries.

2. Introduction of Quality Management of Scientific Projects in IHEP

During the process of big science project and research, IHEP has significant advantages in accelerator physics and technology, human resources, international cooperation and academic exchange. IHEP owns mature model and advanced experience in the quality management of scientific projects.

2.1. Project Management System

Before 2011, the project manager is responsible for the big science project management in IHEP. International cooperation group is formed and fees are under the sponsors' supervision and review. There is a perfect project management system, though without quality management system meeting international standards.

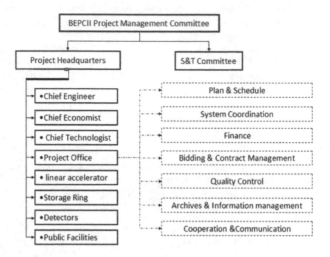

Figure 2. The Organization Chart of the BEPCII Project Management.

In the project management system shown in Fig.2, special-purpose management mechanism such as fund, purchasing, quality, safety and archive is established, with clear responsibilities and authorities. Besides, the internal communication mechanism and interface management mechanism are also set up. CPM Plan is adopted for fund and schedule management. To ensure the quality of the project, during the design and development process, experts are always invited for evaluation. And an international council committee is asked for review in terms of major international cooperation projects.

In fact, the requirements of the project management system have already displayed in the ISO 9001 quality management system. Though without a systematic quality manual and standards and lack of resource, purchasing and archive management. In the project management system, quality management is more focused on the management of various test guidelines and processing of key parts (including outsourced progress)

2.2. Quality Management Systems

The BEPCII project headquarters has placed great important on the quality management and published "BEPCII project management file" in 2002. In the file, responsibilities and rights of personnel, fund management, file number, document signing and alteration, early stages management, bidding and purchasing are described in detail.

At the beginning of 2005, during the construction of BEPCII project, the headquarters built a quality management system according to GB/T19001-2000(idt ISO9001:2000). Although the system doesn't get a national certification, it is completely in accordance with standards of quality management system requirements and it has played a very good effect. In 2009,

BEPCII completed the construction task successfully by time, with high quality and budget under control.

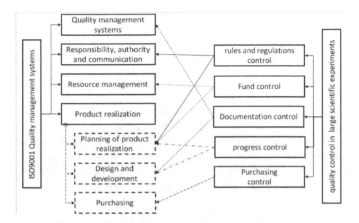

Figure 3. The Relationship between the quality control system in large scientific experiments and ISO9001 Quality management systems.

As described in Fig.3, The quality control in large scientific experiments corresponds with ISO9001 Quality management systems, which is classified according to the production. While, the quality control in large scientific experiments is classified according to the type of different work. The ISO9001 Quality management system is widely adopted by corporations all over the word and it's more normative.

In 2011, IHEP passed a national quality management certification system: GB/T19001-2008(idt ISO90012008). After two years' development of quality management system from its very beginning to being passed, it has confirmed that IHEP has the ability to produce scientific production meeting requirements.

The set up of quality management system makes the project management procedure standard, and promotes the overall management level in IHEP. The clients' needs are fully met and the quality management of IHEP joined the line of international standard management. The role played by quality management in the scientific research, especially in the big science project, is invaluable and imponderable.

3. Quality management in R&D of BESIII detector

The project of BESIII detector began its research and development, according to the scientific project management system and quality management system, like other big science projects.

3.1. Mechanism Management

BESIII detector R&D is part of BEPCII project. So the quality management of the detector research is responsible by the project director. As a whole, BESIII carries out the management system of BEPCII project headquarters strictly and makes some special mechanism to form a mechanism with a clear hierarchy. Quality technician are employed in the project.

BESIII detector R&D project has outlined the responsibilities and rights of each person in charge with an appropriate staffing in the organization. The communication methods of the total and sub system and record control requirements are defined.

The director in charge of sub system is responsible for the implementation of the BESIII research plan, management, arrangement of related resources and coordination with scientific and technical issues. Each division leading person is specifically responsible for the respective task implementation plan. Members in the project cooperate with each other closely at reaching difficult goals. The whole project has the characteristic of unified task, defined responsibilities, reasonable arrangement and integrated resources.

The high energy physics experiment is a complex project, and the communication in different study cells seems more important. The Task Control Form is widely used in study works, and the forms are preserved and archived as records of the system.

Subject				
Send to				
From		Date		
Serial No.		Pages		
Attached				
C.C.				
Content				
Jointly Sign				
validation	Prepared by	Checked by	Examined by	Approved by
Signature				
Date				

Figure 4. The task control form used by different teams.

Researchers in the project communicate with each other in time and have a regular meeting each or twice a week, to make sure the project is under schedule control and discuss some technical problems. Meeting minutes are kept as a reference. Sub-system will report the progress of the project and accept an inspection and evaluation regularly.

3.2. Fund Management

Fund management is important for the whole management of scientific project. Appropriate fund use a basis for carrying out any high energy physics experiment smoothly. As for the R&D of BESIII detector, the experiment design and development planning will affect the rationality of the budget and fund use directly. They are also the important contents in the requirements of the quality management system

Funds come from Chinese Academy Sciences (CAS) allocation and self-provided funds in the BESIII project. At the end of the year, expenses are counted and reported to CAS and the project will receive examination and evaluation.

3.3. Control of documents and records

Control of documents and records is critical whether for scientific project management or for quality management. For high energy physic experiments, large and complicated equipments are usually involved. During the project design and scheme phase, rules for documents and records reserved need to be made clearly and principles for numbering and signing the documents and records need to be described specifically.

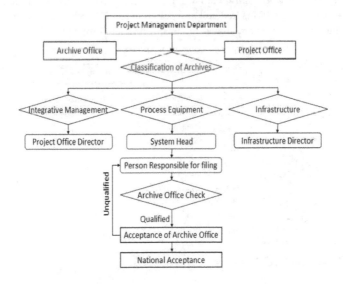

Figure 5. The workflow of archive management.

BEPCII project builds up a special mechanism of file control. Because BESIII is part of the whole project, the rules of document management are in accordance with the requirements of BEPCII. *Documents and records* need to be signed according to the regulations, in accordance with the whole project and effective as well. *Documents and records* need to be preserved and archived on a regular basis.

There are several characteristics in archive management work, especially for the high energy experiments. Firstly, this work must be arranged by the project management department at the beginning of the project. Secondly, the document and records which need to be preserved must be clearly described and the responsibility should be defined at the first time. Thirdly, the archive office, the project office and each member working for the project should cooperate to get the work done quickly and perfectly.

All the quality documents of the whole process of each single detector, from design, research, test, and acceptance are preserved according to the regulations. Technical specifications, interface of different tasks, diagrams, test reports are archived as written documents. Regular meeting minutes are kept also as archives. Those *Documents and records* can be used to track and follow the quality of the product in the whole process.

The running cycle of big science project, just like its construction cycle, is as long as to last more than ten years. Therefore, control of documents and records is very essential for the running and maintenance of the big science project, as an important prop and support.

3.4. Schedule Management

BESIII project has followed Critical Path Method (CPM) to control the schedule of the whole project. The plan in the CPM is in detail and convenient for check. It is easy for revision according to the actual process and make sure it is updated in time within the system.

	Task Name	Start	Finish	2002	2003	2004	2005	2006	2007	2008
116	⊟BEPCII zero-grade CPM project	8/15/2002	12/31/2007							
117	...	8/15/2002	8/24/2005							
118	⊟Facilities installation and commissioning	11/21/2004	11/30/2006							
119	...	11/2 /2004	3/30/2005							
120	⊞Dismantalment and installation of the storage	4/1/2005	12/27/2005							
125	Joint-commissioning of facilities at the storage	1/1/2006	2/9/2006							
126	Beam tuning at the storage ring, Synchrotron Radiation	2/16/2006	9/30/2006							
127	Detector assembling	2/10/2006	9/30/2006							
128	Detector in the colliding point, recovery of the	10/2/2006	10/31/2006							
129	Joint-commissioning of detector, recovery of the	11/1/2006	11/30/2006							
130	Joint-commissioning, trial run	12/1/2006	2/28/2007							
131	High energy physics experiment	3/1/2007	12/31/2007							
132	preperation for the acceptance test/experts' review	10/10/2007	12/31/2007							

Figure 6. BEPCII zero-grade CPM project (partly, 2002).

In order to give a better control of the schedule, CPM is classified. Any sub-system could make its own play and updates in time following the step of the total plan. Therefore inter communication plays an important role in the schedule management. In a word, CPM is a further refinement of the time arrangement of the project design report and makes the management of the project construction effective.

The CPM project is highly in accord with the practical progressand BEPCII zero-grade CPM project is modified frequently. The BEPCII project was finished in 2008 and was finally checked in 2009.

3.5. Purchasing Management

The R&D of large detectors is involved with bulk purchase. In the BESIII project, purchasing management rules are made according to the relevant laws and regulations on acquisition. Purchasing and approval process are defined clearly. Bidding is strictly adopted in the project to save research money. An appropriate regulation in the purchasing process is a guarantee for carrying out the project under the budget..

Abroad purchase has a long life cycle, heads of procurement need to do significant preparatory work in advance, and the heads should be quite familiar with the procurement procedures in order to complete the purchase in time. The purchasing department published the flowchart to facilitate the work.

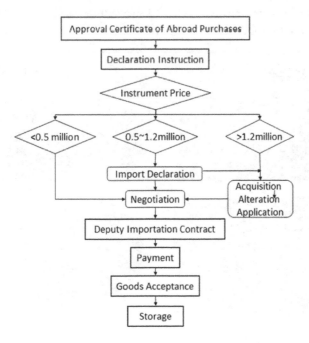

Figure 7. Abroad purchase flowchart

4. BESIII-MUC Quality Management in R&D of BESIII-MUC Detector

4.1. Introduction of BESIII Detector and MUC Detector

The Beijing Spectrometer (BESIII) is designed to measure the properties of the particles produced in the collisions of electrons and positrons at BEPCII. The physics goal of the BESIII experiment is to conduct high statistics and highly precise studies on a number of physics topics in this energy region, including light hadron spectroscopy, charmonium spectra, charm meson decay properties, QCD, tau physics, rare decays, search for glueballs and other non-pure quark states [3].

The BESIII detector will consist of a 1 T superconducting solenoid magnet, a high precision main drift chamber (MDC), Time-Of-Flight counters (TOF), a CsI crystal Electromagnetic Calorimeter (EMC) and a muon identifier chamber (MUC) that is integrated in the iron magnetic field return yoke [7]. The muon identifier is the outer most subsystem of the BESIII detector [8], which is constructed by resistive plate chambers (RPCs, shown in Fig.8.a). 962 RPC are used in the whole MUC detector, which consists of 136 RPC superlayer modules (SM, shown in Fig.8.b). And the Fig.8.c shows the status of the MUC detector when it was finished it's barrel part assemblage. The Fig.8.d shown the designed construct of the BESIII MUC detector with the endcap and barrel parts.

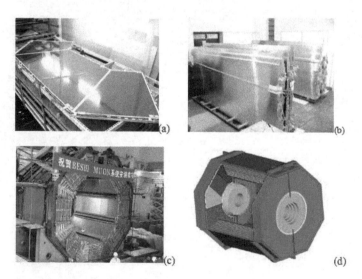

Figure 8. a). The RPC moduls, (b). The Suprlayer Modul, (c). The overview the barrel part of the MUC detector after it's assemblage, (d) The construct of the BESIII MUC detector.

4.2. Quality Management in the R&D of BESIII-MUC Detector

The whole process of R&D of MUC detector include the design of the basic unit RPC, properties investigation, bulk production, SM design; design of MUC detector, installation debugging, running and maintenance.

Throughout the research process, the project director managed the project scientifically and effectively, with each research aspect considered carefully, comprehensively and deeply, and made some achievements. From the pre-research in 2003 to the formal data collection in 2009, more than 30 papers have been published by the research group of MUC, covering the whole research process.

7 papers have been published in *NIMA*, as follows:

1. A new surface treatment for the prototype RPCs[9],

2. Cosmic ray test results on resistive plate chamber for the BESIII experiments [10]

3. The Design and Mass Production on RPC for the BESIII Experiment [11]

4. A monitor for the composition of the gas mixture of BESIII muon chambers [12]

5. First results of the RPC commissioning at BESIII [13]

6. The BESIII Muon Identification System [14]

7. An underground cosmic-ray detector made of RPC [15]

8 papers have been published in *Chinese Physics C,*as follows:

1. Cosmic Ray Test Station for BES@ RPC [16]

2. Research and Development of Large Area Resistive Plate Chamber [17]

3. A Study of RPC Gas Composition using Daya Bay RPCs [18]

4. Quality control and database on RPC for the BES@ experiment [19]

5. Test of BES@ RPC in the avalanche mode [20]

6. Performance Study of RPC Prototypes for the BES@ Muon Detector [21]

7. Study of the RPC-Gd as thremal neutron detector [22]

	Design	Performance Test	Mass Production	Research Work	Application
RPC	1 b	2 a c e f	3 d	4	7 g
SM			6		
MUC			6	5	

Table 1. The analysis of the manuscripts published by MUC group.

As shown in Table 1, it is not difficult to come into conclusion that the whole R&D of MUC detector applied scientific project quality management, which promotes the research work. In the phase of initial RPC research, the key point is on the study of the detector's performance test. It is the phase for building a standard quality management. After the acceptance of RPC and project review, mass production and SM reassembling come into being. In this phase, scientific quality control and management play a key role.

A perfect quality tracking system is established in each session, from the production and test of RPC, assembling and test of modules, to the installation and debugging of MUC detector, to ensure the supervision of the performance of detector is plausible.

Especially for the mass production of RPC and SM, before research and test, a database is built for storage related data and affording date support for quality control and final running & maintenance.

4.3. Summary

All the requirements such as verification, validation, monitoring, measurement, inspection and test activities specific to the detector are described in the design report of the detector in detail. The report plays the same role as in making a particular quality control plan.

□ ■	Design	Prototype	Mass production	Assemblage	Debug	Running
critical characteristic	■	□				
major characteristic	■	■	□			
critical process		■	■			
article inspection	■	■	■			■
quality improvement	■	■		■		
effectiveness			■	■		
traceability			■	■	■	■
preventive action	□	□			■	■
corrective action					■	
quality plan			□	■		

Table 2. Quality management/control factor distribution of MUC detector.

The design report of the detector divide the R&D process into several phases, including concept design, project design, sample trail-manufacture, product research and production, test, installation and debugging. In each phase, review and identification is defined. For important phases, such as aging test, assembly test and system test, detailed guidelines and instructor are written. As shown in Table 2, during the outsourcing process, key parts are defined, and acceptance rules are also clearly described. Control point is set up and design files are carried out strictly to ensure the product quality. More detailed could be found in table 2 for summary.

5. Significance of Scientific Quality Management in Research

5.1. Promote Scientific Projects

We could come into conclusion that scientific quality management can promote scientific projects to proceed successfully, in the following ways:

The schedule of the project could be arranged and controlled well, especially the adoption of CPM, which could provide a time map for the whole project. Throughout the four years' successful implementation and of BEPCII project, CPM plays an important role in the project acceptance in due. CPM was adjusted in time according to the project status, thus effective management and restriction was formed for all the related sub systems in the project.

The project has been implemented within the budget and cost was controlled. Purchasing procedures and approval process were strictly described, which played a role for the fair use of the fund.

Documents and records were kept in detail, as reference in the project to find the source of old problems and avoid new problems. Especially for those big scientific projects which will last more than ten years, files about interface management and quality management and various records are significant for the running and maintenance in the following work. They also act as important reference for the future project construction in high energy physics.

5.2. Promote Scientific Research

Scientific quality management could promote scientific research effectively. At the same time, as the development of scientific research, cooperation among researchers will be increased. It is good for the communication and exchange in the area of quality management and promotes the refining of the quality management system thus.

Experiences in big scientific project are good for the growth of young researchers. With participation in the R&D of big science equipment under quality management system, researchers will learn how to organize and manage scientific programs or projects in future.

In an ongoing scientific project managed launched by IHEP, researchers are from participants in BESIII or DayaBay. Although it is non-international, at the beginning the project is managed as required in strict quality management, just like that in big science project. As the development of the project, communication and cooperation among other institutions both at home and abroad have increased. To coordinate the partnership among different organizations and unites, cooperation group is formed. As shown below, a formality management system and strictness organization is built, which lays a solid foundation for the sustainable development of cooperation group and joint research work in future, whose Organization Chart shown in fig.9 for example.

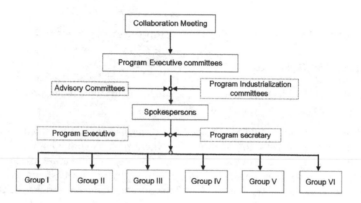

Figure 9. The organization of the BEPCII

6. Conclusion

Quality management plays a significant role both in project management and in the scientific research. With a scientific and comprehensive quality management system, big science project will be duly executed. The level of scientific projects will be greatly improved by the application and popularization of national and international quality standards.

Acknowledgements

In the process of writing this manuscript, we have received much understanding and support from many departments in our institute. We are particularly grateful to those staffs in the IHEP offices, archives, the purchasing department and the project teams for their strongly supported. Special thanks go to Prof. Zhao Jingwei for this support and encouragement to finish this work.

Author details

Xuemin Zhu[1*] and Sen Qian[1*]

*Address all correspondence to: zhuxm@ihep.ac.cn

1 The Institute of High Energy Physics, Chinese Academy of Sciences, China

References

[1] The Institute of High Energy Physics. http://english.ihep.cas.cn/au/bi/.

[2] The BEPCII Project. http://english.ihep.cas.cn/rs/fs/bepc/index.html.

[3] The Beijing Spectrometer. http://bes3.ihep.ac.cn/orga/institute.htm.

[4] European Organization for Nuclear Research. http://public.web.cern.ch/public/.

[5] The Bay Reactor Neutrino Experiment. http://dayabay.ihep.ac.cn/twiki/bin/view/Public/WebHome.

[6] China Spallation Neutron Source (CSNS). http://csns.ihep.ac.cn/english/index.htm.

[7] Tianchi, Z. (2010). Design and construction of the BESIII detector Nuclear. *Nuclear Instruments and Methods in Physics Research A*, 614, 345-399.

[8] Boxiang, Y. (2009). The construction of the BESIII experiment. *Nuclear Instruments and Methods in Physics Research A*, 598, 7-11.

[9] Jiawen, Z. (2005). A new surface treatment for the prototype RPCs. *Nuclear Instruments and Methods in Physics Research A*, 540(2005), 102-112.

[10] Jifeng, H. Cosmic ray test results on resistive plate chamber for the BESIII experiments. *Cosmic ray test results on resistive plate chamber for the BESIII experiments.*

[11] Jiawen, Z. (2007). The Design and Mass Production on RPC for the BESIII Experiment. *Nuclear Instruments and Methods in Physics Research A*, 580, 1250-1256.

[12] Sen, Q. (2008). A monitor for the composition of the gas mixture of BESIII muon chambers. *Nuclear Instruments and Methods in Physics Research A*, 595, 520-525.

[13] Yuguang, X. (2008). First results of the RPC commissioning at BESIII. *Nuclear Instruments and Methods in Physics Research A*, 595, 520-525.

[14] Sen, Q. (2010). The BESIII Muon Identification System. *Nuclear Instruments and Methods in Physics Research A*, 614, 196-205.

[15] Qingmin, Z. (2007). An underground cosmic-ray detector made of RPC. *Nuclear Instruments and Methods in Physics Research A*, 583, 278-284.

[16] Qian, L. (2006). Cosmic Ray Test Station for BES⊛ RPC. *China Physics C (High Energy And Unclear Physics)*, 30(4).

[17] Jiawen, Z. (2003). Research and Development of Large Area Resistive Plate Chamber. *China Physics C (High Energy And Unclear Physics)*, 27(7).

[18] Malie, H. (2010). Study of RPC gas composition using Daya Bay RPCs. *China Physics C (High Energy And Unclear Physics)*, 34(8).

[19] Jifeng, H. (2008). Quality control and database on RPC for the BES⊛ experiment. *China Physics C (High Energy And Unclear Physics)*, 32(3).

[20] Jifeng, H. (2008). Test of BES⊛ RPC in the avalanche mode. *China Physics C (High Energy And Unclear Physics)*, 32(5).

[21] Yuguang, X. (2008). Performance Study of RPC Prototypes for the BES⊛ Muon Detector. *China Physics C (High Energy And Unclear Physics)*, 31(1).

[22] Sen, Q. (2009). Study of the RPC-Gd as thremal neutron detector. *China Physics C (High Energy And Unclear Physics)*, 33(8).

Quality Control in Cosmetics

Chapter 5

Cosmetics' Quality Control

Bruna Galdorfini Chiari,
Maria Gabriela José de Almeida,
Marcos Antonio Corrêa and Vera Lucia Borges Isaac

Additional information is available at the end of the chapter

1. Introduction

The quality of a cosmetic product, in the same way as to other kind of products, is initially defined by the manufacturer that chooses the features that a product should present. On the other hand, the quality control of a product aims to verify if all of these defined features are in accordance with the standard definitions and if it will be maintained during the shelf life of the product (Shewhart, 1980).

The quality control of cosmetics is important to ensure the efficacy and safety of products and its raw-materials. Due to the rapid growth that cosmetic industries have exhibit all over the world, efficient, low cost and rapid methods to assay cosmetics' quality control are a priority. Some current techniques used by the cosmetic industry can be applied to the evaluation of cosmetics' quality control in an efficient manner, such as: rheology, sensory analysis and small angle X-ray scattering (SAXS).

Sensory analysis is a powerful tool, since there is no equipment able to measure the human feelings. It applies experimental design and statistical analysis to obtain information about a product in relation to what people feel when use or consume a product, in other words, it is used to indicate consumer acceptance of a particular product. It can be understood as the discipline that interprets, assess and measures characteristics of a product, after stimulating people in relation to their vital senses, as vision, touch, smell and taste (Stone et al., 1992). It is widely used in food industry and recently, it has also been applied in the cosmetic industry (Almeida et al., 2008; Aust et al., 1987; Backe et al., 1999; Lee et al., 2005; Parente et al., 2005; Wortel et al., 2000).

The sensory analysis can be applied in the research and development of a new cosmetic (Isaac et al., 2012a), in controlling the manufacturing process to evaluate raw-materials quality and, even, to make possible the substitution of a raw-material of a product that is traditional in the market without changes in the product's features (Meilgaard et al., 1991; Muñoz et al., 1993).

The application of sensory analysis could be related to the product control, referring to the storage, packaging and maintenance of sensory quality in relation to time and temperature (Muñoz et al., 1993), since these factors can change a sensory attribute that the product present originally (Zague, 2008) and people who participates of the sensorial panel could realize the changes in the sensorial attributes. Another function of this important tool is to performance comparative tests between competing products.

Another tool that could be applied to evaluate cosmetics' quality control is the rheology, which studies the flow and deformation of fluids. It has been used in research laboratories and industries as a tool for characterizing ingredients and products, and to predict the performance of products and consumer acceptance.

Rheology has been widely used because, by means of this tool, the researcher can determine physicochemical properties of a product. Constructing a rheogram, it is possible to check the flow curve, evaluate if there is a yield stress and a hysteresis area, which appears to be related to the release of drugs and actives. It is also possible to construct a creep and recovery curve obtaining information about viscoelasticity of each system.

Specifically, in relation to the quality control of cosmetics, specifically, rheology can be applied to help in determining the stability of products by means of the apparent viscosity measured periodically in a determined period exposing the samples to stress conditions (high and low temperatures, solar irradiation), and to monitor the flow characteristics during the shelf life or in the stability assay of a product.

The SAXS technique have being used for the analysis of cosmetics, in order to evaluate the presence of liquid crystalline structures, called liquid-crystals, which are known to increase the stability of formulations becoming, therefore, desirable in cosmetics (Makai et al., 2003).

Combining these three tools, it is possible to test the quality of cosmetics with a rich range of data, and obtain a deep characterization of the system. The results contribute to determining product use, or even, they provide indication of what need to be done to develop a product with predetermined characteristics.

2. Sensory analysis

Sensory analysis is defined by Piana et al. (2004) as the examination of a product through the evaluation of the attributes perceptible by the five sense organs (organoleptic attributes), such as color, odor, taste, touch, texture and noise, allowing the establishment of the organoleptic profile of diverse products, including cosmetics.

The sensory analysis was first applied to the food industry, but the high advance in other areas, such as the cosmetic and pharmaceutical industries, and the important data obtained with the sensory analysis, demanded this useful technique to describe what the consumers fell.

An important advantage of the use of sensory analysis in the quality control of a cosmetic product is that it yields a complex analysis in relation to all sensorial attributes that a product could present, it means that, the volunteer who participates of the sensorial panel is able to give information about the fragrance, the sensation, the appearance, the consistence, and other features that this person experience when use such product. The description of these characteristics by means of equipment would be an arduous work and would provide not sufficient or not valuable data when compared to the data provided by the human senses. Beyond that, the acquisition of this equipment could be of high cost when compared to the sensory analyses' costs (Ross, 2009).

The association of data obtained from sensory analysis and instrumental analysis (especially physicochemical analysis) provides great information and a more complete profile of the product (Ross, 2009).

Nowadays, there are companies specialized in perform sensory analysis of cosmetic products, and thus, they could be contracted to perform this study for cosmetic industries that don't have a sector trained to do it.

The sensorial performance of cosmetics is essential to the acceptance of consumers (Almeida et al., 2008; Fouéré et al., 2005; Lee et al., 2005; Proksch, 2005), thus, especial attention should be given to this subject.

The sensorial features of a formulation are mainly related to the raw-materials and package (Dooley et al., 2009). The raw-materials influence directly in what the consumer feels when applies the cosmetic. The emollients, for example, are raw-materials of marked influence in the tactile sense (Parente et al., 2008; Gorcea and Laura, 2010). Other raw-materials are available at the market and are commercialized to be used in formulations as sensorial modifiers. The main representatives of this kind of product are the silicones and Polymethyl Methacrylate (Ozkan et al., 2012).

The package influences in the first impression of the consumer about a product, since the first sense used to choose a cosmetic in the market is the vision. After, the smell is used too. The tact is not involved in the first purchase attitude, but it will define if a consumer will become a loyal consumer.

In this context, it is possible to verify that the sensorial features of a cosmetic are of great importance in the success of it in the market.

Thus, the sensorial analysis could help a company to define the attributes that a product should or not present beyond the characteristics and intensity of these attributes.

Another point is that these desired sensorial characteristics should be maintained during the cosmetic shelf life. To obtain that, the raw-materials used should be of good quality, the manufacture practices should be appropriate, the preservatives used need to be efficient and the formulation should be stable.

In conclusion, the sensorial analysis is an indispensable technique to help the formulator to evaluate the quality of its new product, in relation to its sensorial characteristics and to its stability, testing if the product will keep the nice sensorial feelings that transmit to the consumer during the time of use. This tool is helpful to the research and development area of a company which aims to obtain good quality products of high acceptance by the consumers. The suitable application of sensory evaluation could avoid the outlay of a company with the launching of a product in the market that was rejected by the volunteers of the preliminary study.

Currently, the sensorial analysis have gained more scientific rigor due to the need to offer to the consumers products that meet their expectations and due to the high competition between the major industries of this sector.

To perform the sensorial analysis with rigor and organization, the laboratory destined to it must have the following areas:

A room destined to the analyst who leads the team (Figure 1a)

A conference room (Figure 1b)

A room for the samples preparation (Figure 1c)

An area to the analyses with the volunteers (Figure 1d)

The laboratory should be located in an easy access place.

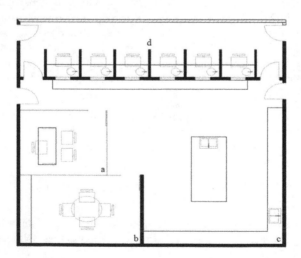

Figure 1. An example of layout of a sensorial analysis laboratory (Isaac et al., 2012a).

The area where will be performed the analyses should be divided in individual cabins (Figure 2) with a window, where the analyst must offer the samples to the volunteer, sink and faucet, to the volunteer use when necessary (Isaac et al., 2012).

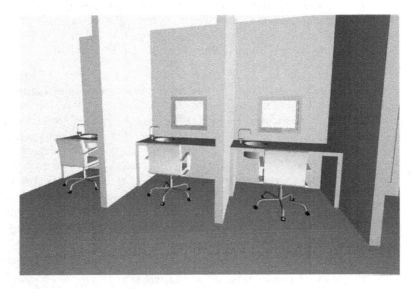

Figure 2. An example of layout of sensorial analysis cabine (Isaac et al., 2012a).

The cabins must be ventilated and odor free, to avoid interferences in the analyses. The temperature and humidity should be controled around 22 ºC and at 45% of humidity (Isaac et al., 2012).

It is recommended that the walls and furniture of the rooms are colored with neutral and light colors to not disturb the attention of the volunteers and to not interfere in the attributes analyzed by the vision, such as color and appearance of the product.

The volunteers should not smoke, should be healthy, with ease of memorization and communication.

In the study, the volunteers judges could be an experienced judge or not, depending on the kind of evaluation and the answers that the professional team needs to obtain. In the case of utilization of sensorial analysis in the quality control of a cosmetic, usually the volunteers are regular users of the product in analysis, since they need to be familiarized with the characteristics of the product and have sensibility to perceive slight modification on it. When the aim of the sensorial analysis is to evaluate the acceptance of a product that should be launched in the market, it is recommended that the volunteers are potencial users of this new product, orienting the formulator to make changes in the formulation and guiding the company to evaluate if the costs of the product launch are recommended or not.

There are four different methods to perform the sensorial analysis that are most used, they are: affective, discriminative, descriptive (Aust et al., 1987) and methods to evaluate the effective of the product.

Independent of the method of sensory analysis suitable for each evaluation, the professional team should use printed questionnaires to obtain the answers from each volunteer. The use of printed questionnaires avoids the contact between the professional and the volunteers preventing that the professional is biased in his responses, beyond that, it facilitates the data collection.

In the elaboration of these questionnaires the professional team should use suitable lexicons for each class of product, for example, the lexicons used to the evaluation of lip products are different from that used for corporal lotions (Dooley et al., 2009). Some researches had developed suitable lexicons for different classes of cosmetic products (Civille and Dus, 1991; Wortel and Wiechers, 2000; Dooley et al., 2009). The manner as the volunteer is questioned is fundamental to obtain the information required from them. An inadequate formulary could invalidate a sensory evaluation. It is interesting also, that a description of all descriptors attributed to the formulation being provided to the volunteer, for example: "Thickness: Viscosity of the cream when picking up from the container", "Ease of spreading: Ease of rubbing the sample over the skin", "Absorption: Ease of absorption of the product through the skin", "Residue: Amount of product left on the skin after application" (Parente et al., 2010).

The affective methods represent the consumer opinion and evaluate how much consumers like or dislike a product. It is a quantitative method that is performed in order to know the consumers preferences (Aust et al., 1987). This technique could be applied in the development of new products and when it is necessary to replace a constituent of a formulation without loss of the product quality. It could be performed in two different ways: offering two different samples to the volunteer asking him about what sample he prefers between them or using a hedonic scale for the volunteer attributes grades of intensity of its acceptation in relation to the sample.

The hedonic scale either can be presented to the panel of evaluators in different manners, as shown in Figure 3.

The affective methods provide quantitative data and allow more than one attribute in each sample being evaluated at the same time.

The discriminative test is better represented by the Triangular test. It allows differentiating one between three different samples and is very useful in shelf life studies and in the quality control of cosmetics. The ideal is to perform this evaluation with twelve to forty volunteers, who will receive the three samples and should indicate the different one between them (Zenebon et al., 2008).

The descriptive tests provide a broad sensory description about the product that is being evaluated (Almeida et al., 2008), helping to predict the consumer acceptance and what consumers think about such product (Almeida et al., 2006; Aust et al., 1987).

Option 1 Do you like the color of the product?

Not at all _____|_____ Enormously

The volunteer will place the vertical stroke on the scale line according to his opinion

Option 2 How much do you like the color of the product?

( ) 1: most pleasant
( ) 2: very pleasant
( ) 3: moderately pleasant
( ) 4: slightly pleasant
( ) 5: neither pleasant nor unpleasant
( ) 6: slightly unpleasant
( ) 7: moderately unpleasant
( ) 8: very unpleasant
( ) 9: most unpleasant

The volunteer will mark with a cross the scale according to his opnion

Figure 3. Examples of presentation of hedonic scale (Olshan et al., 2000; Barkat et al., 2003).

The tests to evaluate the effective of the products should be performed in true conditions of use and the volunteer may use only the product that is being assessed. These tests could be conduct by the evaluation of dermatologists, by the evaluation of volunteers, and even, by the measurement of one parameter by un equipment, such as the equipment that measures hydration, sebum and transepidermal water loss, to define if a product is really effective. Based on these clinical evaluations, a company could create an efficacy claim to the product (Wortel and Wiechers, 2000).

The sensory analysis could be also applied when a cosmetic industry needs to replace a raw-material of a commercialized product without changes in the performance of it. This replacement could be originated by many factors, such as the reduction of costs, problems with the firm who provides this raw-material problems with same raw material which causes irritation, comedogenicity or other problems that affect the consumer. In this field, the sensorial analysis helps the formulator, who proposes different raw materials as substitute, to evaluate if the consumer will notice the adaptation in the cosmetic product.

The statistical analysis is indispensable in the sensory studies. The sensory analysis data should be evaluated transforming them in scores which allows the application of statistical analysis to calculate the mean and standard deviation of the results, and the determination if the difference between the scores obtained is statistically significant. Graphics, tables and preference maps could be elaborated with the results obtained to facilitate the analysis of the data by the professional team.

The sensory analysis is especially indispensable in the industries of fragrances and perfumes, and because of that, high-resolution instrumental methods for evaluation of flavor and aroma have been developed and between them are the breath analysis via mass spectrometry (Dijksterhuis and Piggott, 2001; Ross, 2009). Instrumental measurements are thought to be objective, representing an independent fact or truth, however, the human smell sense is irreplaceable, being considered by Ross (2009) not necessarily valid because instrumental methods cannot account for the complexity of human perception.

Nevertheless, rheological studies have been applied to objectify the sensations when cosmetic emulsions are applied to the skin (Brummer and Godersky, 1999).

3. Rheology

Rheology is a tool widely applied in the food, petrochemical and pharmaceutical industries, but to the cosmetic industry it is incipient yet. Until now, the majority of cosmetic industries use viscometers to guarantee that the viscosity of different batches of a product is maintained.

This chapter was elaborated in order to show that many other rheological characteristics could be used to evaluate and to predict the stability of cosmetic products and could be applied to compare competing products in the market and to assay if a change in the composition will cause alterations that could be perceived by the consumer.

First, it is necessary to define the three parameters of most importance in rheology: shear stress, shear rate and viscosity. Shear stress can be defined as a force applied in an area. Shear rate is the ratio of the velocity of material to its distance from a stationary object (Naé, 1993). The shear rate can be calculated by the ratio between the velocity and the layer or film thickness. In a lipstick application, for example, with a velocity estimated in 5 cm/s and a layer thickness of 0.1 mm, the ratio (shear rate) is 5.10^2 s^{-1}. Finally, the viscosity can be defined as the resistance to flow. Thus, a viscous product presents smaller flow than others.

Concluding, rheology is the study of deformation and flow of materials under external forces. Some equations and the units of these parameters are (Naé, 1993):

$$\sigma = F/A \qquad\qquad (1)$$

Where:

σ = shear stress (Pa = kg.m^{-1}.s^{-2})

F = force (N or kg.m.s^{-2})

A = area (m^2)

The viscosity can be defined as the ratio between shear stress and shear rate:

$$\eta = \sigma/\dot{\gamma} \qquad\qquad (2)$$

Where:

= viscosity

= shear stress (Pa)

$\dot{\gamma}$ = shear rate (s⁻¹)

Since the unit of shear stress is Pa and the unit of deformation is s⁻¹, the unit of viscosity is Pa.s. These parameters are involved in scientific measurements of rotational assays.

Using controlled shear rate and measuring shear stress is possible to carry out rotational assays, and determine flow curves and describe the models: Newtonian or non-Newtonian and, among the last one, plastic, pseudoplastic, dilatant, tixotropic and reopetic fluids. Newtonian fluids are materials that present constant viscosity, independent of time and temperature. These materials present flow curves with proportionality between shear stress and shear rate. The Figure 4 represents the flow curve of a Newtonian material.

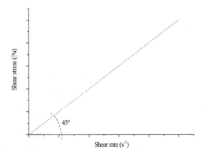

Figure 4. Flow curve of a Newtonian material.

In the case of non-Newtonians materials, this proportionality between shear stress and shear rate does not happen.

If in the beginning of the flow curve there is an increasing in the shear stress but the shear rate is equal to zero, and after to it is verified a Newtonian flow, this material is called plastic. This initial shear stress with shear rate equal to zero is called yield value and it represents the shear stress necessary for the material flow. The Figure 5 represents a plastic material. The yield value is related to the energy required to deform the material sufficiently so that they can flow. The value of the yield stress can be determined by measuring the deformation of the material as a function of the applied stress (Abdel-Rahem et al., 2005).

For non-Newtonian materials time-dependents, if the viscosity decreases with the shear rate, the material is called pseudoplastic and if the viscosity increases, the material is called dilatant. On the other hand, if the material is time-independent, it will be called tixotropic if the viscosity decreases with the shear rate or reopetic if the viscosity increases with the shear rate (Naé, 1993). When the ascending and the descending curves of the flow curve do not overlap it shows thixotropy which is a desirable feature for cosmetics and semisolid drug carriers for topical application (Lippacher et al., 2004). The Figures 6, 7, 8 and 9 represent the flow curves of non-Newtonian materials (Naé, 1993).

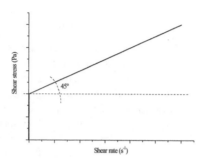

Figure 5. Flow curve of a plastic material.

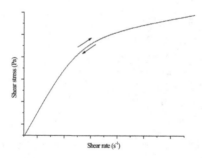

Figure 6. Flow curve of a pseudoplastic material.

For screening purposes and in the initial phases of the formulation development, the rheological tests proved to be very useful for the study of stability.

In a stability assay to determine the shelf life of a recently developed product, the formulation should be exposed to stress conditions, such as storage at -5 °C, 45 °C, and cycles of -5 °C during 24 hours followed by exposure to 45 °C during more 24 hours. This procedure is done in order to induce the appearance of instability signals in the formulations, where can be cited the darkening of the formulation, the precipitation of a constituent, the phase separation in the case of emulsions, and other signals. These stressing conditions are kept for a period around 2 or 3 months.

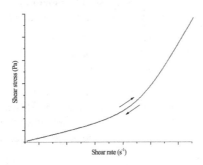

Figure 7. Flow curve of a dilatant material.

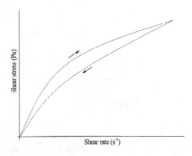

Figure 8. Flow curve of a thixotropic material.

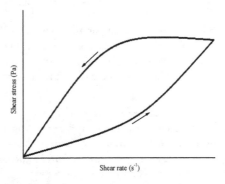

Figure 9. Flow curve of a reopetic material.

It is usually measured the viscosity of the stressed formulations periodically during the stability assay. It could be done by means of a viscometer or by using a rheometer.

With a viscometer, it is possible to carry out rotational assays or measurements by steady-state flow. On the other hand, the rheometer allows the development of oscillatory assays or dynamic measurements (Biradar, 2009).

When using an oscillatory rheometer it is necessary to carry out a flow curve assay and determine the apparent viscosity of the formulation in a defined shear rate. It is recommended to use the higher shear rate in the ascendant curve of the flow curve, since in this point the sample is in a suitable condition, it means that the formulation is not starting to flow and is not excessively sheared (Figure 10).

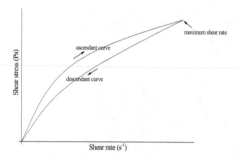

Figure 10. Example of a flow curve indicating the condition to the measurement of apparent viscosity.

In some papers, the flow curves have been plotted as viscosity as a function of shear stress instead of the traditional approach of plotting it versus shear rate because has been previously found that such curves are more discriminating and give better results for evaluation (Roberts, 2001; Samavati, 2011).

After obtaining, periodically, the minimum apparent viscosity of the samples exposed to stress conditions during a period, they should be compared with the initial value, and also compared the viscosity values of the control with the samples exposed to stress conditions, which allows the verification of the increase, decrease or maintenance of this attribute of the formulations.

Further exploiting the same assay, it is possible to calculate the hysteresis area of the formulation in each flow curve performed during the stability assay. The hysteresis loop areas can be obtained through a three-step experiment: upward curve, plateau, downward (Benchabane and Bekkour, 2008) and represents a way to measure, indirectly, the spreadability of the formulation, so it is possible to define if the formulation losses or gains easiness on spreadability during the shelf life. How much bigger is the hysteresis area, higher is the spreadability.

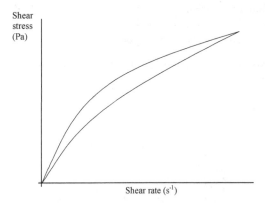

Figure 11. Flow curve with hysteresis area.

Using the flow curve is possible to compare two samples in relation to its hysteresis area and viscosity. A simple way to verify what formulation have a higher viscosity is by simple observation of the rheogram, since the curve that forms a bigger inclination in relation to the *x* axis of the graphic is the one with higher viscosity. On Figure 12 is showed an example of it, where sample 2 is more viscous than sample 1. It happens because the tangent of the angle formed is correspondent to the viscosity of the formulation in each shear rate.

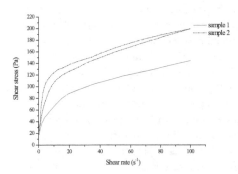

Figure 12. Comparison between flow curves of different samples (a thixotropic and a plastic fluid).

Beyond the different sensorial features caused by the differences in viscosity is known that the viscosity of emulsioned systems is one of the factors that retards or avoids the phase separation processes. The coalescence of dispersed phase can be due to the emulsifier agent and can be related to an instability because of low viscosity of dispersed phase (Corrêa & Isaac, 2012). This low viscosity can occur because of high shear stress (Samavati et al., 2011).

In general, for emulsioned systems, the continuos phase is shear thinning, which means that its viscosity decreases with the increasing on shear rate and viscoelastic, which means that it has viscous and elastic components (Tadros, 2004).

An example of the verification of differences in viscosity and thixotropy between two samples is shown on Figure 13.

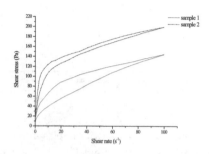

Figure 13. Comparison between flow curves of different samples.

Sample 1 is less viscous but more thixotropic than formulation 2. This simple verification gives to the analyst wide information, depending on what he needs.

Lescanne et al. (2004) studied organogels and aging properties of them. Organogels can be obtained by precipitation processes. These authors verified that, when aggregates are formed by the cooling rate, can be observed a elastic behavior, however, these aggregates can be aligned in the direction of the flow without lost the structure and when the flow is stopped, the aggregates are quickly rearranged and it inducing an thixotropic behavior. When the hot solution is introduced between the flat and the conical plates of the rheometer cell it is cooled to 5 °C with a cooling rate of 20°C/min, during the first hour of the gel life, it was measured the elastic properties of a gel as a function of time just after the cooling. Five minutes after its formation, the gel was submitted to a periodic stress (0.5 Pa) at a constant frequency (f = 1Hz). The authors showed that the shear moduli are constants and the aging phenomenon did not modify the elastic properties at least in a period of 1 h. However, when more than a week of aging is waited the samples lost most of its elastic properties.

The flow curve is a rotational assay, but using a rheometer it is possible to perform oscillatory assays too. Among the oscillatory assays are stress sweep and the frequency sweep assays.

The elastic (storage) modulus G' and the viscous (loss) modulus G'' are determined as a function of frequency or stress. The elastic modulus is a measure of energy stored and recovered per cycle of deformation and represents the solid-like component of a viscoelastic material. If a sample is elastic or highly structured then the elastic modulus will be high. The viscous modulus is a measure of the energy lost per cycle and represents the liquid-like component. If a sample is viscous the viscous modulus will be high.

In the stress sweep analyses, the structure of the sample is progressively destroyed by applying oscillations with an increasing stress amplitude at a fixed frequency (Callens et al., 2003). The linear viscoelasticity region occurs over that region of strain where the complex modulus is independent of the strain (Hemar, 2000). The linear viscoelastic region is determined by the maximum stress which can be applied without affecting G' and G''. Furthermore, the relative magnitude of the moduli is a qualitative indication for the structure in the sample. Two different situations can occur: G' > G'' for a network consisting of secondary bonds and G' ≤ G'' for a physically entangled polymer solution (Callens et al., 2003).

Frequency sweep tests are performed in the linear viscoelastic region of each sample, keeping the structure of the system intact during the measurement. By performing such small stress amplitude oscillations at a whole range of frequencies, the type of network structure can be revealed. The main difference between a network of secondary bonds and one of physical entanglements is located in the low frequency range: in an entangled network the polymers can disentangle if the available time is long enough (low frequency). In a network with secondary bonds the bonds are fixed irrespective of the time scale. This results for an entangled solution in a limiting slope of 2 for G' and 1 for G'' at low frequency in a log-log plot of moduli versus frequency, while at intermediate frequency a plateau develops. For a network of secondary bonds an almost constant value of G' and G'' is observed over the whole frequency range, with the value of G' exceeding that of G''(Callens et al., 2003; Madsen et al., 1998).

The stress sweep is important to evaluate the linear viscoelastic region of a sample that is a range of shear stress in which the formulation does not suffer profound alterations on it structure, being not disrupted. When a shear stress of the linear viscoelastic region is applied in an oscillatory assay, only the intermolecular and interparticle forces are being evaluated (Martin, 1993). To determine the linear viscoelastic region, the oscillating stress sweeps are carried out for the most extreme values. These measurements are used to determine where the reological properties are independent of the applied stress and the identify the critical rheological properties (Tuarez, 2011).

Knowing the values of shear stress that do not cause the disrupt in the formulation by means of the stress sweep, the analyst could perform a frequency sweep of the formulation. The frequency sweep is carried out in a constant shear stress found in the linear viscoelastic region. With this assay it is possible to evaluate the elastic or storage modulus (G') and the viscous or loss modulus (G''). The cosmetic excipients most used, emulsions and gels, are often viscoelastic samples. The viscoelastic samples when evaluated by means of the frequency sweep present G' and G'' values. When the G' value is higher than G'' it is an indicative that the formulation is more elastic than viscous. It is a characteristic of gels.

Emulsions which exhibits G' values higher than G'' (Figure 14) are described as more stable than formulations with G'' values higher than G' (Figure 15), since they tends to recovery its initial structure faster and more efficiently than the others, and are less susceptible to the gravitational forces which retards or avoids the coalescence process and the phase separation of emulsions (Alam and Aramaki, 2009). So, the G' values higher than G'' in emulsions is a desirable feature, being an indicative of stability of the cosmetic system.

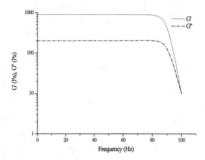

Figure 14. A frequency sweep example (G'>G'').

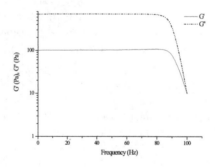

Figure 15. A frequency sweep example (G''>G').

Another assay that could be conducted using an oscillatory rheometer is the creep and recovery assay. It is done by submitting the samples to a constant shear stress during a period, and after, removing this shear stress and monitoring the formulation in relation to the deformation (measured by the compliance - J) during the same period. The compliance parameter is the resulting strain divided by the applied stress (Koop, 2009; Toro-Vazquez et al., 2010). If the compliance parameter is the relationship between strain and the applied stress, the strain is dimensionless and stress is measured in Pa, then, the compliance can be measured in 1/Pa.

In the example showed on the Figure 16 the samples were submitted to a shear stress during 300 seconds, and after removing this shear stress it was monitored during more 300 seconds.

Analyzing the result obtained in the first 300 seconds is verified that sample 1 exhibited lower compliance values than sample 2, which represents a higher difficult on being deformed than sample 1. The difficult on being deformed is always linked to higher viscosity values.

In the second part of the assay, where the shear stress imposed to the sample is removed, represented in the graphic by the time 301 to 600 seconds, is verified the viscoelastic properties of the samples. Formulations that are able to recovery its initial structure or part of it exhibit a gradually decrease in the compliance values. On Figure 17 there is an example of a formulation that is not a viscoelastic sample, it means that it do not exhibits storage modulus, and is not able to recovery its structure when the shear stress is ceased.

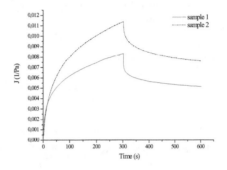

Figure 16. A creep and recovery example of viscoelastic samples.

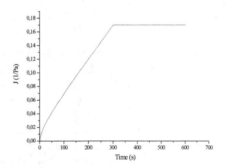

Figure 17. A creep and recovery example of a non-viscoelastic sample.

In addition, the rheology can be used to evaluate the stability over the time by dynamic and oscillatory rheological measurements (Pénzes et al., 2004; Vasiljevic et al., 2006) and the release of active principles. According to Martinez et al. (2007), the transdermal absorption of topically administered drugs depends on the rate of release and the permeability of them into the skin and also of the viscosity of the formulation (Martinez et al., 2007).

Thus, it is possible to say that different categories of products should present peculiar rheological properties inherent to its application (Gregolin et al., 2010).

In this way, the rheology can influence the diffusion coefficient, altering the release and permeation of cosmetics active substances (Welin-Berger et al., 2001; A-sadutjarit et al., 2005; Vasiljevic et al., 2006). Some authors have related the influence of rheological characteristics on the release profiles and consequently in the permeation of active substances in the skin; thus, the addition of thickening agents or attainment of a weak-gel because of physical entanglement of polymer chains must be considered in the choice of cosmetics bases (Spiclin, et al., 2003). Thus, rheology can help in the assay of release and permeation in the skin. Some studies have been published about it.

So, in a short way, the rheology is a valuable tool that helps in the quality control of cosmetics, being used in the stability tests, in the comparison between competing samples, in the comparison between an original product and a product with an alteration in a constituent, and in the development of new products, aiming to develop cosmetic with rheological characteristics which indicate stability.

4. Small Angle X-ray Scattering (SAXS)

The use of this technique in determining the quality control of a cosmetic is closely related to the stability of the product, which could be improved with the presence of liquid crystals.

Liquid crystals are described as a state of matter between solids and liquids, it means that, they are fluid like liquids but are organized like solids, being called mesophases (Marsh, 1973; Kelker and Hatz, 1980; Müller-Goymann, 2004). These organization contributes to the highly stability of systems.

The formation of liquid crystals in emulsions could be induced by some components present in this system, such as surfactants (Müller-Goymann, 2004). So, what happens is that it is possible to find a peculiar system that is not a simple emulsion and not a genuine liquid crystal, but an emulsioned system that contains liquid crystals, commonly lamellar structures, that are formed around of the inner phase of the emulsion (Oka et al., 2008), making difficult the coalescence, flocculation and the separation of the oily and water phases, what makes the system formed more stable than a simple emulsion (Figures 18 and 19). Flocculation is defined as the formation of aggregates of droplets of an emulsion under the influence of interparticle colloidal forces which are net attractive (Dickinson, 1992) and the formation of lamellar structures avoid or prevent the occurrence of this phenomenon. The formation of lamellar structures is essential to obtain emulsified oil/water systems finely dispersed, with balanced hydrophilic-lipophilic properties, resulting in minimal interfacial tension between aqueous and oily phases, thus contributing to the stability of the system (Engels et al., 1995). Previous studies have also shown that it is possible to make correlation between SAXS and rheological analysis, since were verified that the thicker the interlamellar water layers, the higher the viscosity of the cream (Eccleston et al., 2000). Thus, liquid crystals could be responsible by the emulsion stabilization and by the increasing in the viscosity (Klein, 2002), being the presence of this structures desirable in cosmetic emulsions which could be an indicative of quality of them.

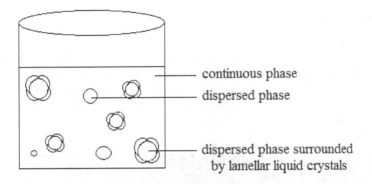

Figure 18. Scheme of a cosmetic emulsion containing liquid crystals.

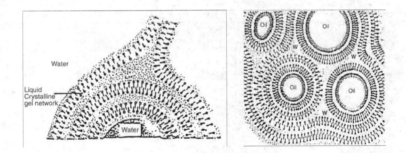

Figure 19. Schemes of the microscopic visualization of lamellar gel networks surrounding emulsion droplets proposed by Klein (2002).

This kind of structure is more commonly found in cosmetics due to the high diversity of components used in it in order to obtain a moisturizer, emollient, humectant, good sensory and, above all, stable cosmetic. In other pharmaceutical forms, usually are used a less diversified composition, which gives a system easier to understand, described as emulsion or liquid crystal, or even, a gel, a suspension, etc. The quantity of these lamellar structures, found in cosmetic emulsions, probably is dependent of three main factors: the raw-materials, the amount of it used and the process of preparation, where should be cited, the temperature and the speed of agitation.

In cosmetics, other kinds of systems could be used, such as genuine liquid crystals aiming to explore its characteristics of controlled delivery systems.

There are different kinds of liquid crystals and different classifications, but this chapter has not the function of describe them, since it have been done by many authors (Bechtold, 2005; Formariz et al., 2005; Atkins and Jones, 2006), the aim was to demonstrate the importance of these structures in the maintenance of the cosmetics' quality. Nevertheless, according to the literature data (Klein, 2002) and to our experience in this subject, it is possible to say that the lamellar arrangement is the most commonly found in cosmetic emulsions.

An initial analysis of the presence of liquid crystals in a cosmetic emulsion could be done using a polarized light microscope, but it should be confirmed and better analyzed by means of Small Angle X-Ray Scattering. When a microscope slide containing a sample of the system is studied and it presents structures that reflect the incident light, it is an evidence of the presence of liquid crystals (Figure 20). So, they should be submitted to SAXS analysis to confirm this expectation (Savic et al., 2011).

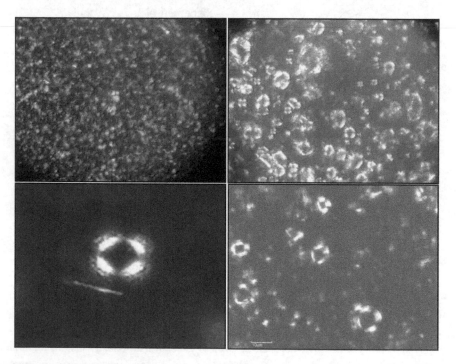

Figure 20. Photomicrographs of liquid-crystal present in emulsions evaluated by polarized light microscope.

The SAXS method requires a synchrotron light source that is formed by means of a particle accelerator, and using a monochromatic beam, that is used to irradiate the sample. After that, the scattering of the rays in small angle should be analyzed (Glatter and Kratky, 1982; Urban, 2004; Koch, 2010). Liquid crystals can be analyzed by SAXS since they are able to disperse the X-rays focused on it. In the SAXS line is used an X-rays detector and an multichannel analyzer to capture the intense of the SAXS measures ($I(q)$) in function of the modulus of the scattering vector (q) (Glatter and Kratky, 1982; Molina et al., 2006; Koch, 2010).

Analyzing the data obtained (Figure 19), the d value obtained represents the distance between the particles able to scatter the X-rays. It is calculated by the equation: $d = 2\pi / q\ max$, where $q\ max$, is the maximum intensity of scattering (Craievich, 2002). The relation between the d values obtained indicates the type of arrangement found in the system (Glatter and Kratky, 1982; Craievich, 2002; Alexandridis et al., 1998).

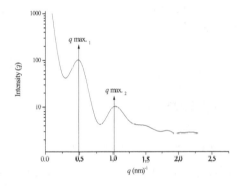

Figure 21. Hypothetical SAXS curve.

In the case of the hypothetical curve showed in Figure 19, d_1 / d_2 would result in 2, which describe lamellar structures (Alexandridis et al., 1998).

Beyond the advantages already mentioned, in a research conducted by Moaddel and Friberg (1995), the authors showed that the presence of lamellar liquid crystals in an emulsion avoids the water evaporation rate in this system, thus contributing in another way to the stability and maintenance of the cosmetic quality.

According to the advantages obtained with the presence of liquid crystals, these mesophases can be of great importance to the Cosmetic Industry in the development of very stable cosmetics and, the SAXS technique, an efficient tool to confirm the presence of these desirable structures that helps in the maintenance of cosmetics' quality control.

Camerel et al. (2003) pointed the importance in correlate the microstructure of a colloidal suspension with its rheological behavior to define its better use in industry and in life, beyond that, according to these authors there are few reports correlating these analyses.

Our research group has invested in researches to assess the stability of cosmetics (Isaac et al., 2008); evaluating of the influence of the addition of thickening agents in creams using rheological measurements (Isaac et al., 2012a); evaluating the thickeners' influence on the rheological properties of a cosmetic (Isaac et al., 2012b,c); proposing alternative methods to assay the efficacy and safety of them (Chiari et al., 2012a; Chiari et al., 2012b) and using of the sensory analysis in the cosmetics development (Isaac et al., 2012a) which, in different points of view of what was demonstrated in this chapter, also influence in the product quality.

5. Conclusion

This chapter aimed to show the facility that some simple or advanced techniques already used, sometimes to other finalities, could offer to the quality control of cosmetic products. The sensory analysis, rheology and SAXS technique have earned attention due to the important contribution that they can offer to the cosmetic area.

Author details

Bruna Galdorfini Chiari, Maria Gabriela José de Almeida, Marcos Antonio Corrêa and Vera Lucia Borges Isaac*

*Address all correspondence to: veraisaac@fcfar.unesp.br

Faculdade de Ciências Farmacêuticas, UNESP - Univ Estadual Paulista, Departamento de Fármacos e Medicamentos, Laboratório de Cosmetologia – LaCos, Araraquara, Laboratório de Cosmetologia, São Paulo, Brazil

References

[1] Abdel-Rahem, R., Gradzielski, M., & Hoffmann, H. (2005). A novel viscoelastic system from a cationic surfactant and a hydrophobic counterion. Journal of Colloid and Interface Science, 288, 570–582.

[2] Alam, M.M., & Aramaki, K. (2009). Glycerol effects on the formation and rheology of hexagonal phase and related gel emulsion, J. Colloid Interface Sci., 336, 820-826.

[3] Alexandridis, P., Olsson, U., & Lindman, B. (1998). A record nine different phases (four cubic, two hexagonal, and one lamellar lyotropic liquid crystalline and two micellar solutions) in a ternary isothermal system of an amphiphilic block copolymer and selective solvents (water and oil). Langmuir, 14, 2627-2638.

[4] Almeida, I.F., Gaio, A.R., & Bahia, M.F. (2006). Estimation of hedonic responses from descriptive skin sensory data by chi squared minimization. J. Sens. Stud., 21(1), 2-19.

[5]   Almeida, I.F., Gaio, A.R., & Bahia, M.F. (2008). Hedonic and descriptive skinfeel analysis of two oleogels: comparison with other topical formulations. J. Sens. Stud., 23(1), 92-113.

[6]   A-Sadutjarit, R., Sirivat, A., & Vayumhasuwan, P. (2005). Viscoelastic properties of carbopol 940 gels and their relationships to piroxicam diffusion coefficients in gel bases. Pharmaceutical Research, 22(12), 2134-2140.

[7]   Atkins, P., & Jones, L. (2006). Princípios de química: questionando a vida moderna e o meio ambiente. Porto Alegre: Bookmam. 3ed., p. 293-295 and 300-302.

[8]   Aust, L.B., Oddo, P., Wild, J.E., Mills, O.H., & Deupree, J.S. (1987). The descriptive analysis of skin care products by a trained panel of judges. J. Soc. Cosmet. Chem., 38, 443-448.

[9]   Backe, I., Meges, S., Lauze, C., Macleod, P., & Dupuy, P. (1999). Sensory analysis of four medical spa spring waters containing various mineral concentrations. Int. J. Dermatol., 38(10), 784-786.

[10]   Barkat, S., Thomas-Danguin, T., Bensafi, M., Rouby, C., & Sicard, G. (2003). Odor and color of cosmetic products: correlations between subject judgement and autonomous nervous system response. International Journal of Cosmetic Science, 25, 273-283.

[11]   Bechtold, I. H. (2005). Liquid crystals: A complex system of simple application. Rev. Bras. Ensino Física, 27(3), 333-342.

[12]   Benchabane, A., & Bekkour, K. (2008). Rheological properties of carboxymethyl cellulose (CMC) solutions. Colloid Polymer Science, 286, 1173-1180.

[13]   Biradar, S.V., Dhumal, R.S., & Paradkar, A. (2009). Rheological investigation of self-emulsification process. Journal of Pharmacy and Pharmaceutical Science, 12(1), 17-31.

[14]   Brummer, R., & Godersky, S. (1999). Rheological studies to objectify sensations occurring when cosmetic emulsions are applied to the skin. Colloids and Surfaces A: Physicochemical and Engineering Aspects, 152, 89-94.

[15]   Callens, C., Ceulemans, J., Ludwig, A., Foreman, P., & Remon, J.P. (2003). Rheological study on mucoadhesivity of some nasal powder formulations. European Journal of Pharmaceutics and Biopharmaceutics, 55, 323-328.

[16]   Camerel, F., Gabriel, J.C.P., Batail, P., Panine, P., & Davidson, P. (2003). Combined SAXS – Rheological studies of liquid-cristalline colloidal dispersions of mineral particles. Langmuir, 19, 10028-10035.

[17]   Chiari, B.G., Magnani, C., Salgado, H.R.N., Côrrea, M.A., & Isaac, V.L.B. (2012a). Estudo da segurança de cosméticos: presente e futuro. Revista Brasileira de Ciências Farmacêuticas Básica e Aplicada, 33(2).

[18]   Chiari, B.G., Martini, P.C., Moraes, J.D.D., Andréo, R., Corrêa, M.A., Cicarelli, R.M.B., & Isaac, V.L.B. (2012b). Use of HepG2 cells to assay the safety of cosmetic active substances. International Journal of Research in Cosmetic Science, 2(2), 8-14.

[19] Civille, C.V., & Dus, C.A. (1991). Evaluating tactile properties of skincare products: A descriptive analysis technique. Cosmet. Toilet., 106, 83–88.

[20] Corrêa, M.A., & Isaac, V.L.B. (2012). Emulsões. In: CORRÊA, M.A. Cosmetologia: ciência e técnica. São Paulo: Medfarma, p. 337-381.

[21] Craievich, A. F. (2002). Synchrotron SAXS studies of nanostructured materials and colloidal solutions. Materials Research Rev., 5(1), 1-11.

[22] Dickinson, E. (1992). Structure and composition of adsorbed protein layers and the relationship to emulsion stability. J. Chem. Soc. Faraday Trans., 88(20), 2973-2983.

[23] Dijksterhuis, G. B., & Piggott, J. R. (2001). Dynamic methods of sensory analysis. Trends in Food Science and Technology, 11, 284-290.

[24] Dooley, L.M., Adhikari, K., & Chambers IV, E. (2009). A general lexicon for sensory analysis of texture and appearance of lip products. J. Sens. Stud., 24(4), 581-600.

[25] Eccleston, G.M., Behan-Martin, M.K., Jones, G.R., & Towns-Andrews, E. (2000). Synchrotron X-ray investigations into the lamellar gel phase formed in pharmaceutical creams prepared with cetrimide and fatty alcohols. International Journal of Pharmaceutics, 203, 127–139.

[26] Engels, T., Förster, T., & Von Rybinski, W. (1995). The influence of coemulsifier type on the stability of oil-in-water emulsions. Colloids Surfaces A: Physicochemical and Engineering Aspects, 99, 141-149.

[27] Formariz, T.P., Urban, M.C.C., Da Silva Júnior, A.A., Gremião, M.P.D., & De Oliveira, A.G. (2005). Microemulsões e fases líquidas cristalinas como sistemas de liberação de fármacos. Revista Brasileira de Ciências Farmacêuticas, 41(3), 301-313.

[28] Fouéré, S., Adjadj, L., & Pawin, H. (2005). How patients experience psoriasis: results from a European survey. J. Eur. Acad. Dermatol. Venereol., 19(3), 2-6.

[29] Glatter, O., & Kratky, O. (1982). Small-Angle X-ray Scattering, Academic Press, New York.

[30] Gorcea, M., & Laura, D. (2012). Evaluating the physiochemical properties of emollient esters for cosmetic use. Cosmetics and Toiletries, 125(12), 26-33.

[31] Gregolin, M.T., Chiari, B.G., Ribeiro, H.M., & Isaac, V.L.B. (2010). Rheological Characterization of hydrophilic gels. Journal of Dispersion Science and Technology, 31, 820-825.

[32] Hemar, Y., & Horne, D.S. (2000). Dynamic rheological properties of highly concentrated protein-stabilized emulsions. Langmuir, 16(7), 3050-3057.

[33] Isaac, V.L.B., Cefali, L.C., Chiari, B.G., Almeida, M.G.J., Ribeiro, H. M., & Corrêa, M.A. (2012c) Effect of various thickening agents on the rheological properties of O/W emulsions containing non-ionic emulsifier. Journal of Dispersion Science and Tech-

nology.   Available   at: http://www.tandfonline.com/doi/full/
10.1080/01932691.2012.695952

[34] Isaac, V.L.B., Cefali, L.C., Chiari, B.G., Oliveira, C.C.L.G., Salgado, H.R.N., & Corrêa,
      M.A. (2008). Protocolo para ensaios físico-químicos de estabilidade de fitocosméticos.
      Rev. Ciênc. Farm. Básica Apl., 29(1), 81-96.

[35] Isaac, V., Chiari, B.G., Magnani, C., & Corrêa, M.A. (2012a). Análise sensorial como
      ferramenta no desenvolvimento de cosméticos. Revista de Ciências Farmacêuticas
      Básica e Aplicada, 33 (in press).

[36] Isaac, V.L.B., Moraes, J.D.D., Chiari, B.G., Guglielmi, D.A.S., Cefali, L.C., Rissi, N.C.,
      & Corrêa, M.A. (2012b). Determination of the real influence of the addition of four
      thickening agents in creams using rheological measurements. Available at: http://
      www.tandfonline.com/doi/full/10.1080/01932691.2012.683759

[37] Kelker, H., & Hatz, R. (1980). Handbook of Liquid Crystals, Verlag Chemie, Wein-
      heim, Germany.

[38] Klein, K. (2002) Liquid crystals and emulsions: a wonderful marriage. Chapter 26, p.
      265-269. In: Skin Barrier: Chemistry of Delivery Systems. Available at: http://
      www.alluredbooks.com/sample_pages/skin_barr_chem_skin_deli_syst_ch26.pdf.
      Acessed on july, 2012.

[39] Koch, M.H.J. (2010). SAXS Instrumentation for Synchrotron Radiation then and now.
      XIV International Conference on Small Angle Scattering (SAS09). Journal of Physics.
      Conference Series 247.

[40] Koop, H.S., Praes, C.E.O., Reicher, F., Petkowicz, C.L.O., & Silveira, J.L.M. (2009).
      Rheological behavior of gel of xanthan with galactomannan: effect of hydroalcoholic-
      ascorbic acid. Materials Science and Engineering C, 29, 559-63.

[41] Lee, I-S., Yang, H-M., Kim, J-W., Maeng, Y-J., Lee, C-W., Kang, Y-S., Rang, M-J., &
      Kim H-Y. (2005). Terminology development and panel training for sensory evalua-
      tion of skin care products including aqua cream. J. Sens. Stud., 20(5), 421-433.

[42] Lescanne, M., Grondin, P., D'Aléo, A., Fages, F., Pozzo, J.L., Moundain Monval, O.,
      Reinheimer, P., & Colin, A. (2004). Thixotropic organogels based on a simple N-hy-
      droxyalkyl amide: rheological and aging properties. Langmuir, 20(8), 3032-3041.

[43] Lippacher, A., Müller, R.H., & Mäder, K. (2004). Liquid and semisolid SLNe disper-
      sions for topical application: rheological characterization. European Journal of Phar-
      maceutics and Biopharmaceutics, 58, 561–567.

[44] Madsen, F., Eberth, K., & Smart, J.D. (1998). A rheological assessment of the nature of
      interactions between mucoadhesive polymers and a homogenized mucus gel. Bioma-
      terials, 19, 1083-1092.

[45] Makai, M., Csányi, E., Németh, Z.S., Pálinkás, J., & Erós, I. (2003). Structure and drug
      release of lamellar liquid crystals containing glycerol. Int. J. Pharm., 256, 95–107.

[46] Marsh, H. (1973). Carbonization and liquid-crystal (mesophase) development: Part 1. The significance of the mesophase during carbonization of coking coals. Fuel, 52, 205-212.

[47] Martin, A. (1993). Physical Pharmacy, fourth ed., Lea & Febiger, Philadelphia.

[48] Martinez, M.A.R., Gallardo, J.L.V., Benavides, M.M., López-Duran, J.D.G., & Lara, V.G. (2007). Rheological behavior of gels and meloxicam release. International Journal of Pharmaceutics, 333, 17-23.

[49] Meilgaard, M., Civille, G.V., & Carr, B.T. (1991). Consumer test and in-house panel acceptance tests. In: Meilgaard, M., Civille, G.V., Carr, B.T. Sensory evaluation techniques. Florida: CRC Press, p. 142-7, 281.

[50] Moaddel, T., & Friberg SE. (1995). Phase equilibria and evaporation rates in a four component emulsion. J. Disp. Sci. Technol., 16, 69-97.

[51] Molina, C., Dahmouche, K., Hammer, P., Bermudez, V.Z., Carlos, L.D., Ferrari, M., Montagna, M., Gonçalves, R.R., De Oliveira, L.F.C., Edwards, H.G.M., Messaddeq, Y., & Ribeiro, S.J.L. (2006). Structure and Properties of Ti^{4+}-Ureasil Organic-Inorganic Hybrids, J. Braz. Chem. Soc., 17(3), 443-452.

[52] Müller-Goymann, C.C. (2004). Physicochemical characterization of colloidal drug delivery systems such as reverse micelles, vesicles, liquid crystals and nanoparticles for topical administration. European Journal of Pharmaceutics and Biopharmaceutics 58, 343–356.

[53] Muñoz, A.M., Civille, G.V., & Carr, B.T. (1993). Sensory evaluation in quality control. New York: Van Nostrand Reinhold, p. 240.

[54] Naé, H.N. (1993). Introduction to rheology. In: Laba, D. Rheological propertie of cosmetics and toiletries. New York: Marcel Dekker, 426 p.

[55] Oka, T., Miyahara, R., Teshigawara, T., & Watanabe, K. (2008). Development of novel cosmetic base using sterol surfactante. I. Preparation of novel emulsified particles with sterol surfactant. Journal of Oleo Science, 57(10), 567-575.

[56] Olshan, A.A., Kohut, B.E., Vincent, J.W., Borden, L.C., Delgado, N., Qaqish, J., Sharma, N.C., & Mcguire, J.A. (2000). Clinical effectiveness of essential oil-containing dentifrices in controlling oral malodor. American Journal of Dentistry, 13, 18C-22C.

[57] Ozkan, S., Gillece, T.W., Senak, L., & Moore, D.J. (2012). Characterization of yield stress and slip behaviour of skin/hair care gels using steady flow and LAOS measurements and their correlation with sensorial attributes. International Journal of Cosmetic Science, 34, 193–201.

[58] Parente, M.E., Ares, G., & Manzoni, A.V. (2010). Application of two consumer profiling techniques to cosmetic emulsions. Journal of Sensory Studies, 25, 685-705.

[59] Parente, M.E., Gámbaro, A., & Ares, G. (2008). Sensory characterization of emollients. Journal of Sensory Studies 2, 149–161.

[60] Parente, M.F., Gambaro, A., & Solana, G. (2005). Study of sensory properties of emollients used in cosmetics and their correlation with physicochemical properties. J Cosmet Sci., 56(3), 175-182.

[61] Pénzes, T., Csóka, I., & Eros, I. (2004). Rheological analysis of the structural properties effecting the percutaneous absorption and stability in pharmaceutical organogels. Rheological Acta, 43, 457-63.

[62] Piana, M.L., Oddo, L.P., Bentabol, A., Bruneau, E., Bogdanov, S., & Guyot Declerck, C. (2004). Sensory analysis applied to honey: state of the art. Apidologie, 35, S26–S37.

[63] Proksch, E., & Lachapelle, J.M. (2005). The management of dry skin with topical emollients: recent perspectives. J. Dtsch. Dermatol. Ges., 10(5), 768-774.

[64] Roberts, G.P., Bames, H.A., & Carew, P. (2001). Modelling the flow behavior of very shear-thinning liquids. Chem. Eng. Sci., 56, 5617-5623.

[65] Ross, C.F. (2009). Sensory science at the humane-machine interface. Trends in Food Science & Technology, 20, 63-72.

[66] Samavati, V., Emam-Djomeh, Z., Mohammadifar, M.A., Omid, M., & Mehdinia, A.L.I. (2011). Stability and rheology of dispersions containing polysaccharide, oleic acid and whey protein isolate. Journal of Texture Studies, p. 1-14.

[67] Savic, S., Lukic, M., Jaksic, I., Reichl, S., Tamburic, S., & Müller-Goymann, C. (2011). An alkyl polyglucoside-mixed emulsifier as stabilizer of emulsion systems: The influence of colloidal structure on emulsion skin hydration potential. Journal of Colloid and Interface Science, 358, 182-191.

[68] Shewhart, W.A. (1980). Economic control of quality of manufactured product, American Society for Quality Control.

[69] Spiclin, P, Homar, M, Valant, A.Z., & Gasperlin, M. (2003). Sodium ascorbyl phosphate in topical microemulsions. International Journal of Pharmaceutics, 256, 65-73.

[70] Stone, H.S., & Sidel, J.L. (1992). Sensory evaluation practices. San Diego, CA: Academic Press.

[71] Tadros, T. (2004). Application of rheology for assessment and prediction of the long-term physical stability of emulsions. Advances in Colloid and Interface Science, 108 – 109, 227–258.

[72] Toro-Vazquez, J.F., Morales-Rueda, J., Ajay Mallia, V., & Weiss, R.G. (2010). Relationship between molecular structure and thermo-mechanical properties of candelilla wax and amides derived from (R)-12-hydroxystearic acid as gelators of safflower oil. Food Biophysics, 5, 193-202.

[73] Tuarez, E.P., Sadtler, V., Marchal, P, Choplin, L., & Salager, J.L. (2011). Making use of formulation-composition map to prepare highly concentrated emulsions with particular rheological properties. Ind. Eng. Chem. Res., 50, 2380-87.

[74] Urban, M. C. C. (2004). Desenvolvimento de sistemas de liberação micro e nanoestru-
     turados para administração cutânea do acetato de dexametasona. 2004. Dissertação
     (Mestrado em Ciências Farmacêuticas) - Faculdade de Ciências Farmacêuticas, Uni-
     versidade Estadual Paulista Júlio de Mesquita Filho, Araraquara.

[75] Vasiljevic, D., Parojcic, J., Primorac, M., & Vuleta, G. (2006). An investigation into the
     characteristics and drug release properties of multiple W/O/W emulsion systems
     containing low concentration of lipophilic polymeric emulsifier. International journal
     of Pharmaceutics, 309, 171-177.

[76] Welin-Berger, K., Neelissen, J.A.M., & Bergenstahl, B. (2001). The effect of rheological
     behavior of a topical anaesthetic formulation on the release and permeation rates of
     the active compound. European Journal of pharmaceutical Sciences, 13, 309-18.

[77] Wortel, V.A.L., & Wiechers, J.W. (2000). Skin sensory performance of individual per-
     sonal care ingredients and marketed personal care products. Food Qual. Pref.,
     11(1-2), 121-127.

[78] Zague, V., Nishikawa, D.O., Silva, D.A., Baby, A.R., Behrens, J.H., Kaneko, T.M., &
     Velasco, M.V.R. (2008). Influence of storage temperature on cooling intensity of topi-
     cal emulsions containing encapsulated menthol. J. Sens. Stud., 23(1), 26-34.

[79] Zenebon, O., Pascuet, N.S., & Tiglea, P. (2008). Métodos físico-químicos para análise
     de alimentos. Instituto Adolfo Lutz (São Paulo). On line version. Available at: http://
     www.crq4.org.br/sms/files/file/analisedealimentosial_2008.pdf

Sops: What Are They Good For?

Chapter 6

Standard Operating Procedures (What Are They Good For ?)

Isin Akyar

Additional information is available at the end of the chapter

1. Introduction

Standardization is defined as an activity that gives rise to solutions for repetitive application to problems in various disciplines. Generally, the activity constitutes the process of establishing (determining, formulating, and issuing) and implementing standards. Thus, standards are the perfect result of a standardization activity and inside the context of quality systems consist of quality documents or documents related to the quality system. High levels of quality are important to accomplish Company business objectives. Quality, a source of competitive benefit, should stay a symbol of Company products and services. High quality is not an additional value; it is an important elementary necessity. Each employee in all organizational units is responsible for guaranteeing that their work processes are effective and continually getting better. Top management should provide the training and an appropriate motivating environment to support teamwork both inside and across organizational units for employees to advance processes. Ultimately, everyone in an institution is responsible for the quality of its products and services. An institution in the role of a sponsor of clinical trials can best achieve its business objectives by establishing and managing robust quality systems with their integral quality documents including standard operating procedures (SOPs) (Manghani, K. 2011). The Quality Management system must evolve by trial and error, with enlarging experience, by group discussions and with changing understanding. In the beginning, attention will be focused on basic operational SOPs, afterwards moving to record keeping (as more and more SOPs are issued) and filling gaps as practice admits missing links in the chain of Quality Assurance. Essentially problems will turn up. One way to react to them is to talk with people in other laboratories who have faced similar problems. It should not be forgotten that Quality Management is a tool rather than a goal. The goal is quality performance of the laboratory. The philosopher Kant saw autonomy as self-government originning from morality, with morality proceeding from knowledge and self-discipline. Conger & Kanungo noted that an appropriate level of authority, discretion, formalization, and rule structure is a requirement for worker empowerment, which we see as consistent with the concept of self-government. Merriam-Webster defined autonomy as 'the quality or state of being self-governing; especially: the right of self-government; self-directing freedom and especially moral independence'. Necessitated SOP use will be absolutely related to the sense of self-determination experienced by workers. Worker participation in SOP advancement and clarification controls the affiliation between required SOP use and the sense of self-determination experienced by workers.

Standard Operating Procedures (SOP) is a process document that describes in detail the way that an operator should perform a given operation. SOPs involve the purpose of the operation, the equipment and materials required, how to perform the set-up and operations required for the process, how to perform the maintenance and shutdown operations carried out by the worker, a description of safety issues, trouble-shooting, a list of spare parts and where to find them, illustrations, and checklists. The SOP is one of many process documents which is needed for consistent operation of a given process, with other documents involving process flow charts, material specifications, and so forth.

The purpose of SOPs today is to guarantee that all workers are performing tasks in the same way, which is a needed for condition to get expected output from the process. When all workers perform their tasks constantly, it becomes possible to run controlled experiments to test the impact of changing various process parameters. When a process change is shown to improve process performance, SOPs are updated and workers are trained to the new procedures. All over the process, it is adorable to involve workers in SOP development and to praise worker ideas for the SOP improvement. For constant organizational advance, organized processes need to be constantly improved, hence necessitating ideas from those workers using those procedures. Ideas are not creative simply because they deviate from organized knowledge; ideas are creative when they are novel and suitable to the task at hand. Workers may have many ideas; nevertheless, what they choose to do with their ideas will depend on various organizational and individual-difference factors. The most important factor, however, for the advancement of creative behaviours is worker intrinsic motivation– a sine qua non of worker creative contribution. By the help of confirmatory factor analysis, the Spreitzer construct validated the four dimensions of intrinsic motivation (i.e. psychological authorization): (a) Competence (example item includes 'I am confident about my ability to do my job'); (b) Meaning (example item includes 'The work I do is very important to me'; (c) Impact (example item includes 'I have a great deal of control over what happens in my department'; (d) Self-determination (example item includes 'I can decide on my own how to go about doing my work'). Furthermore, Spreitzer argued and empirically established that an antecedent condition to innovation (i.e. creativity) and effectiveness is intrinsic motivation (De Trevil et al. 2005).

2. Overview

The quality documents constitudes of Company policies, quality management plan, SOPs, working instructions, conventions, guidelines, forms, templates, logs, tags and labels. They are organized by consensus and approved by a nominated body and they provide for common and repeated use, rules, guidelines or characteristics for activities or their results with a view to promote transparency, consistency, reproducibility, interchangeability and to facilitate communication. The hierarchy and types of quality documents relevant to quality systems will depend upon Company business objectives and business model. SOPs are Level 2 quality documents and, along with other related quality documents, guarantee the efficacy and effectiveness of quality systems (Manghani, K. 2011). Standard operating procedures (SOPs) are a vital component in any quality management system (Hattamer-Apostel, R. 2001). Every good quality system is based on its Standard Operating Procedures (SOPs) (Saxena). The advancement and use of SOPs are a necessary part of a successful quality system as it supplies individuals with the information to carry out a job adequately, and aids precision in the quality and integrity of a product or end-result (United States Environmental Protection Agency, 2007). They assign all processes involved in an organization (Frank, D. 2010). A quality system is defined as the organizational structure, responsibilities, processes, procedures and resources for implementing quality management (Manghani, K. 2011).

Standard Operating Procedures are sets of instructions having the force of a directive, covering those features of operations which lend themselves to a definite or standardized procedure without loss of effectiveness (Saxena).

The purpose of a SOP is to reach out the operations correctly and always in the same manner. A SOP should be available at the place where the work is done". SOPs assist the progress of constant application of processes and procedures so even when there are changes in personnel, organizations avoid inconsistencies and safety risks (Frank, D. 2010). Standard operating procedures or SOPs are written step-by-step procedures that quality control (QC), quality assurance (QA), and production units use in order to assure the accuracy and precision of the quantitative experimental results and materials that they generate and provide in support of other units. SOP's are needed to guarantee the continuity of processes to obtain quality performance and quality products/preparations (Natural Resources Management and Environment Dept.). SOP's are alive documents that detail written instructions describing specific steps to follow in all activities under defined conditions (Jain, SK. 2008). They are used to accomplish standardization when performing specific functions and is used to set out the way practice and procedures necessitated to be performed. SOPs are written instructions and records of procedures agreed and adopted as standard practice (Cardiff University, 2009). SOP's are necessary to guarantee the progression of processes to accomplish quality performance and quality products/preparations (Jain, SK. 2008). A Standard Operating Procedure (SOP) document is a routine or repetitive activity followed by an organization. SOPs describe both technical and administrative operational elements of an organization that would be managed under a Quality Assurance Project Plan and under an organization's Quality Management Plan (Almeida S.L.), (United States Environmental Protection Agency 2001).

SOPs are determined to be specific to the organization whose activities are defined and assist that organization to maintain their quality control and quality assurance processes (United States Environmental Protection Agency 2001).

All organizations, businesses, etc. should have SOPs (Jain, SK. 2008). SOPs support employees with the information necessitated to perform their jobs regularly and help guarantee consistency in the quality of performance (Frank, D. 2010). SOPs are used by the governmental agencies, private industry, and academic laboratories by scientists and engineers from all of the science, technology, engineering, and mathematical disciplines. SOPs can also be intensely valuable in academic laboratories and can be employed anytime there is process that likely more than one person will use in a research group (Natural Resources Management and Environment Dept.). SOPs are mainly associated with specific documentation necessities. It should not be forgotten that "If you don't document, it didn't happen! (Jain, SK. 2008). The International Conference on Harmonization Good Clinical Practice (ICH GCP) guideline ascertaines SOPs as "detailed, written instructions to achieve uniformity of the performance of a specific function". SOPs must be well written in order to supply an efficacious control of good clinical practice (GCP) and prevent errors from occurring, thereby lessening waste and rework. Poorly written SOPs are a source of misinformation. To be user friendly, they should be absolute, unambiguous and must be written in plain language. SOPs are controlled documents and are best written by persons involved in the activity, process or function that is required to be specified or covered in the SOP. SOPs must be reviewed prior to their approval for release, for adequacy, completeness and compliance with Company standards and all applicable legal, ethical and regulatory requirements. They must be checked out and updated as necessitated over their life cycle and any changes made to the SOPs must be re-approved. They must bear a revision status on them and their distribution must continually be documented and controlled. When obsolete SOPs are needed to be hold for any purpose, they should be suitably identified to prevent unintended use. Only relevant SOPs in their current version must be available at points of use and must remain legible. SOPs are mandatory for the implementation of GCP and other GxPs, namely, cGMP (Good Manufacturing Practice) and GLP (Good Laboratory Practice), within the scope of quality systems; therefore, it is well said that without SOPs there are no GxPs: no SOPs, no quality systems, and no GxPs (Manghani, K. 2011). SOPs are necessary for a clinical research organization whether it concerns a pharmaceutical company, a sponsor, a contract research organization, an investigator site, an Ethics Committee or any other party involved in clinical research to achieve maximum safety and efficiency of the performed clinical research Operatings. It is therefore a must that all people and sites involved in clinical studies (both at the sponsor and at the investigative sites) have suitable SOPs in place so as to conduct clinical research and to ensure compliance with the current regulations.

The presence of these quality documents is important when regulatory inspections (FDA, EMEA) take place since the most frequent reported deficiencies during inspections are the lack of written SOPs and/or the failure to adhere to them. The risk of GMP non-compliance is high at organizations with a poor suitability of specific SOPs and also if at all they are achiavable the staff or the people for whom they were written are not either following them. It therefore becomes very essential for the personnel to be trained on these SOPs so that they are absolutely aware of why and how SOPs can play important role in fulfilling the specific organizatory requirements from WHO, FDA, EMEA or other national health authorities. Health authorities world wide like the FDA or EMEA expect pharmaceutical, cosmetic and food producers to describe their manufacturing processes in written SOPs (GMP7.com). An organization's SOP manual is an important training document and provides workers with increased confidence, motivation and a sense of achievement (Frank, D. 2010). A SOP is a compulsory instruction. If deviations from this instruction are allowed, the conditions for these should be documented including who can give permission for this and what exactly the complete procedure will be. The original should rest at a secure place while working copies should be authenticated with stamps and/or signatures of authorized persons. The advancement and use of *SOPs* are a basic part of a successful quality system. It supplies information to perform a job regularly, and constantly in order to access pre-determined specification and quality end-result.

SOP clarifies the followings; what is the objective of SOP (Purpose), what are applicability and use of SOP (Scope)?, who will perform tasks (Responsibility), who will ensure implementation of procedure (Accountability), how tasks will be performed (Procedure).

Responsibility	Responsible
Identifying the need for development or revision of a standard operating procedure (SOP) and to convey that need to their immediate supervisor and/or the QA Manager (QAM).	Staff
An individual SOP to include sufficient detail that the process or procedure can be followed by another person when needed.	Author
Requesting peers to review the SOP to determine whether it contains sufficient detail.	Author
Reviewing and approving the SOP prior to its use.	Immediate supervisor and the QA Manager
Ensuring that the procedure or process follows the details noted in the individual SOP and to detail in writing when the SOP or a component of that SOP has not been followed.	Staff and the QAM
Ensuring that all routine operations and activities in their area are documented by SOPs.	Manager
Overseeing the appropriate preparation, numbering, retention, indexing, revision, and use of SOPs.	QAM
(United States Environmental Protection Agency, 2007).	

Table 1. Responsibility distribution in SOP.

Procedures are not an end in themselves - they do not ensure good performance or results. More important are well-designed systems and processes, qualified employees, and a motivating company culture. Procedures provide process people – environment but do not create processes, qualified people, or a good working environment (Jain, SK. 2008). The responsibility distribution in a SOP is shown in Table 1.

3. Purpose

The purpose of SOP is to assign the procedures for the preparation, approval, distribution, amendment and storage of Standard Operating Procedures (Cardiff University, 2009). The purpose or objective of the procedure should express and expand well written title (Jain SK., 2008). SOPs serve as frame for organizational action – support direction and structure. They tell what, how, when, why, and who. (Iowa State University, 2010). In order to be active, SOPs need to define not only what needs to be, but who is qualified to carry it out, and under what conditions the procedure can be performed reliably (Levine D.I., 2010). They should aid constant conformance support data quality. They should be determined to be specific to the organization and assist that organization to obtain their quality control and quality assurance processes and ensure compliance (Almeida S.L.) SOPs specify the commonly recurring work processes that are to be conducted or followed inside an arrangement. They approve the way activities are to be performed to alleviate constant conformance to technical and quality system necessities and to provide data quality. They may define, for example, basic programmatic actions and technical actions such as analytical processes, and procedures for maintaining, calibrating, and using equipment. If not written appropriately, SOPs are of limited value. Additionally, the best written SOPs will fail if they are not followed. Therefore, the use of SOPs needs to be checked out and re-enforced by management, alternatively the direct supervisor. Current copies of the SOPs also need to be readily accessible for reference in the work areas of those individuals absolutely carrying out the activity, either in hard copy or electronic format, otherwise SOPs serve little purpose (United States Environmental Protection Agency, 2007).

4. Benefits

The improvement and use of SOPs promotes quality through consistent implementation of a process or procedure within the organization reduced work effort, along with advanced data comparability, credibility, and legal defensibility (Almeida S.L.) The details in an SOP *standardize* the process and support step-by-step how-to instructions that enable *anyone* within your operation to perform the task in a consistent manner (Iowa State University, 2010). They abbreviate difference and advance quality through constant impact of a process or procedure inside the organization, although there are temporary or permanent personnel changes.

SOPs can signify agreement with organizational and governmental needs and can be used as a part of a personnel training program, since they should supply detailed work instructions. It minimizes opportunities for miscommunication and can address safety concerns.

When historical data are being estimated for current use, SOPs can also be very important for reconstructing project activities when no other references are accessible. Besides, SOPs are commonly used as checklists by inspectors when auditing procedures. Eventually, the benefits of a valid SOP are decreased work effort, along with developed comparability, credibility, and legal defensibility.

The advancement and use of SOPs is a basic part of a successful quality system. It supplies individuals with the information to perform a job regularly and aids constancy in the quality and integrity of a product or end-result through constant implementation of a process or procedure inside the arrangement.

SOPs can also be used as a part of a personnel training program, hence they should support detailed work instructions. When historical data are being assessed for current use, SOPs can be beneficial for reconstructing project activities. Additionally, SOPs are commonly used as checklists by inspectors when auditing procedures. Finally, the benefits of a valid SOP are minimized work effort, together with improved data comparability, credibility, and legal defensibility. SOPs are necessary even when published methods are being administered because cited published methods may not include appropriate information for conducting the procedure in-house.

For example, if the SOP is written for a standard analytical method, the SOP should designate the procedures to be followed in greater detail than appear in the published method, detailing how, if at all, the SOP differs from the standard method and any options, changes or alterations that the organization follows (United States Environmental Protection Agency, 2007). The significance regularly set up and managed quality control and quality assurance systems with their integral well-written SOPs and other quality documents for the achievement of Company business objectives cannot be ignored. They serve as a passport to success by assisting the Company to accomplish high-quality processes, procedures, systems, and people, with eventual high-quality products and services and enhancement of the following: Customer satisfaction, and therefore, customer loyalty and repeat business and referral; timely registration of drugs by eliminating waste and the requirement for rework; operational results such as revenue, profitability, market share and export opportunities; alignment of processes with achievement of better results; understanding and motivation of employees toward the Company quality policy and business objectives, as well as participation in continuous quality improvement initiatives; and confidence of interested parties in the effectiveness and efficiency of the Company as demonstrated by the financial and social gains from Company performance and reputation (Manghani, K. 2011). Benefits of SOPs are shown in Table 2.

Benefit	Explanation
To provide people with all the safety, health, environmental and functional information necessitated to perform a job properly	Placing value only on production while disregarding safety, health and environment is costly finally. It is better to train employees in all aspects of doing a job than to face accidents, fines and litigation later
To guarantee that production operations are performed constantly to obtain quality control of processes and products.	Consumers, from individuals to companies, want products of consistent quality and specifications. SOPs specify job steps that help standardize products and consequently quality.
To guarantee that processes continue uninterrupted and are completed on a prescribed schedule.	By following SOPs, you help to guarantee against process shut-downs caused by equipment failure or other facility damage
To guarantee that no failures occur in manufacturing and other processes that would harm anyone in the surrounding community.	Following health and environmental steps in SOPs guarantees against spills and emissions that threaten plant neighbors and create community outrage
To guarantee that acknowledged procedures are followed in compliance with company and government regulations.	Well-written SOPs help to gurantee that government regulations are satisfied. They also show a company's good-faith intention to operate perfectly. Failure to write and use good SOPs only signals government regulators that your company is not serious about compliance.
To serve as a training document for teaching users about the process for which the SOP was written.	Thorough SOPs can be used as the basis for supplying standardized training for employees who are new to a particular job and for those who need re-training.
To serve as a checklist for co-workers who observe job performance to reinforce proper performance.	The process of actively caring about fellow workers involves one worker coaching another in all aspects of proper job performance. When the proper procedures are outlined in a good SOP, any co-worker can coach another to help improve work skills.
To serve as a checklist for auditors.	Auditing job performance is a process similar to observation mentioned in the previous item only it usually involves record keeping. SOPs should serve as a strong basis when detailed audit checklists are developed.
To serve as an historical record of the how, why and when of steps in an existing process so there is a factual basis for revising those steps when a process or equipment are changed.	As people move from job to job inside and between companies, unwritten knowledge and skills disappear from the workplace. Regularly maintained written SOPs can chronicle the best knowledge that can serve new workers when older ones move on.
To serve as an explanation of steps in a process so they can be reviewed in accident investigations.	Although accidents are unfortunate, view them as opportunities to learn how to improve conditions. A good SOP gives you a basis from which to being investigating accidents
(Jain, SK. 2008)	

Table 2. Benefits Of SOPs.

5. Writing style

SOPs should be written in a step-by-step, easy-to-read format by subject-matter experts who know the processes and the structure of the organization (Frank, D. 2010). They should be written by individuals aware of the activity and the organization's internal structure. These individuals are basically subject-matter experts who actually perform the work or use the process. A team accession can also be followed, particularly for multi-tasked processes where the experiences of a number of individuals are critical (United States Environmental Protection Agency, 2007).

Well-written SOPs should first shortly define the purpose of the work or process, involving any regulatory information or standards that are suitable to the SOP process, and the scope to show what is covered. Any specialized or different terms either in a separate definition section or in the suitable discussion section should be explained.

The information presented should be clear and easy to understand. The active voice and present verb tense should be used. SOP shall be simple and short. Information should be transported clearly and absolutely to remove any doubt as to what is needed. Flow charts should be used to illustrate the process being defined (Jain SK., 2008), (United States Environmental Protection Agency, 2007). (United States Environmental Protection Agency, 2001), (Almeida S.L.). It may be helpful to include additional experts to help gather information and to review, test and approve draft SOPs (Frank D., 2010).

The most commonly used method of task analysis is *Hierarchical Task Analysis (HTA)*. Operating instructions should be close to the user and kept up to date. The following issues should be considered in evaluating operating procedure documentation:

1. There should be no easier, more dangerous opportunities than following the procedure.

2. There should be an appropriate QA system in place to guarantee that the procedures can be kept up to date and that any errors are rapidly detected and corrected.

3. The procedures should not be needlessly prescriptive. The best way of guaranteeing that procedures do not become overly prescriptive is through involving the operator during the design stage.

4. Procedures should contain information on the necessities for the wearing of personal protective equipment during the task.

5. Any risks to the operator should be documented at the start of the procedure, based on a risk assessment of the task.

6. An appropriate method of coding each procedure should be used.

7. Each time a procedure is produced it should be dated.

8. There should be no uncertainty between which procedures apply to which situations.

9. Procedures do not always have to be paper based.

10. At the start of the procedure an overview of the task should be provided.

11. Prerequisites should presented clearly at the start of the procedure to guarantee that the operator can check that it is safe to proceed.

12. The most important information on the page should be defined and this should be designed to be the most prominent information.

13. Separate headings should be used to discriminate apparently between sub tasks.

14. Any warnings, cautions or notes should be placed immediately prior to the instruction step to which they refer.

15. Language should be kept as simple as possible, i.e. use nomenclature familiar to the operator.

16. The nomenclature should be consistent with that on controls or panels.

17. Symbols, colours, and shapes used for graphics should conform to industry standards (Health and Safety Executive).

6. Preparation of SOP

When actualizing a SOP one can choose number of different ways to organize and format them. There are some factors which determine what type of SOP to use or create: How many decisions will user need to make during process? How many steps and sub steps are there in procedure? Routine procedures that are short and necessitate few decisions can be written using simple steps format. Long procedures consisting of more than 10 steps, with few decisions should be written along with graphical format or hierarchical steps. Procedures that necessitate many decisions should be written along with flow chart. Requirement for document identification and control, accountability and traceability responsibility must be involved with every SOP; this can be obtained by supporting constant format.

The need for an SOP or the revision of an existing one should be identified by informing the appropriate supervisor. Written instructions on standardized procedures supply guidance to guarantee that activities are conducted in a constant way, hence leading to reliable product and service quality. SOPs should be prepared in full compliance with guidelines and organizations and must mirror current organizational practices (Hattamer-Apostel, R. 2001). Ideally, SOP's should be written by teams that involve some or all of the following people: Those who will perform the job, those who will perform maintenance on equipment involved in an SOP, engineers or others who design equipment and processes, technical initiator, safety personnel, environmental personnel, equipment manufacturers (Jain, SK. 2008).

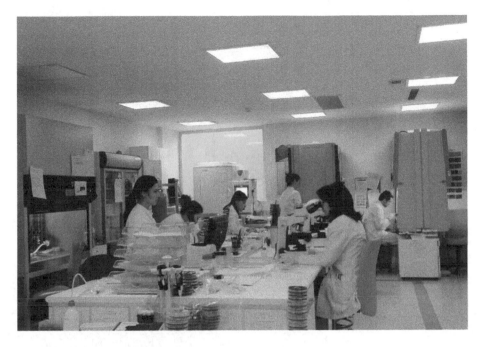

Figure 1. A SOP should be written by a team in that field.

7. Implementing SOP

The most substantial step for administering the SOP in working area, train or retrain the user. Every one should follow the procedure accurately with each and every step in detail, it is very significant to train the user otherwise individual may interpret meaning in different ways.

The trainer should share the reason WHY, SOP must performed correctly while training the user. People can follow better when they understand significance of procedure. Trainer should explain and demonstrate how each step in the SOP will be performed and should assure them this will increase Quality of product by providing safety and accuracy which will ultimately increase the confidence of the user.

The people in the writing team can write or edit parts of an SOP independently and then one person can combine the individual contributions. After combination the SOP should be circulated the draft SOP for review among the initiator before editing a final draft for review by supervisors and subsequent supervised testing by employees. Ideally a writing team should meet at least once in the beginning of a project to establish writing objectives, targets and responsibilities, but then can work semi-independently with one person serving as coordinator. SOPs should be checked out by several people qualified to assess the SOP in terms of its completeness and clarity of subject matter.

SOPs should at least mention:

a. who can or should make which type of SOP;

b. to whom proposals for a SOP should be submitted, and who estimates the draft;

c. the procedure of approval;

d. who decides on the date of implementation, and who should be informed;

e. how revisions can be made or how a SOP can be withdrawn.

It should be organized and recorded who is responsible for the proper distribution of the documents, the filing and administration (e.g. of the original and further copies). Finally, it should be indicated how frequently a valid SOP should be periodically evaluated (usually 2 years) and by whom. Only officially issued copies may be used, only then the use of the proper instruction is guaranteed (United States Environmental Protection Agency, 2007).

8. SOP Review and approval

SOPs should be reviewed (that is, validated) by one or more individuals with appropriate training and experience with the process (Almeida S.L.).

It is especially helpful if draft SOPs are completely tested by individuals other than the original writer before the SOPs are finalized. The completed SOPs then must be checked out and approved by peer reviewers, the QA Manager, and appropriate management prior to the use of the SOP. A set format in styling, information necessitated, and a numbering system is required, as well as biannual or annual review to ensure that the procedure is up-to-date. An archival system is needed to ensure that an historical record can be maintained and only current SOPs are available for staff use (United States Environmental Protection Agency, 2007).

The finalized SOPs should be approved as described in the organization's Quality Management Plan or its own SOP for preparation of SOPs. Generally the immediate supervisor, such as a section or branch chief, and the organization's quality assurance officer review and approve each SOP. Signature approval indicates that an SOP has been both reviewed and approved by management. When practical, use of electronic signatures, as well as electronic maintenance and submission, is an acceptable substitution for paper.

SOP general form defines an integrated system of management activities involving planning, implementation, documentation, assessment, and improvement to ensure that a process, or item, is of the type and quality needed for the project (United States Environmental Protection Agency, 2007), (Jain, SK. 2008).

9. Revising SOPS

If the SOP does not definitely describe the procedure, then the SOP must be revised. Any change in the procedure must be included into the SOP. Nevertheless, prior to any change to the SOP, management must be advised of, and approve, the change.

If there are some errors in the finalized SOPs, such as typographical errors, printing errors, e.g., wrong page numbers or misaligned sentences) or any errors that do not affect the scope of the procedure, they may be correctly immediately and reprinted. These types of errors do not require full SOP revision, thus a revision number will not be generated and management approval is not needed. If the error occurs on the signature page then the signature page will be resigned. These types of corrections will be traceable since the historical file will reflect all corrections including typographical errors. Specifically, the historical SOP file will contain both the SOP with the correct page(s) as well as the page(s) containing the error. The page with the error will not be removed from the historical file. Additions can be made to an SOP via a clarification or an addendum. Explanations and addenda must be attached to the appropriate SOP until such time that the SOP can be revised. Usually, the revision will be organized during the biannual review process. When the SOP is revised, the revision number is updated. Revisions, explanations, and addenda are prepared by appropriate personnel, but must be approved by management. An SOP can be eliminated when it is no longer applicable. Management must approve the elimination of an SOP. Two or more SOPs can be consolidated; in this case one SOP supersedes the other, but management approval is required for consolidation of procedures. The signed revised SOP must be sent to the historical file for archiving (United States Environmental Protection Agency, 2007).

10. Frequency of revisions & Reviews

SOPs necessitate to remain current to be useful. The review process should not be overly cumbersome to encourage timely review. Therefore, whenever procedures are changed, SOPs should be updated and re-approved. If desired, only the pertinent section of an SOP can be modified and indicate the change date/revision number for that section in the Table of Contents and the document control notation.

SOPs should also be reviewed systematically on a periodic basis, e.g. every 1-2 years, to ensure that the policies and procedures remain current and suitable, or to decide whether the SOPs are even needed. The review date should be added to each SOP that has been reviewed. If an SOP defines a process that is no longer followed, it should be removed from the current file and archived (Almeida S.L.) The frequency of review should be indicated by management in the organization's Quality (Jain, SK., 2008).

11. Checklists

SOPs should describe how the checklist is to be prepared or on what it is to be based (Almeida S.L.)

Many activities use checklists to guarantee that steps are followed in order. Checklists are also used to document completed actions. Any checklists or forms involved as part of an activity should be referenced at the points in the procedure where they are to be used and then attached to the SOP (United States Environmental Protection Agency, 2007).

In some cases, detailed checklists are prepared specifically for a given activity. In those cases, the SOP should describe, at least generally, how the checklist is to be prepared, or on what it is to be based. Copies of specific checklists should be then maintained in the file with the activity results and/or with the SOP.

Many activities use checklists to guarantee that steps are followed in order. Checklists are also used to document completed actions. Any checklists or forms involved as part of an activity should be referenced at the points in the procedure where they are to be used and then attached to the SOP. In some cases, detailed checklists are prepared specifically for a given activity. In those cases, the SOP should describe, at least generally, how the checklist is to be prepared, or on what it is to be based. Copies of specific checklists should be then maintained in the file with the activity results and/or with the SOP. Remember that the checklist is not the SOP, but a part of the SOP (Jain SK., 2008).

12. Document Control

Each organization should develop a numbering system to systematically identify and label their SOPs, and the document control should be described in its Quality Management Plan. Usually, each page of an SOP should have control documentation notation. A short title and identification (ID) number can serve as a reference designation. The revision number and date are very useful in identifying the SOP in use when reviewing historical data and is critical when the requirement for observable records is included and when the activity is being reviewed (United States Environmental Protection Agency, 2007).

13. SOP Document Tracking and Archival

The organization should sustain a master list of all SOPs. This file or database should show the SOP number, version number, date of issuance, title, author, status, organizational division, branch, section, and any historical information regarding past versions. The QA Manager (or designee) is usually the individual responsible for sustaining a file listing all current quality-related SOPs used inside the organization. If an electronic database is used, automatic "Review SOP" notices can be sent. Note that this list may be used also when audits are being considered or when questions are raised as to practices being followed within the organization.

The Quality Management Plan should indicate the individual (s) responsible for assuring that only the current version is used. That plan should also designate where, and how, outdated versions are to be maintained or archived in a manner to prevent their continued use, as well as to be available for historical data review.

Electronic storage and retrieval mechanisms are generally easier to access than a hard-copy document format. For the user, electronic access can be limited to a read-only format, thereby protecting against unauthorized changes made to the document (United States Environmental Protection Agency, 2007).

14. SOP General Format

This term describes an integrated system of management activities involving planning, implementation, documentation, assessment, and improvement to ensure that a process, or item, is of the type and quality needed for the project (Levine, D.I. 2010).

How should a SOP be organized? A SOP should be organized to ensure ease and efficiency in use and to be specific to the organization which develops it. There is no one 'correct' format; and internal formatting will vary with each organization and with the type of SOP being written.

How much detail needs to be included in a SOP? A SOP should be written with sufficient detail so that someone with a basic understanding of the field, can successfully reproduce the activity or procedure when unsupervised (United States Environmental Protection Agency, 2007).

The QA systems in place will be covered in general by 'standard operating procedures' (SOP) and will be made up of the following essential components:

SOI's should be organized to guarantee ease and efficiency in use and to be specific to the organization which develops it. There is no one "correct" format; and internal formatting will vary with each organization and with the type of SOP being written. Where possible break the information into a series of logical steps to avoid a long list. The level of detail provided in the SOP may differ based on, e.g., whether the process is critical, the frequency of that procedure being followed, the number of people who will use the SOP, and where training is not routinely available. A generalized format is discussed next (Levine, D.I. 2010).

Organization shall have SOP on Preparation, approval, revision and control of standard Operating Procedure for more excellent control and management of SOPs. Before finalizing and distributing SOPs, organizations should get the documentation reviewed and validated by people with training and experience on the processes. If the SOP does not definitely define the procedure, then the SOP must be revised. Any change in the procedure must be included into the SOP. After all, prior to any change to the SOP, management must be advised of, and approve, the change. Finalized SOPs, containing typographical errors, printing errors, e.g., wrong page numbers or misaligned sentences) or any errors that do not act on the scope of the procedure may be corrected immediately and reprinted.

An organization's SOPs should be written in a format that is tailored to the organization type and its unique requirements. In general, administrative/programmatic SOPs will consist of five elements: Title page, Table of Contents, Purpose, Procedures, Quality Assurance/Quality Control, and Reference (Frank, D. 2010). General SOP format is shown in Table 3.

Element	Explanation
Title page	The SOP should be arranged to guarantee ease and efficiency in use and to be specific to the organization (Almeida S.L.) Each SOP produced will be issued with a unique SOP number for reference purposes. This will be located in the table on the front page and in the footer of the document. This number will state where the SOP originated, the year it was produced, the SOP number and also state the version number. The SOP reference and effective date should be included in the footer on each page of the SOP. The first page or cover page of each SOP should contain the following information: a title that clearly identifies the activity or procedure, an SOP identification (ID) number, date of issue and/or revision, the name of the applicable agency, division, and/or branch to which this SOP applies, and the signatures and signature dates of those individuals who prepared and approved the SOP. Electronic signatures are satisfactory for SOPs obtained on a computerized database. (Jain SK., 2008), (United States Environmental Protection Agency, 2001), (Almeida S.L.), (Frank D., 2010). The Author shall be the individual primarily responsible for writing the SOP. **Chapter pages:** Chapter pages can help divide content by area or task type. Chapter pages serve as mini title pages introducing each section and indicate dates for the most recent revisions. **Title** – a clear, brief title describing the aim of the SOP and the conditions under which it can be accurately used (Levine D.I., 2010).The title should use directive language to declare what is being done to what (United States Environmental Protection Agency, 2007). Each SOP should be given a unique name which captures the significance of the practice described (Levine D.I. ,2010).
Table of Contents	Table of contents is not required if SOP is three pages or less. A table of contents may be necessitated for quick reference, particularly if the SOP is long, for locating information and to designate changes or revisions made only to certain sections of an SOP. Denotes changes or revisions made only to certain sections of a SOP (Almeida S.L.), (United States Environmental Protection Agency, 2007).
Definitions	There should be a part defining any words, phrases, or acronyms having special meaning or application (United States Environmental Protection Agency 2001).
Purpose	Each chapter should first briefly describe the purpose of the work or process, including any regulatory information or standards that are appropriate to the process (Levine, D.I. 2010). It is recommended to include criteria for the control of the described system during operation.
Procedures	In general there are four major types of procedure: Procedures that supply general operating guidance; an aid to meeting operating aims; mandatory and prescribe behaviour; and used as a training tool. The key to any program striving for quality is the set of Standard Operating Procedures (SOPs) that describe how work is to be done. The procedure section will identify how the aims will be achieved. This will clearly indicate a step by step description of how the procedure to be followed. Steps should include products and equipment required, possible obstacles, personnel qualifications and safety considerations. For lengthy process descriptions, a flow chart might be necessary to define processes that often involve interferences or variances.

Procedures | If calculations are involved in analyzing the data, then an example of the calculation should be
(continued) | provided. Figures and tables showing laboratory apparatus, representative data, etc. can be included
here (Levine, D.I. 2010).

Once the necessity for a particular SOP is organized, it should be drafted immediately. SOPs are drafted by laboratory or supervisory staff qualified to perform the procedure. Next the SOP is reviewed by other staff, where possible, and then approved by the QA Manager (QAM) and management, such as immediate supervisor. Circulation to staff members for review/comment is advisable prior to acquiring management approval. The SOPs should be written to define study methods or procedures in sufficient detail so as to guarantee the quality and integrity of the data or procedure to be followed. When writing SOPs, the detail used may include both procedural requirements (exact instructions) and guidance information (general information) on the procedure. Procedural requirements must be followed accurately, while guidance information is used to help perform the procedure; it is not a mandatory requirement and, therefore, it does not have to be followed exactly. Procedural requirements can be distinguished from guidance elements, based on the context they are used. Office standard format for margins, font, and font size should be followed. Official SOPs will have a colored header and footer on each page, dated signatures on the front title page, and be printed on ivory colored paper with a watermark. An outline format should be used and include alpha and/or numeric characters are to be included to indicate levels of information (United States Environmental Protection Agency, 2007).

A SOP should be written as soon as the need for a standard written procedure for an activity is required (Cardiff University, 2009). How much someone knows about an entire process or job affects the way he or she does that job. Incorporate safety, health and environment into the traditional how-to-operate or how-to-do steps. Based on best practice/standards, the procedure should be written in specific detail to ensure that the procedure can be repeated in a reproducible fashion to include the order of steps that should be followed, the times allowed for each step (as needed) and the temperatures at which the steps are performed.

It should be kept in mind that many people do not read all the steps before starting on step one. A SOP should be written as long as necessary for a specific job. People tend to ignore long SOPs because they cannot remember more than 6 to 12 steps. If the SOP goes beyond 10 steps, the following solutions should be considered; The long SOPs should be broken into several logical sub-job SOPs, an accompanying shortened SOP should be written that lists only the steps but not detailed explanations of those steps, and the long-form SOP should be made as a training document or manual to supplement the shorter sub-job SOPs mentioned earlier (Jain, SK. 2008).

All SOPs before implementation or after revision will be approved by the management committee before implementation. Previous versions of all documentation will be stored electronically, with only the current versions available in the biorepository file.

All SOPs will be checked out on an annual basis by the management committee. Protective equipment that should be worn by staff when performing the procedure described. A list of the equipment needed to perform the procedure. All materials and supplies should be recorded. The date the procedure was first introduced as well as the date of the most recent version. The date format should be based on the ddmmyyyy system where d represents day, m represents month and y represents year.

Procedures **(continued)**	Personnel Qualifications/Responsibilities (identifying any special qualifications users should have such as certification or training experience and/or any individual or positions having responsibility for the activity being described)(United States Environmental Protection Agency 2001)
	Any related SOPs (of operations used in the present SOP); possible safety instructions should be added.
	Generally there are four types of procedure: (Health and Safety Executive).
	General operating guidance procedures
	Procedures that an aid providing procedures to meeting operating aims
	Mandatory and behaviour prescribing procedures.
	Training tool procedures
	Scope and Applicability–under what specific conditions can this protocol be used reliably; are there any known interferents or other limitations on the protocol's effective use?
	Introduction–Appropriate background information on the system, methods, and instruments are used. The background section should plan the procedure and the specific aim of the SOP.
	Materials and Supplies–There should be a list of any reagents involving names of suppliers used in this procedure. If the suppliers are obscure sources, a list of addresses and contact information should be supplied as well. **Cautions** – If there are some specific health and safety precautions they should be considered. For example, should gloves be worn? If so, what kind? How should spills, if they occur, be cleaned up? Are there any special procedures that should be followed in order to safely dispose of waste? (Levine, D.I. 2010). Some SOPs should be written for people who perform under different interpersonal circumstances, people who work alone, two or more people who work together as a team, for people who will control other people doing a job, for people who not familiar with rules generally understood by your employees (Jain, SK. 2008).
	Well-written SOPs should first briefly describe the purpose of the work or process, including any regulatory information or standards that are appropriate to the SOP process, and the scope to indicate what is covered. Diagrams and flow charts should be used to help to break up long sections of text and to briefly summarize a series of steps for the reader(Almeida S.L.)
	The age, education, knowledge, skill, experience and training, and work culture of the individuals should be considered who will be performing the SOP steps.
	Criteria, checklists, or other standards should be applied during the procedure such as citing the document as guidance for reviewing SOPs Records Management (specifically,e.g.,as forms to be used and locations of files.
	Once writing of an SOP have been completed, there should be several workers test it and give you feedback.
Health and Safety Warnings	Primarily for technical SOPs
Cautions	Primarily for technical SOPs
Interferences	Primarily for technical SOPs

Quality Assurance/ Quality Control	The preparation of appropriate QC procedures (self-checks, such as calibrations, recounting, reidentification) and QC material (such as blanks - rinsate, trip, field, or method; replicates; splits; spikes; and performance evaluation samples) that are needed to display successful performance of the method should be defined. All SOPs should be checked out annually to certify all SOPs are in line with current processes, guidelines and regulations. They should be checked out in regards with the review date assigned and recorded on the front page of each SOP. The designated individuals will approve all SOP amendments. All significant amendments will be required 2 months in advance of the annual review. Any control steps and provisions for review or oversight should be defined prior to acceptance of the product or deliverable. This can involve test plans such as verification and validation plans for software or running a "spell-check" program on the finished document (United States Environmental Protection Agency 2001). Finally, next all appropriate QA and quality control (QC) activities for that procedure should be defined, and list any cited or significant references (United States Environmental Protection Agency, 2007). Before finalizing and distributing SOPs, organizations must get the documentation reviewed and validated by people with training and experience on the processes. Additionally, it is a good idea to have the SOPs tested by staff who will be asked to comply with them. By following these steps, the author can identify missing information or needed revisions. Once SOPs are approved, they should be made readily available to facility management, building occupants and cleaning employees. The SOP will require final approval and authorization. The signature on an SOP will authoise the associated forms which should show an identical issue date to the SOP. When an SOP is issued and become effective, adequate time is required for training purposes. Finally, SOPs must remain current, so they should be updated and re-approved at least annually or whenever procedures change. Though the SOP development process takes time and effort, it can provide significant improvement to a cleaning organization's operational results and workers' understanding and job performance (Frank, D. 2010). All SOPs are reviewed by the applicable supervisor at least every two years in order to maintain their relevancy. Names of those individuals who have reviewed and approved the SOP for use in the laboratory. Signatures and dates should be supplied whenever possible as well. For those SOPs which do not necessitate a revision, documentation attesting to that fact must be submitted to the QAM who in turn initials and dates the table located at the bottom of the title page of the original SOP (United States Environmental Protection Agency, 2007). All SOPs require version control to ensure that individuals are using the correct verision of SOP. It is good to practice to assign a document a version number, in the format N. n where N represents a finalized document and n represents draft versions. Each new, approved and finalized document a major verison number.... should be assigned. When taking a document for revision or as draft, assign a new minor version. During the review cycle assign each new revision of the draft the next minor version, upon approval/finalization of the document assign the next major version (United States Environmental Protection Agency 2001), (Natural Resources Management and Environment Dept.).
References	References relating to the development of the SOP are required to be listed. These may include other SOPs, regulatory guidelines and published papers etc. Documents listed in the SOP must be recorded in the appendices and listed accordingly (United States Environmental Protection Agency 2001).

Contact list	It should involve contact details for relevant individuals such as author of document.
Appendices	This section should list appendices of other SOPs referenced in the document, or related to the procedure.
Distribution	Once approved the original paper SOP folder, it will also contain supporting documentation relating to each approved SOP for referencing purposes. An electronic copy of the SOP will be held. Approved SOPs will be distributed in hard copy to PDs and will be published. The paper version of the abandoned SOP will be filled into the archived SOP folder. All SOPs will be checked out and approved annually before it is superseded, unless a specific reason for a 6 month review can be justified. All SOPs must be kept for the duration of the project. When the Sop fulfils all the necessary requirements it is printed. The author hands over the manuscript (or the floppy disk with text) to the SOP administrator who is responsible for the printing. The number of copies is decided by him/her and the author. Copying SOPs is forbidden. Extra copies can be obtained from the SOP administrator. The author (or his successor) signs all copies in the presence of the administrator before distribution. As the new copies are distributed the old ones (if there was one) are taken in. For each SOP a list of holders is made. The holder signs for receipt of a copy. The list is kept with the spare copies. Users are responsible for proper keeping of the SOPs. If necessary, copies can be protected by a cover or foil, and/or be kept in a loose-leaf binding. Appropriate SOPs will be placed in green binders to be found in a designated spot in each work area, e.g., laboratory, equipment rooms, the library, etc., and shall be available to staff and managers. These binders will not be located in the supervisor's office. Removal of an individual SOP requires completion of the sign-out located on the insider of the binder. The binder must not be removed from its designated spot by anyone other than the QAM or laboratory director. It is the responsibility of the QAM to update each binder as individual SOPs are revised. The staff is required to read any revised SOP within 7 working days of issuance if the SOP is applicable to their work. Reading of the updated SOP requires signature on the SOP review sheet (United States Environmental Protection Agency, 2007).
Archiving	Proper archiving is essential for good administration of SOPs. All operating instructions should be kept up-to-date and be accesible to personnel. Good Laboratory Practice requires that all documentation pertaining to a test or investigation should be kept for a certain period. SOPs belong to this documentation. An historical file is created for each SOP that is approved by management and will be maintained in the company's archives by the QAM. The historical file will consist of the original signed SOP and all subsequent modifications thereof. Official SOPs will have both colored header and footer lines, and be printed on watermarked ivory colored paper. All copies of the original will be black and white, initialed, numbered, and placed in the appropriate binder located in each office. If a procedure is incorporated into another SOP (superseded), a copy of the superseded version is placed in the historical file of both SOPs (United States Environmental Protection Agency, 2007).

Table 3. General SOP Format.

15. Types of SOP

Several categories and types of SOPs can be distinguished. The name "SOP" may not always be appropriate, e.g., the description of situations or other matters may better designated *protocols, instructions* or simply *registration forms*. Also *worksheets* belonging to an analytical procedure have to be standardized (to avoid jotting down readings and calculations on odd pieces of paper) (Almeida S.L.)

Some of the most important SOP types:

- Fundamental SOPs. These give instructions how to make SOPs of the other categories.

- Methodic SOPs. These describe a complete testing system or method of investigation.

- SOPs for safety precautions

- Standard procedures for operating instruments, apparatus and other equipment.

- SOPs for analytical methods.

- SOPs for the preparation of reagents.

- SOPs for receiving and registration of samples.

- SOPs for Quality Assurance.

- SOPs for archiving and how to deal with complaints.

Generally the SOPs may be written for any repetitive technical activity, as well as for any administrative procedure (Almeida S.L.).

SOPs may be written for any repetitive technical activity, as well as for any authoritative or functional programmatic procedure, that is being followed inside an organization. General guidance for preparing both technical and administrative SOPs follows and examples of each are located in the Appendix (United States Environmental Protection Agency, 2007).

16. Guidelines for Technical SOP Text

Technical SOP and Administrative SOP are typical structures of SOPs. Technical and administrative SOPs need to involve the specific steps aimed at initiating, coordinating, and recording and/or reporting the results of the activity, and should be tailored only to that activity.

A technical SOP is a standard operating procedure which involves environmental data generation, manipulation, or accumulation, e.g., an analytical process. Technical SOPs can be written for a wide variety of activities.

Examples are SOPs instructing the user how to perform a specific analytical method to be followed in the laboratory or field (such as field testing using an immunoassay kit), or how to collect a sample in order to preserve the sample integrity and representativeness (such as collection of samples for future analysis of volatile organic compounds or trace metals), or how to conduct a bioassessment of a freshwater site. Technical SOPs are also needed to cover activities such as data processing and evaluation (including verification and validation), modeling, risk assessment, and auditing of equipment operation. Citing published methods in SOPs is not always acceptable, because cited published methods may not contain pertinent information for conducting the procedure-in-house. Technical SOPs need to include the specific steps aimed at initiating, coordinating, and recording and/or reporting the results of the activity, and should be tailored only to that activity. Technical SOPs should fit within the framework presented here, but this format can be modified, reduced, or expanded as required.

17. Guidelines for Administrative or Fundamental Programmatic SOP

An administrative SOP is a standard operating procedure which does not include environmental data manipulation activities, e.g., how to conduct an inspection. As with the technical SOPs, these SOPs can be written for a wide variety of activities, e.g., reviewing documentation such as contracts, QA Project Plans and Quality Management Plans; inspecting (auditing) the work of others; determining organizational training needs; developing information on records maintenance; validating data packages; or describing office correspondence procedures.

Administrative SOPs need to include a number of specific steps aimed at initiating the activity, coordinating the activity, and recording and/or reporting the results of the activity, tailored to that activity. For example, audit or assessment SOPs should specify the authority for the assessment, how auditees are to be selected, what will be done with the results, and who is responsible for corrective action. Administrative SOPs should fit within the framework presented here, but this format can be modified, reduced, or expanded (United States Environmental Protection Agency, 2007).

18. Conclusion

Eventually, SOPs serve as a fundamental means of communication for all levels of the organization. Not only do they include employees departmentally, but they also allow management and employees to gain a cross-functional view of the organization. This attitude encourages employees to think about how process change may affect other functional areas. A good system forces employee to think through processes and examine how procedure might influence product, personnel, production, and equipment. *It should not be forgotten that the "Best written SOPs will fail if they are not followed"* (Hattamer-Apostel, R. 2001), (Jain, SK. 2008).

What happens to workers' intrinsic task motivation and creativity when they are required to follow SOPs in completing their tasks? Job design and work motivation theory literatures have suggested a negative relationship; the OM literature has suggested a positive relation. We suggest that the discussion has been hindered by differences in conceptualizing required SOP use, by not explicitly incorporating the multidimensional nature of intrinsic motivation into the analysis, by an ambiguous definition of autonomy, and by ignoring important contextual moderators. When these three elements are included in the discussion, we showed that the relationship between required SOP use and intrinsic motivation could theoretically be positive. Finally, our model high- lights the importance of worker participation. Production pressures, high capacity utilization, and lack of management – especially supervisor – support are likely to reduce opportunities for worker participation, and hence lower intrinsic motivation and creativity (De Trevil et al. 2005).

Example SOP

TITLE: Preparation of the Perfect Cup of Coffee by the Drip Method

Date of Preparation: 11/29/05; *Date of Revision:* N/A; *Revision No.:* N/A

Submitted by: Ay Dot Student; *Approved by:* Professor Ex

Purpose: Provide an example of a standard operating protocol or SOP that can be appreciated by undergraduate research students from all academic disciplines.

Scope and Applicability: The following protocol can be used wherever quality coffee beans, good drinking water, and a drip coffee maker are available.

Introduction: Coffee is the beverage of choice of many college students. Properly prepared the beverage provides an invigorating and revitalizing effect. One of the most frequently used methods of preparation is the drip method. In this method, water, heated to near boiling temperatures, is slowly added to finely ground coffee beans held in a filter unit. The coffee beverage is collected below the filter unit in a glass carafe. Today this procedure is frequently accomplished using a semi-automated process in an electronic coffee maker. The procedure below outlines a reliable method for preparing drip coffee using any commercially available drip coffee maker, high quality ground coffee beans, and filtered water.

References: For information on coffee beans, the standard methods of preparation of coffee, and recipes see:

Materials and Supplies: Freshly ground Starbucks® coffee (any flavor you prefer; medium grind works best with most commercial coffee makers), commercial 4-c drip coffee maker including filter (gold mesh preferred but high quality paper filter may be used), good quality drinking water (Polar Springs®, Brita®-filtered, or similar quality source recommended), coffee cup, and additives (as desired: sugar or sugar alterative, cream or milk).

Cautions: Hot coffee can scald and burn. Water is an electrical conductor. If spills occur during the brewing process, wait until the brewing process is complete, turn of the electricity, and disconnect the unit from the electricity before attempting to clean up any spills. Accidental spills may be cleaned up with a kitchen sponge and dish washing detergent such as ….®. Used coffee grounds can be disposed of in the regular trash. Be sure to carefully read the directions that accompanied your coffee maker unit before attempting to use it. In particular, it is important to find out if your unit has (1) a pause feature that will allow you to remove the carafe while the coffee is brewing; and (2) an auto-off feature that turns off the heater unit located beneath the carafe at a set time after the coffee has been brewed.

Personnel Qualifications: No special knowledge or training is required to make coffee. However, due to the potential risk of burns, it is recommended that anyone performing this procedure who is less than ten years old be actively supervised by an adult.

Protocol

1. Make sure that the coffee maker is off. Locate water reservoir unit on coffee maker and carefully add 4-cups of clean drinking water to the reservoir. Note that the outside or inside of most quality coffee makers' water reservoir units are marked for the user's convenience.

2. Locate the coffee filter assembly on the coffee unit. If you are preparing the standard 4-c carafe of coffee, carefully measure one coffee measure of ground coffee into your units coffee filter assembly. Note that one standard coffee measure is equivalent to 1/8-c of coffee. Close the coffee filter assembly.

3. Plug in the coffee maker and turn the unit on. Wait until the carafe located beneath the coffee filter unit is filled with coffee. Note that some units may have a "pause" feature that will allow you to temporarily remove the carafe and pour a cup of coffee while the unit is working. If you are unfamiliar with your unit, be sure to wait until the unit is done filtering before attempting to remove the carafe.

4. If coffee spills beneath the base of the carafe unit, be sure to turn off the unit and disconnect the electricity before attempting to clean up the spill.

5. Pour yourself a cup of coffee. Most coffee units will keep the carafe warm for a set period of time before turning off automatically. Some however, do not turn off automatically. Be sure to read your coffee maker's instructions beforehand. If in doubt, be sure to turn off the electricity to your unit after the brewing process is complete. (Levine D.I et al, 2010)

Author details

Isin Akyar*

Address all correspondence to: isinakyar@gmail.com

Acibadem University Faculty of Medicine Department of Microbiology, Turkey

References

[1] Almeida-Lynne, Sherri. Guidance for Preparing Standard Operating Procedures ppt. Available at: http://www.google.com.tr/#hl=tr&safe=active&output=search&sclient =psy-ab&q=Guidance+for+Preparing+Standard+Operating+Proced.

[2] Cardiff University (2009). Standard operating procedure for the use or storage of human tissue for the purposes of research or education. Available at: http://www.cf.ac.uk/govrn/cocom/resources/standard%20Operating%20procedures.pdf.

[3] De Trevil, Suzanne., Antonakis, John., & Edelson, Norman. (2005). Can Standard Operating Procedures be Motivating? Reconciling Process Variability Issues and Behavioural Outcomes. *Total Quality Management,* 16(2), 231-41.

[4] Frank, Dave. (2010). How to write SOPs that help increase consistency and improve performance quality in Standard Operating Procedures: A Writing Guide. Available at: http://www.cmmonline.com/management-training/article/standard-operating-procedures-a-writing-guide.

[5] GMP7.com (GMP online consultancy). What is a standard operating procedure? Available at: http://www.gmp7.com/whatisastandardoperatingprocedure_cm 380.html.

[6] Hattamer-Apostel, Rita. (2001). Standard operating procedures-a novel perspective. *The Quality Assurance Journal*, 5(4), 207-219, DOI:10.1002/qaj.155, available at:, http://onlinelibrary.wiley.com/doi/10.1002/qaj.155/abstract?systemMessage=Wiley+Online +Library+will+be+disrupted+3+Mar+from+.

[7] Health and Safety Executive. Operating procedures. Available at: http://www.hse.gov.uk/comah/sragtech/techmeasoperatio.htm.

[8] Iowa State University (2010). Hotel, restaurant and management extension. Available at: http://www.extension.iastate.edu/HRIM/HACCP/restaurants.htm.

[9] Jain, Sanjay Kumar. (2008). Standard operating procedures (SOP) - Back Bone of Pharmaceutical Industries. Pharma info.net Available at: http://www.pharmainfo.net/reviews/standard-operating-procedures-sop-back-bone-pharmaceutical-industries.

[10] Levine, David I., & Toffel, Michael W. (2010). Quality management and job quality: How the ISO 9001 standard for quality management systems affects employees and employers. *Journal Management Science*, 56(6), 978-96.

[11] Manghani, Kishu. (2011). Quality assurance: Importance of systems and standard operating procedures. *Perspect Clin Res.*, 2(1), 34-37, Doi: 10.4103/2229-3485.76288.

[12] Natural Resources Management and Environment Dept. Guidelines for quality management in soil and plant laboratories. FAO corporate document repository. Available at: http://www.fao.org/docrep/W7295E/w7295e04.htm.

[13] Saxena, Akanksha. SOP Writing for Clinical Trials: Staff Training Aspects. International Biopharmaceutical Association Publication. Available at: http://www.ibpassociation.org/IBPA_articles/sop_writing.htm.

[14] United States Environmental Protection Agency (2001). Guidance for Preparing Standard Operating Procedures (SOPs)." 10 Aug. 2010. United States Environmental Protection Agency. EPA QA/G-6. Available at: http://www.cluin.org/download/toolkit/thirdednew/guidanceprepsops.pdf.

[15] United States Environmental Protection Agency (2007). Guidance for Preparing Standard Operating Procedures (SOPs) EPA QA/G-6. Available at: http://www.epa.gov/quality/qs-docs/g6-final.pdf.

Quality Control in Clinical Laboratory Medicine

Chapter 7

Quality Assurance in Antimicrobial Susceptibility Testing

Onur Karatuna

Additional information is available at the end of the chapter

1. Introduction

Most of the clinically important bacteria causing infections in humans are capable of exhibiting resistance to antimicrobial agents commonly used for the treatment. Therefore, upon isolation of the organism in the clinical microbiology laboratory, characterization frequently also employs tests to detect its antimicrobial susceptibility. Thus, the report produced by clinical microbiology laboratory for the physician, also includes organism's susceptibility profile to different antimicrobials along with its identification [1]. Antimicrobial susceptibility testing (AST) is performed on bacteria that are isolated from clinical specimens to determine if the bacterial etiology of concern can be killed or inhibited by antimicrobial drugs that are potential choices for therapy, at the concentrations of the drugs that are attainable at the site of infection using the dosing regimen indicated in the drug product's labeling. The results of AST are generally reported with interpretive categories. The category "susceptible" indicates that the bacteria are inhibited by the usually achievable concentrations of antimicrobial agent when the dosage recommended to treat the site of infection is used. The "intermediate" category defines the bacteria for which the response rates to usually attainable blood and tissue levels of antimicrobial agent are lower compared to susceptible isolates. The intermediate category plays the role of a buffer zone between the susceptible and resistant categories, but also indicates a number of other possibilities; the antimicrobials which are concentrated at the site of infection may be regarded as options for treatment (e.g., nitrofurantoin for the urinary tract infections). The "resistant" category, however, defines the bacteria which are not inhibited by the usually achievable concentrations of the agent with normal dosage regimens and that the clinical efficacy of the agent against the isolate may not be sufficient [2]. Clinicians consider these interpretations to determine which antimicrobial agent might be effective in treating the particular patient. The primary role of routine microbiology laboratories is to provide accurate and timely antimicrobial susceptibility test results for guiding the treatment of infectious diseases. In order to achieve that, the microbiologist should inform the clinician about whether an infectious agent is present in the patient's specimen and which antimicrobial agent should provide the optimum therapy. Although the importance of antimicrobial susceptibility testing is well established, the procedure itself is very sensitive to changes in the environment and test conditions. Therefore, it is crucial that each variable in the procedure should be standardized and carefully controlled. With more reliable susceptibility results, infectious disease specialists and public health leaders can be able to recognize emerging resistance and novel resistance patterns. Additionally, the results of AST can be applied to define the agent of choice for empirical therapy, establish institutional or nationwide policies for prescribing of antibiotics, conduct epidemiological studies or resistance surveillance, and to evaluate the efficacy of newly developed agents. Owing to numerous variables that may affect the results, rigorous quality control is of utmost importance for susceptibility testing. Properly performed quality control would aid in providing accurate, reproducible and timely results. In this chapter the components of a quality assurance program for antimicrobial susceptibility testing will be highlighted.

2. Overview of the antimicrobial susceptibility testing methodologies

Fleming was first to report the inhibitory effect of penicillin on agar by observing a zone of growth inhibition of staphylococcal colonies grown next to a *Penicillium* contaminant on an agar plate. Fleming also made two significant contributions to the field of AST in the 1920s. In 1924, he introduced the use of the ditch plate technique for evaluating antimicrobial qualities of antiseptic solutions [3]. Fleming's second contribution to modern AST was the development of broth dilution technique using turbidity as an end-point determination [4]. Filter paper disks incorporating penicillin were utilized by Vincent & Vincent for assaying this newly discovered compound in 1940s [5]. Agar dilution AST method was also described in the 1940s [6]. At an early stage, it was realized that there were many variables affecting AST methods [7]. In 1961, World Health Organization (WHO) published a report on standardization of AST methodology [8]. The broad application of AST was introduced to clinical laboratories by the efforts of Bauer, Kirby and co-workers, with the method known as Kirby-Bauer disk diffusion method which is still the most widely used AST technique in the world [9]. Bergeron & Ouellette highlighted the shortcomings of the phenotypic approach to AST and concluded that different bacterial species have different susceptibilities to the same antibiotic, and that there is no international aggreement on breakpoints for interpretation of antimicrobial susceptibility tests [10]. The need for developing standardized AST methods became a necessity soon after antibiotics became commercially available. During World War II, following penicillin, other antibiotics were discovered and used. Altough these new antibiotics were regarded as "wonder drugs" at the time of their introduction, emergence of resistant strains followed. With the emergence of bacterial resistance to antimicrobials and the changing properties of different bacteria to different classes of antimicrobials, the need for the performance of AST on pathogens became a practical necessity.

Nationwide attempts were made to standardize AST methodologies; Clinical and Laboratory Standards Institute (CLSI, formerly NCCLS) (USA) [11], Werkgroep Richtlijnen Gevoeligheidsbepalingen (Netherlands) [12], Comité de l'Antibiogramme de la Société Française de Microbiologie (France) [13], the Swedish Reference Group for Antibiotics (Sweden) [14], Deutsches Institut für Normung (Germany) [15], the British Society for Antimicrobial Chemotherapy (UK) [16], they all published guidelines to improve the methodology and interpretation of AST. Recently, the European Committee on Antimicrobial Susceptibility Testing (EUCAST), a non-profit organization under the auspices of European Society of Clinical Microbiology and Infectious Diseases (ESCMID), developed and published AST guidelines. Breakpoint and QC tables for disk diffusion and minimum inhibitory concentration (MIC) testing can freely be accessed on organization's website [17].

In clinical laboratories, widely adopted AST methods are disk diffusion and broth dilution methods. In disk diffusion method, disks impregnated with antimicrobial agents are used. The disks are placed onto agar plates which are preinoculated with the suspension of the microorganism being tested. The basic principle of the disk diffusion method is the diffusion of the antimicrobial agent into the medium which occurs when the disks come into contact with the moist surface of the plate. The concentration of the agent reduces logarithmically as the distance from the disk is increased. After the incubation period the plates are observed for the circular inhibiton zone created around the disk which is due to the inhibitory effect of the antimicrobial agent on the microorganism. Within the zone the concentration of the agent is sufficient to inhibit growth, whereas at the point where concentration of the agent is no longer enough to inhibit growth, the organism is able to grow and forms a lawn of bacteria around the disk. To interprete the test results, the radius of the inhibition zone is measured and compared against the predefined values provided by the guidelines [18]. The most widely used guidelines are the CLSI and EUCAST guidelines [2, 17]. CLSI divides the results into three categories for most of the organism-agent combinations; susceptible, intermediate and resistant, whereas EUCAST uses only two categories, susceptible and resistant.

In the dilution methods, however, the susceptibility of the microorganisms to antimicrobial agents is determined whether in tubes (macrobroth dilution method) or in microtube wells molded into a plastic plate (microbroth dilution method). Both broth dilution methods use the same principle; first serial two-fold dilutions of the antimicrobial agent to be tested are made in the tubes/wells containing broth, and then same amount of bacterial suspension is distributed on each tube/well. At the end of the incubation period, the tubes/wells are examined for turbidity which is the indicator of bacterial growth in broth. The tubes/wells remain clear where the concentration of the agent is high enough to inhibit the bacterial growth, whereas at lower concentrations of the agent, the bacteria may grow which causes the tube/well become turbid. The lowest concentration of antimicrobial agent that prevents the *in vitro* growth of bacteria is defined as the minimal inhibitory concentration (MIC) [18]. As in the disk diffusion method, the MIC values are compared against the predefined values provided by the guidelines and their intrepetive category is determined and reported.

3. Quality assurance program for antimicrobial susceptibility testing

Clinical microbiology laboratories are an integral part of the total healthcare delivery system. Quality assurance (QA) is the overall process by which a laboratory can verify that a laboratory does its job well. While QA and quality control (QC) share the similar purposes, their meanings and functions are different [19]. QA can be defined as the overall program by which the quality of the test results can be guaranteed [20]. It evaluates and ensures that procedures provide relevant and timely data in the delivery of healthcare services. QA is primarily concerned with broader measures and monitors the performance of laboratory in total and covers all three phases of testing; pre-analytical, analytical and post-analytical. QC, in the other hand, is responsible for monitoring of the analytical phase of testing only and ensures that the daily tests are working properly [21]. QC and QA, only together provide measures for controlling how correct the tests are being performed because QC by itself often does not detect problems in time to prevent harmful results. For example, if >5% of *Enterobacter, Serratia,* or *Citrobacter* isolates are susceptible to ampicillin, it likely indicates a problem with insufficient inoculum [22]. Although daily or weekly QC test results are in acceptable limits, such an error can be overlooked until enough data have been accumulated and evaluated which can sometimes take weeks.

Standard processes are required to establish quality measures to be monitored. Standardization of AST has been achieved by CLSI, and in part by EUCAST. The processes defined in CLSI guidelines help clinical laboratories to perform QC tests, measure their results and provide corrective action recommendations covering a broad spectrum of error types. Each laboratory should establish its own quality requirements for testing processes. Only with established quality goals, laboratories can determine whether acceptable quality is being achieved, identify processes that are not performing satisfactorily and are in need of improvement, or to plan new processes to reach a specified level of quality [21]. And to ensure that all the established quality goals are achieved, a comprehensive QA program should be functional in a clinical laboratory.

The major components of a comprehensive QA program for AST, with the relative amount of effort required to be spent on each component given in parantheses, can be listed as follows [23]:

- Clinically relevant testing strategies (15%)

- Testing of reference QC strains (15%)

- Technical competency (15%)

- Organism antibiogram verification (15%)

- Supervisor review of results (15%)

- Procedure manual (10%)

- Cumulative antibiogram (5%)

- Proficiency surveys (5%)

- Other (5%)

The goals of the QC program as set by the CLSI [24, 25] includes to monitor the following:

- the precision (repeatability) and accuracy of AST procedures

- the performance of reagents used in the tests

- the performance of persons who carry out the tests and read the results

The continuous monitorization of the performance is best achieved, but not limited to, by the testing of QC strains.

3.1. Developing relevant antimicrobial susceptibility testing strategies

Only organisms likely to be the cause of an infection should be tested for antimicrobial susceptibility which necessitates the differentiation should be done between the normal flora that resides at the site of the infection and the actual organism causing the infection. Some important factors are to be considered to decide which bacterium or bacteria from a clinical specimen must be included in the AST; such as the body site from which the organism was isolated, the presence of other bacteria and the quality of the specimen from which the organism was grown, the host's status, the ability of the bacterial species to cause infection at the body site from which the specimen was obtained, etc. [1, 26].

3.2. Selecting antimicrobials to test and to report

Each laboratory is unique in its capability, resources, level of experience or institutional needs. Therefore, the decision of which antimicrobials to test depends on each laboratory's specifications and cannot be generalized. The decision involves the opinions of infectious diseases specialist and the pharmacist and should also be in concordance with the hospital formulary. Generally, a laboratory defines 10 to 15 antimicrobial agents for routine testing against various organisms or organism groups, which is called antimicrobial panel or battery. In CLSI's M100 documents Table 1A (Suggested Groupings of Antimicrobial Agents With FDA Clinical Indications That Should Be Considered for Routine Testing and Reporting on Nonfastidious Organisms by Clinical Microbiology Laboratories in the United States) is a valuable source of information to refer to when such tables are to be created at the local level [2]. Because the identity of the bacterial isolate is often not known at the time the AST is performed, some drugs, which are inappropriate to report for that particular isolate, may be tested. These results, however, should be supressed in the final report.

The goal of the clinical microbiology laboratory is to create a report which will direct the clinician to use the least toxic, most cost-effective and most clinically effective agent that is available. This is accomplished by using the selective-reporting protocol provided by the CLSI. CLSI categorizes antimicrobial agents generally into four groups, Group A, B, C and U. Group A includes the primary agents whose results to be reported first. The results of

Group B drugs should be selectively reported because these are generally broader spectrum agents. However, if the isolate is resistant to the primary agents, the patient cannot tolerate drugs in Group A, the infection has not responded to the therapy with the primary agents, a secondary agent would be a better clinical choice for the particular infection or that the patient has organisms isolated from another site also, and a secondary agent might be more appropriate for treating both organisms, then the results of Group B drugs can be reported [26]. Group C includes alternative or supplemental agents for special cases; such as resistant strains, for patients allergic to primary drugs, for treatment of unusual isolates or for epidemiological purposes. And finally, Group U, includes the agents that are used only or primarily in the treatment of urinary tract infections (e.g., nitrofurantoin, norfloxacin).

Selective-reporting, also called cascade-reporting, improves the clinical relevance of the reports produced and minimizes the selection of multiresistant strains by avoiding the use of broad spectrum agents when narrow spectrum option is susceptible.

3.3. Standardization of the antimicrobial susceptibility testing methodology

The procedural steps of each method must be followed strictly in order to obtain reproducible results. Standardization of AST methodology helps to optimize bacterial growth conditions so that the inhibition of growth can be attributed to the antimicrobial agent and the effects of nutrient limitations, temperature differences or other environmental conditions can be eliminated. And it also optimizes conditions for maintaining antimicrobial integrity and activity so that the failure to inhibit bacterial growth can be attributed to the organism's resistance mechanisms [1].

The standardized components of AST include:

Bacterial inoculum size: Preparation of the inoculum is one of the most critical steps in any susceptibility test method. Inoculum suspensions are prepared using either a log-phase or direct-colony suspension. When direct-colony suspension method is used, 4 to 5, fresh (16- to 24-hour old) colonies, rather than a single colony, should be selected to minimize the possibility of testing a susceptible colony only and missing the resistant mutants dispersed in other colonies. McFarland turbidity standards are used to standardize the number of bacteria in the inoculum. McFarland standards can be prepared by adding specific volumes of 1% sulfuric acid and 1.175% barium chloride to obtain a barium sulfate solution with a specific optical density. The most commonly used is the McFarland 0.5 standard, which provides turbidity comparable with that of a bacterial suspension containing approximately $1.5 \ 10^8$ CFU/mL (CFU: colony-forming unit). Once standardized, the inoculum suspensions should be used within 15 minutes of preparation. False-susceptible results may occur if too few bacteria are tested, and false-resistant results may be the outcome of testing too many bacteria [26].

Growth medium: The most frequently used growth media are Mueller-Hinton broth and Mueller-Hinton agar. The standardized variables regarding these media should include; its formulation, pH, cation concentration and thymidine content, thickness of agar (disk diffusion test), and supplements such as blood and serum.

Incubation conditions (atmosphere, temperature, duration): Different organisms require different incubation conditions. Moreover, some antimicrobial agents require different incubation length or temperature than the other disks used for the same organism (e.g., oxacillin with *Staphylococcus* spp.). The user should refer to CLSI M100 tables which give detailed testing conditions for each organism or organism group [2].

Antimicrobials concentrations to be tested: The contents of antimicrobial disks in disk diffusion test and concentrations of antibiotic solutions to be tested in dilution tests are also included in CLSI documents [2].

3.4. Quality control testing with reference quality control strains

Routine QC testing with a range of QC strains is the backbone of the internal QC testing. QC strains are well characterized organisms with defined susceptibility or resistance mechanisms to the antimicrobial agent(s) tested. Testing of QC strains helps to concurrently monitor the performance of the test and ensures that the test is being performed properly. The results obtained with the QC strains should be in predefined, acceptable ranges; for disk diffusion test, between the predefined inhibition zone diameters, and for MIC tests in predefined MIC ranges. If deviations from the acceptable limits are observed, it indicates unacceptable performance and the source(s) of the error should be investigated. CLSI recommends to use various QC strains for different aspects of AST. The list of QC strains can be found in the M100 tables which are updated on a yearly basis. Because of the introduction of new drugs, the changes effecting the existing drugs, or the emergence of new resistance mechanisms which should be investigated by the laboratory, the users are always referred to the latest update available. The QC strains recommended by CLSI are divided in two as being regular „QC strains" and „supplemental QC strains". Each laboratory performing AST with CLSI's reference methods should include QC strains in regular QC tests, however, the supplemental strains are only required if they are used to assess a new test, for training new personnel, investigation of special susceptibility or resistance characteristics, etc., and are not required to be included in the routine QC of AST [2].

CLSI's European counterpart, EUCAST, also publishes guidelines for the use of QC strains for AST, however, compared with the comprehensive battery of QC strains suggested by the CLSI, EUCAST is limited to six QC strains at the moment [27]. The guidelines of EUCAST are continously evolving and on areas where EUCAST's experience is not able to cover yet, EUCAST does not refrain from making referrals to relevant CLSI documents. However, one big difference between the QC strains recommended by CLSI and EUCAST is that, EUCAST's recommendation for *Haemophilus influenzae* NCTC 8468 in contrast to CLSI's *H. influenzae* ATCC® 49247. The strain EUCAST chose as a QC strain is susceptible to β-lactam antibiotics whose inhibition zones are easier to read than the ATCC® strain which is a β-lactamase negative, ampicillin resistant (BLNAR) strain. The suggested QC strains by CLSI with their specifications are listed in Table 1 [2].

QC Strain	Test(s), for which strain is primarily used
Escherichia coli ATCC® 25922	Disk diffusion and MIC of *Enterobacteriaceae, Pseudomonas aeruginosa, Acinetobacter spp., Burkholderia cepacia, Stenotrophomonas maltophilia*
	MIC of other non-*Enterobacteriaceae*
	Screening and confirmatory tests for ESBLs (negative)
	Disk diffusion and MIC of *Neisseria meningitidis* (for ciprofloxacin, nalidixic acid, minocycline, and sulfisoxazole)
Escherichia coli ATCC® 35218	Disk diffusion and MIC for β-lactam/β-lactamase inhibitor combination drugs of *Enterobacteriaceae, Pseudomonas aeruginosa, Acinetobacter spp., Burkholderia cepacia, Stenotrophomonas maltophilia, Staphylococcus spp.*
	MIC for β-lactam/β-lactamase inhibitor combination drugs of other non-*Enterobacteriaceae*
	Testing of amoxicillin-clavulanic acid for *Haemophilus spp.*
Klebsiella pneumoniae ATCC® 700603	Screening and confirmatory tests for ESBLs (positive)
Klebsiella pneumoniae ATCC® BAA-1705	Confirmatory test for suspected carbapenemase production in *Enterobacteriaceae* (MHT positive)
Klebsiella pneumoniae ATCC® BAA-1706	Confirmatory test for suspected carbapenemase production in *Enterobacteriaceae* (MHT negative)
Pseudomonas aeruginosa ATCC® 27853	Disk diffusion and MIC of *Pseudomonas aeruginosa, Acinetobacter spp., Burkholderia cepacia, Stenotrophomonas maltophilia*
	MIC of other non-*Enterobacteriaceae*
Staphylococcus aureus ATCC® 25923	Disk diffusion of *Staphylococcus spp.* and *Enterococcus spp.*
	Screening test for β-lactamase production of *Staphylococcus aureus* group and coagulase negative *Staphylococci* (negative)
	Screening test for *mecA*-mediated oxacillin resistance using cefoxitin in *Staphylococcus aureus* group and coagulase negative *Staphylococci* (*mecA* negative; disk diffusion susceptible)
	Screening test for inducible clindamycin resistance in *Staphylococcus aureus* group and coagulase negative *Staphylococci* with disk diffusion (D-zone test) (negative)
	Screening test for high-level mupirocin resistance in *Staphylococcus aureus* group (*mupA* negative; disk diffusion susceptible)
Staphylococcus aureus ATCC® 29213	MIC of *Staphylococcus spp.*

QC Strain	Test(s), for which strain is primarily used
	Screening test for β-lactamase production in *Staphylococcus aureus* group and coagulase negative *Staphylococci* (positive)
	Screening test for oxacillin resistance in *Staphylococcus aureus* group (susceptible)
	Screening test for *mecA*-mediated oxacillin resistance using cefoxitin in *Staphylococcus aureus* group (*mecA* negative; MIC susceptible)
	Screening test for inducible clindamycin resistance in *Staphylococcus aureus* group, coagulase negative *Staphylococci* and *Streptococcus* spp. β-hemolytic group with broth microdilution (no growth)
	Screening test for high-level mupirocin resistance in *Staphylococcus aureus* group (*mupA* negative; MIC susceptible)
Staphylococcus aureus ATCC® 43300	Screening test for oxacillin resistance in *Staphylococcus aureus* group (resistant)
	Screening test for *mecA*-mediated oxacillin resistance using cefoxitin in *Staphylococcus aureus* group (disk diffusion and MIC) and coagulase negative *Staphylococci* (disk diffusion) (*mecA* positive)
Staphylococcus aureus ATCC® BAA-976	Screening test for inducible clindamycin resistance in *Staphylococcus aureus* group, coagulase negative *Staphylococci* and *Streptococcus* spp. β-hemolytic group with broth microdilution (no growth)
Staphylococcus aureus ATCC® BAA-977	Screening test for inducible clindamycin resistance in *Staphylococcus aureus* group, coagulase negative *Staphylococci* and *Streptococcus* spp. β-hemolytic group with broth microdilution (growth)
Staphylococcus aureus ATCC® BAA-1708	Screening test for high-level mupirocin resistance in *Staphylococcus aureus* group (*mupA* positive; disk diffusion and MIC resistant)
Enterococcus faecalis ATCC® 29212	MIC of *Enterococcus spp.*
	Screening test for vancomycin MIC ≥8 µg/mL in *Staphylococcus aureus* group (susceptible)
	Screening test for high-level aminoglycoside resistance in *Enterococcus spp.* (disk diffusion, broth microdilution, agar dilution: susceptible)

QC Strain	Test(s), for which strain is primarily used
	Screening test for vancomycin resistance in *Enterococcus spp.* (agar dilution: susceptible) checking that medium is acceptable for testing sulfonamides, trimethoprim, and trimethoprim/sulfamethoxazole
Enterococcus faecalis ATCC® 51299	Screening test for vancomycin MIC ≥8 µg/mL for *Staphylococcus aureus* group (resistant)
	Screening test for high-level aminoglycoside resistance in *Enterococcus spp.* (broth microdilution, agar dilution: resistant)
	Screening test for vancomycin resistance in *Enterococcus spp.* (agar dilution: resistant)
Haemophilus influenzae ATCC® 49247	Disk diffusion and MIC of *Haemophilus spp.* (BLNAR; β-lactamase negative, ampicillin resistant)
Haemophilus influenzae ATCC® 49766	Disk diffusion and MIC of *Haemophilus spp.* with selected cephalosporins (β-lactamase positive)
Haemophilus influenzae ATCC® 10211	Checking growth capabilities of medium used for disk diffusion and MIC tests for *Haemophilus* spp.
Neisseria gonorrhoeae ATCC® 49226	Disk diffusion and MIC of *Neisseria gonorrhoeae* (CMRNG; chromosomally mediated (penicillin) resistant *N. gonorrhoeae*)
Streptococcus pneumoniae ATCC® 49619	Disk diffusion and MIC of *Streptococcus pneumoniae* (penicillin intermediate), *Streptococcus* spp. β-hemolytic group *Streptococcus* spp. viridans group and *Neisseria meningitidis*
	Screening test for inducible clindamycin resistance in *Streptococcus* spp. β-hemolytic group with disk diffusion (D-zone test) and broth microdilution (negative)
Bacteroides fragilis ATCC® 25285	MIC of anaerobes
Bacteroides thetaiotaomicron ATCC® 29741	MIC of anaerobes
Clostridium difficile ATCC® 700057	MIC of anaerobes
Eubacterium lentum ATCC® 43055	MIC of anaerobes

Table 1. Quality Control Strains Suggested for Antimicrobial Susceptibility Testing by CLSI

3.5. Selection, obtaining and maintenance of reference QC strains

When selecting QC strains for routine internal QC testing; the strains that most closely resemble the patient's isolate should be tested [23]. This will provide that the drugs planned to be tested for the patient can be concomitantly tested with the QC strain. Additionally, same materials and testing conditions used for the clinical isolates can be evaluated. Before obtaining the QC strains, laboratories should decide which strains do fit best to the laboratory's procedures. For example, if a laboratory does not perform Modified Hodge Test (MHT) to confirm suspected carbapenemase production in *Enterobacteriaceae*, the *Klebsiella pneumoniae* ATCC® BAA-1705 (MHT-positive) and *Klebsiella pneumoniae* ATCC® BAA-1706 (MHT-negative) strains are not necessary for that particular laboratory. QC organisms susceptible to the tested antimicrobials are generally used but resistant QC strains are also necessary when testing for special resistance mechanisms.

The QC strains can be obtained from various suppliers and in many formats. What important is, no matter in what format the strain has been received, the initial reconstitution should be performed according to supplier's recommendations. For long term storage, stock cultures can be stored in a suitable stabilizer (e.g., trypticase soy broth with 10 to 15% glycerol, 50% fetal calf serum in broth, defibrinated sheep blood or skim milk) at -20°C or below (preferably at -60°C or below). To obtain working control cultures, subcultures from the permanent stock culture are made onto agar plates. Isolated colonies (4 to 5) are selected and subcultured to an agar slant (trypticase soy agar slants for non-fastidious organisms and chocolate agar slants for fastidious organisms) and incubated overnight. These working cultures on agar slants are stored at 2 – 8°C, for no more than three successive weeks. New working control cultures should be prepared at least monthly from permanent stock cultures. Prior to QC testing, growth from an agar slant is subcultured to agar plates and incubated overnight. To use for QC testing, 4 to 5 isolated colonies from the plate are selected. A new working culture should be prepared each day the QC test is being performed [2, 23].

Working control cultures can be used to monitor precision (repeatability) and accuracy of the AST as long as no significant change in the mean zone diameter or MIC value, not attributable to faulty methodology, is observed. Laboratories usually do not have problems with the maintenance of susceptible QC strains owing to the stability of these strains, however, QC strains with particular resistance mechanisms are harder to maintain since they may be less genetically stable. Repeated subcultures can cause the loss of resistance mechanisms and unsatisfactory performances can be experienced. Documented problems have arisen with the QC strains which carry their specific resistance mechanism on a plasmid (e.g., *E. coli* ATCC® 35218 and *K. pneumoniae* ATCC® 700603) [2]. Suboptimal storage conditions and repeated cultures may cause the spontaneous loss of the plasmid encoding the β-lactamase and off-the-limit results may be encountered.

3.6. Frequency of QC testing

Appropriate QC organisms should be tested daily for all antimicrobial agents routinely included in the antimicrobial battery until a laboratory achieves "satisfactory performance". CLSI makes the definition of "satisfactory performance" as obtaining unacceptable results in no more than 1 out of 20 or 3 out of 30 results obtained in consecutive test days for each antimicrobial agent/organism combination. Once this satisfactory performance is obtained, a laboratory can convert from daily QC testing to weekly QC testing. As long as all QC test results are within the acceptable limits, the laboratory can continue weekly testing, however on occasions when a modification in the test is made, consecutive QC testing is required (Table 2., adapted from reference 2).

Day(s)*	Modification in the Test
1	Start to use new shipment or lot number of disks/MIC panels or prepared agar plates
	Start to use disks from a new manufacturer
	Expand or reduce the dilution range in MIC testing
	Repair of instrument that affects the AST results
5	Start to use prepared agar plates (disk diffusion), broth or agar (MIC) from a new manufacturer
	Convert inoculum preparation/standardization method from visual adjustment of turbidity to use a photometric device which has its own QC protocol
	Update of the software which affects the AST results
20 or 30	Use new method for MIC test (e.g., convert from visual reading to instrument reading of panel, convert from overnight to rapid MIC test)
	Use new manufacturer of MIC test
	Change method of measuring zones in disk diffusion test (e.g., start using an automated zone reader)
	Convert inoculum preparation/standardization method to a method that is dependent on user technique

* Number of days of consecutive QC testing required

Table 2. Required Quality Control Frequency after Modifications in the Test

For both, disk diffusion and MIC testing, addition of any new antimicrobial agent to the existing panel requires 20 or 30 consecutive days of satisfactory testing before it can be tested on a weekly schedule.

3.7. Corrective action

Corrective action is defined as the "action to eliminate the cause of a detected nonconformity or other undesirable situation" [28] and in regard to AST, is needed whenever any of the weekly QC results are not within the acceptable limits. The factors causing for the deviation in the results are various but can be divided in two as being results due to identifiable errors and results with no error identified [24, 25]. Identifiable errors, also named obvious errors, are easy to detect and also easy to correct. Most usual reasons causing for identifiable errors include; use of the wrong disk, use of the wrong QC strain, contamination of the strain or media, use of the wrong incubation temperature or conditions. If the reason causing the out-of-range results is one of the identifiable errors, the test must be carried out again the day the error is observed. If results of the repeat test are in acceptable limits, no further corrective action is necessary. On the other hand, if the reason causing for the error cannot be identified, the test must be carried out again the day the error is observed, preferably with a new working culture or subculture, but should also be monitored for a total of five consecutive test days. During five consecutive days, if all results are within the acceptable limits no additional corrective action is required. However, if any of the results are outside the acceptable limits, additional corrective action is required. At this point, a systematic error, rather than a random should be suspected and the components of AST should be thoroughly investigated. The reasons include; wrong measurement, clerical errors, problems in the adjustment of turbidity, past expiration date materials, failure in providing proper growth conditions (temperature, atmosphere), improper storage of disks, contamination of QC strain, loss of characteristics, inoculum prepared from an old plate (> 24 hours), etc.. In order to start to routine QC testing, satisfactory performance for another 20 or 30 consecutive days is required once the reason causing the error is detected and corrected.

When an out-of-range QC results necessitates a corrective action, the factors listed in Table 3 should be considered for troubleshooting (Table 3., adapted from references 24 and 25).

QC Strain	Use of the wrong QC strain
	Improper storage
	Inadequate maintenance (e.g., use of the same working culture for >1 month)
	Contamination
	Nonviability
	Changes in the organisms (e.g., mutation, loss of plasmid)
Testing supplies	Improper storage or shipping conditions
	Contamination
	Use of a defective agar plate (too thick or too thin)
	Inadequate volume of broth in tubes or wells
	Use of damaged plates, panels, cards, tubes (e.g., cracked, leaking)
	Use of expired materials
Testing process	Use of the wrong incubation temperature or conditions
	Inoculum suspensions were incorrectly prepared or adjusted
	Inoculum prepared from a plate incubated for the incorrect length of time
	Inoculum prepared from differential or selective media containing anti-infective agents or other growth-inhibiting compounds
	Use of wrong disk/reagents, ancillary supplies
	Improper disk placement (e.g., inadequate contact with the agar)
	Incorrect reading or interpretation of test results
	Transcription error
Equipment	Not functioning properly or out of calibration (e.g., pipettes)

Table 3. Factors Frequently Causing Out-of-range Results

3.8. Documentation of the quality control test results

Results from all QC tests should be documented on a QC log sheet [23]. On this log sheet information regarding the following are required: the date, the technician who performed the test, antimicrobial agents used (potency, lot, expiration date, etc.), media used (lot, expiration date, etc.). Once the log sheet has been filled by the technician who performed and read the test, a second technician, or the supervisor, should check the results. Also, corrective actions taken, if any, and their outcomes should be noted.

A useful and simple way of monitoring QC results is to use the Shewhart diagram, in which the daily readings are plotted on a chart with upper and lower control limits marked [29]. It provides the visual assessment of the results but can also provide in depth information if a more formal mathematical approach is followed [20]. An example of presenting daily QC results on a Shewhart diagram is given in Figure 1. The famous rules of Westgard and Klee [30] can be easily adopted to the QC of disk diffusion test in which the control diameters are treated as mean ±2 SD [20].

One QC result lies outside the limits (Westgard rule 1_{2s}): It is a warning, whether it's a random error or the beginning of an emerging problem. Routine test results for that day may be reported if there is no other evidence of problems in the current tests. It does not require corrective action by itself, unless the result is far out of range or there are other indications of a problem.

Two consecutive QC results are outside the limits in the same side of the mean of the range (Westgard rule 2_{2s}): Indicates an error in the test methodology (a systematic error), corrective action is required.

Ten consecutive QC results falling on one side of the mean (Westgard rule 10_x): Results may be accepted but this likely indicates a systematic problem which should be acted on.

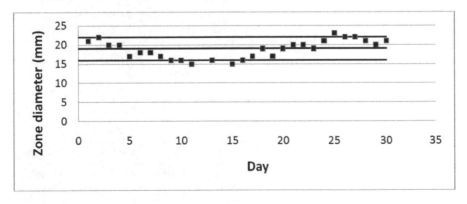

Figure 1. Example for daily disk diffusion QC results for *Escherichia coli* ATCC® 25922 vs. ampicillin plotted on a Shewhart diagram (acceptable zone limits: 16 – 22 mm).

3.9. Organism - Antimicrobial susceptibility test result verification

One of the most widely used supplemental QC measure is the use of susceptibility test results to verify results generated on patient results. Species with „typical" antibiograms are useful in verification of the identification as well as the susceptibility results. CLSI suggests some results to be confirmed before they are reported, these mostly include rare resistance phenotypes. The rare resistance phenotypes are divided in three categories; Category I; not reported or only rarely reported to date, Category II; uncommon in most institutions, and Category III; may be common, but is generally considered of epidemiological concern. Since category I includes the least encountered and most significant results, it is highly important to detect these results before being reported unnoticed and to follow the necessary steps for the verification. Unusual resistance phenotypes which require confirmation are given in Table 3 (adapted from reference 2).

Category	Observed susceptibility result
I	NS to carbapenems, extended-spectrum cephalosporins or fluoroquinolones in *H. influenzae*
	NS to extended-spectrum cephalosporins, meropenem or minocycline, R to ampicillin or penicillin in *N. meningitidis*
	NS to linezolid or vancomycin in *S. pneumoniae*
	NS to ampicillin, penicillin, extended-spectrum cephalosporins, daptomycin, ertapenem, meropenem, linezolid or vancomycin in β-hemolytic group *Streptococcus*
	NS to daptomycin, ertapenem, meropenem, linezolid, or vancomycin, R to quinupristin-dalfopristin in viridans group *Streptococcus*
II	I or R to carbapenems in *Enterobacteriaceae*
	I or R to 3rd generation cephalosporins or fluoroquinolones in *Salmonella* and *Shigella* spp.
	R to colistin/polymyxin in *A. baumannii*
	I or R to colistin/polymyxin in *P. aeruginosa*
	I or R to trimethoprim-sulfamethoxazole in *S. maltophilia*
	R to amoxicillin-clavulanic acid, R to ampicillin without accompanying β-lactamase production in *H. influenzae*
	NS to extended spectrum cephalosporins in *N. gonorrhoeae*

Category	Observed susceptibility result
	I to ampicillin, penicillin, I or R to rifampin, NS to azithromycin in *N. meningitidis*
	R to linezolid, NS to daptomycin for *Enterococcus* spp.
	NS to daptomycin, R to linezolid, I or R to quinupristin-dalfopristin, vancomycin MIC = 4 µg/mL or vancomycin MIC ≥ 8 µg/mL for *S. aureus*
	NS to daptomycin, I or R to quinupristin-dalfopristin or vancomycin, R to daptomycin in coagulase-negative *Staphylococcus* spp.
	I or R to fluoroquinolone, imipenem, meropenem, quinupristin-dalfopristin, rifampin in *S. pneumoniae*
	I or R to quinupristin-dalfopristin in β-hemolytic group *Streptococcus*
III	R to amikacin, gentamicin, and tobramycin in *Enterobacteriaceae*
	I or R to extended spectrum cephalosporins in *E. coli*, *Klebsiella* spp. or *P. mirabilis*
	I or R to carbapenem in *A. baumannii*
	R to amikacin, gentamicin, and tobramycin, or carbapenem in *P. aeruginosa*
	I or R to fluoroquinolone in *N. gonorrhoeae*
	I or R to chloramphenicol or fluoroquinolone in *N. meningitidis*
	R to vancomycin or high-level aminoglycoside in *Enterococcus* spp.
	R to oxacillin in *S. aureus*
	R to amoxicillin, penicillin or extended spectrum cephalosporins in *S. pneumoniae* using nonmeningitis breakpoints

NS; nonsusceptible, I; intermediate, R; resistant

Table 4. Unusual Resistance Phenotypes Which Require Confirmation

The general approach to be followed is, for all three categories, to confirm the identification of the organism and the AST. If the results are confirmed, the infection control should be informed about the case.

3.10. Real-time review of results

Accuracy of the susceptibility test results should be continously monitored. This is mostly accomplished by daily reviewing of the data that is being produced. Profiles which are likely, somewhat likely, somewhat unlikely and nearly impossible should be identified, whether manually or with the help of a software programmed to recognize different patterns of susceptibility data [1]. Prompt recognition of unusual resistance or inconsistent susceptibility helps the laboratory to timely confirm the susceptibility results. In order to confirm the results, first step is to exclude the transcriptional and reading errors and make sure of the purity of the inoculum which has been tested. If no errors are found in the previous steps, the identification of the organism should be confirmed and the susceptibility test be repeated, preferably with another method. In cases where no errors are detected and the unusual resistance is confirmed, the clinician may be warned and measures can be taken to limit the spread of this unusual resistance.

3.11. Education

Education is an important component of the QA process. Having knowledge about the methods also provides the understanding of their limitations and pitfalls. A well-educated technician may timely recognize atypical results and is aware of the approach to follow for the resolution and avoidance of errors [20]. A very efficient way of training in-service personnel is the end-point interpretation control [24, 25]. Laboratory workers, who perform AST, are provided with a set of selected disk diffusion plates and are asked to read the results. The recorded results are then compared by an experienced reader, e.g., the laboratory director, and the individual performances of each technician is evaluated and if necessary, corrected. It significantly helps to minimize variation in the interpretation of zone sizes among laboratory workers.

3.12. External quality assessment

In external quality assessment (EQA) programs, a central laboratory distributes test strains with known susceptibility profiles to all participant laboratories. Each participating laboratory tests and reports the results to the central laboratory. Once all the results are returned from participants, the central laboratory evaluates the results and prepares a feedback report. The benefit of participating in such program is that each individual laboratory can assess ist own performance compared with other laboratories, at national and international levels, it functions as an educational tool, and also provides the evidence of performance required by the accrediting bodies. On the other hand, the number of strains distributed in a year is relatively small, which brings the disadvantage of the rare errors going unnoticed [20]. Also, in contrast to internal QC, which is capable of acting on problems encountered on daily basis, it takes quite a while for the EQA feedback reports to be sent to the participating laboratories, thus corrective action is delayed.

3.13. Internal quality assessment

Internal quality assessment (IQA) is a complementary activity to EQA in which routine tests are repeated on the same day as the original, but this time, with the identity of the specimen blinded. After the reports are produced, the results are compared and discrepancies noted. This activity helps to monitor the precision and accuracy of the test procedure and may highlight problem areas not detected by other QC methods. It monitors not only the performance of the test and reagents, but also the performance of the persons carrying out the tests [20]. The EQA and the IQA are complementary activities, while IQA focuses on monitoring a single laboratory on a daily basis, EQA compares the performance of different laboratories and is important for maintaining long-term accuracy of the AST methods employed [21].

3.14. Proficiency testing programs

They are a type of EQA in which simulated patient specimens are sent to participating laboratories. Again, the reports are produced by each laboratory, and returned to the central laboratory for evaluation. In the United States, government mandates that clinical laboratories be accredited and licensed. The government and licensing agencies are using proficiency testing as an objective method for the accreditation of laboratories [21]. In 1988, the U.S. Congress passed the Clinical Laboratory Improvement Amendment (CLIA '88) which mandated proficiency testing (PT) as a major part of the laboratory accreditation process [31]. The initial CLIA '88 proposal called for two PT specimens per year but final legislative rule, published in 2003, expanded this to study five samples three times per year. The definition of failure is defined as two of five incorrect results on two of the three consecutive PT surveys [32].

4. Quality control of automated antimicrobial susceptibility test systems

According to the work load and the resources a laboratory has, a laboratory can choose to use one of many types of commercial automated antimicrobial susceptibility test systems. Most of these systems use the principle of turbidimetric detection of bacterial growth in a broth medium by use of a photometer which periodically examines the test wells [26]. The most widely used systems in the world are VITEK 2 System (bioMérieux Vitek, Hazelwood, MO), BD Phoenix System (BD Diagnostic Systems, Sparks, MD), MicroScan WalkAway SI (Siemens Healthcare Diagnostics, Sacramento, CA) and TREK Sensititre (ARIS 2X, Trek Diagnostic Systems, Cleveland, OH). Each device has its own QC procedure and commercial susceptibility testing devices are not addressed in CLSI standards. CLSI only describes methods regarding generic reference procedures, however these reference methods are used by the US Food and Drug Administration before clearence is given to a commercial system for marketing in the US to evaluate its performance.

5. Conclusion

Although great improvement has been done in AST methodology and automated susceptibility systems have been introduced which provide same-day results, it should be considered that there are still many variables not covered by the standard methods. First of all, the laboratory test conditions are far different from *in vivo* conditions where the organism and the antimicrobial agent do actually interact. Factors, such as bacterial inoculum size, pH, cation concentration and oxygen tension differ greatly depending on the site of infection [1]. In spite of all these limitations, the clinical microbiology laboratory should follow the most up-to-date guidelines to serve the patients in the best possible way. With a well constructed QA program in operation, a laboratory should aim to ensure that the right test is carried out on the right specimen, and that the right result and right interpretation is delivered to the right person at the right time.

Author details

Onur Karatuna

Acibadem University, Istanbul, Turkey

References

[1] Laboratory Methods and Strategies for Antimicrobial Susceptibility Testing. (2007). In: Forbes B. A., Sahm D. F., Weissfeld A. C. (ed.) Bailey & Scott's Diagnostic Microbiology. 12th ed. St. Louis, MO: Mosby Elsevier; 187-214.

[2] CLSI. (2012). Performance Standards for Antimicrobial Susceptibility Testing; Twenty-Second Informational Supplement. CLSI document M100-S22. Wayne, PA: Clinical and Laboratory Standards Institute.

[3] Fleming, A. (1924). A comparison of the activities of antiseptics on bacteria and on leucocytes. Proceedings of the Royal Society of London, Series B 96, 171-80.

[4] Fleming, A. (1929). On the antibacterial action of cultures of a penicillium, with special reference to their use in the isolatation of B. influenzae. British Journal of Experimental Pathology 110, 226-36.

[5] Vincent, J. G., Vincent, H. V. (1944). Filter paper disc modification of the Oxford cup penicillin determination. Proceedings of the Society for Experimental Biology and Medicine 55, 162-4.

[6] Schmith, K., Reymann, F. E. (1940). Experimentelle og kliniske undersogelser over gonococcers folsomhed overfor sulfapyridin. Nordisk Medicin 8, 2493-9.

[7] Waterworth, P. M. (1951). A comparative study of methods of testing sensitivity to antibiotics and of the factors influencing the results. Journal of Medical Laboratory Technology 9, 65-85.

[8] World Health Organization. (1961). Standardization of Methods for Conducting Microbic Sensitivity Tests. Second Report of the Expert Committee on Antibiotics. WHO Technical Report Series, No. 210. WHO, Geneva.

[9] Bauer, A. W., Kirby, W. M. M., Sherris, J. C., Turck, M. (1966). Antibiotic susceptibility testing by a standardized single disk method. American Journal of Clinical Pathology 45, 493-6.

[10] Bergeron, M. G., Ouellette, M. (1998). Preventing antibiotic resistance through rapid genotypic identification of bacteria and of their antibiotic resistance genes in the clinical microbiology laboratory. Journal of Clinical Microbiology 36, 2169-72.

[11] National Committee for Clinical Laboratory Standards. (1975). Performance Standards for Antimicrobial Disk Susceptibility Tests; Approved Standard M2-A7 ASM-2. NCCLS, Villanova, PA.

[12] Werkgroep Richtlijnen Gevoeligheidsbepalingen Report. (1990). Standaardisatie van Gevoeligheidsbepalingen. WRG, Bilthoven.

[13] Comité de l'Antibiogramme de la Société Française de Microbiologie. (1996). Clinical Microbiology and Infection 2, Suppl 1, S1-49.

[14] The Swedish Reference Group for Antibiotics. (1997). A revised system for antibiotic sensitivity testing. Scandinavian Journal of Infectious Diseases Suppl. 105.

[15] Deutsches Institut für Normung. (2000). Methoden zur Empfindlichkeitsprüfung von bakteriellen Krankheitserregern (außer Mykobakterien) gegen Chemotherapeutika DIN 58940.

[16] Andrews, J. M. For the BSAC Working Party on Susceptibility Testing. (2000). BSAC standardized disc susceptibility testing method. Journal of Antimicrobial Chemotherapy 48, Suppl. 1, 43-57.

[17] European Comittee on Antimicrobial Susceptibility Testing – EUCAST. (2012). http://www.eucast.org (accessed 30 July 2012).

[18] Antimicrobial Susceptibility Testing. (2006). In: Winn W., Allen S., Janda W., Koneman E., Procop G., Schreckenberger P., Woods G. (ed.) Koneman's Color Atlas and Textbook of Diagnostic Microbiology. 6th ed. Baltimore, MD: Lippincott Williams & Wilkins; 945-1021.

[19] August M. J., Hindler J. A., Huber T. W., Sewell D. L. (1990). Cumitech 3A. Quality Control and Quality Assurance Practices in Clinical Microbiology. Coordinating ed. Weissfeld S. A. Washington, D.C.: American Society for Microbiology.

[20] King A., Brown D. F. J. (2001). Quality assurance of antimicrobial susceptibility testing by disc diffusion. Journal of Antimicrobial Chemotherapy ,48, Suppl. S1, 71-6.

[21] Westgard J. O., Klee G. G. (2006). Quality Management. In: Burtis C. A., Ashwood E. R., Bruns D. E. (ed.) Tietz Textbook of Clinical Chemistry and Molecular Diagnostics. 4th ed. St. Louis, MO: Elsevier Saunders; 485-529.

[22] Washington J. A. (1988). Current problems in antimicrobial susceptibility testing. Diagnostic Microbiology and Infectious Diseases 9, 135-8.

[23] Rankin I. D. (2005). Quality Assurance/Quality Control (QA/QC) In: Coyle M. B. (ed.) Manual of Antimicrobial Susceptibility Testing. 1st ed, Washington, D.C.: American Society for Microbiology; 63-89.

[24] CLSI. (2012). Performance Standards for Antimicrobial Disk Susceptibility Tests; Approved Standard–Eleventh Edition. CLSI document M02-A11. Wayne, PA: Clinical and Laboratory Standards Institute.

[25] CLSI. (2012). Methods for Dilution Antimicrobial Susceptibility Tests for Bacteria That Grow Aerobically; Approved Standard-Ninth Edition. CLSI document M07-A9. Wayne, PA: Clinical and Laboratory Standards Institute.

[26] Marsik F. J. (2011). Antimicrobial Susceptibility Testing. In: Mahon C. R., Lehman D. C., Manuselis G. (ed.) Textbook of Diagnostic Microbiology. 4th ed. Maryland Heights, MO: Saunders Elsevier; 276-314.

[27] European Comittee on Antimicrobial Susceptibility Testing. (2012). EUCAST recommended strains for internal quality control. Version 2.1, valid from 2012-06-29. http://www.eucast.org/fileadmin/src/media/PDFs/EUCAST_files/Disk_test_documents/EUCAST_QC_tables_2.1_120629_errata.pdf (accessed 30 July 2012).

[28] ISO. (2000). Quality Management Systems–Fundamentals and Vocabulary. ISO 9000. Geneva: International Organization for Standardization.

[29] Shewhart W. A. (1931). Economic control of quality of the manufactured product. New York: Van Nostrand.

[30] Westgard J. O., Barry P. L., Hunt M. R., Groth T. A. (1981). A multirule Shewhart chart for quality control in clinical chemistry. Clinical Chemistry 27, 493-501.

[31] US Department of Health and Human Services. (1992). Clinical Laboratory Improvement Amendments of 1988; Final Rules and Notice. 42 CFR Part 493. The Federal Register 57, 7188-288.

[32] US Centers for Medicare & Medicaid Services (CMS). (2003). Medicare, Medicaid, and CLIA Programs: Laboratory Requirements Relating to Quality Systems and Certain Personnel Qualifications. Final Rule. The Federal Register 16, 3640-714.

Chapter 8

Postmortem DNA: QC Considerations for Sequence and Dosage Analysis of Genes Implicated in Long QT Syndrome

Stella Lai, Renate Marquis-Nicholson,
Chuan-Ching Lan, Jennifer M. Love, Elaine Doherty,
Jonathan R. Skinner and Donald R. Love

Additional information is available at the end of the chapter

1. Introduction

Long QT syndrome is a rare disorder of cardiac ion channels, characterised by a prolonged QT interval and T-wave abnormalities on electrocardiogram (ECG) and the occurrence of the ventricular tachycardia *torsade de pointes*. Sodium, potassium or calcium channels present in heart muscle may be affected, altering the regulation of electrical current in the cells [1-3]. Individuals with this condition will be predisposed to cardiac events such as arrhythmias and polymorphic ventricular tachycardia, which may lead, if untreated, to sudden cardiac death [2,3]. Thirteen genes are associated with the condition, and hundreds of mutations have been identified [3-5]. Currently, more than 95% of the pathogenic mutations listed in disease databases (Gene Connection For the Heart, http://www.fsm.it/cardmoc/; online Human Gene Mutation Database, www.hgmd.cf.ac.uk/) are sequence variants (including point mutations and small insertions or deletions), but the importance of whole or multi-exon deletions and duplications has more recently been recognised [6] and it is now recommended to use both sequence and dosage techniques in order to provide comprehensive analysis [3].

In New Zealand, the majority of specimens referred for Long QT syndrome diagnostic testing are retrieved after death. Postmortem specimens are often difficult to handle as they are usually either tissue samples or severely haemolysed blood. The extracted DNA is frequently of low quality, due to the presence of unwanted material such as short fragments produced by degradation and chemical modifications from oxidation and hydrolysis processes [7]. As a result, only short sequences can be reliably amplified [7]. Moreover, capillary-based sequencing, the gold standard first-line diagnostic test for Long QT syndrome, is very sensitive to the presence of contaminants, such as proteins, RNA and residual salt. The presence of such contaminants leads to poor quality electropherograms for analysis, which tend to be compromised by the presence of dye blobs, C-shoulders and a variable degree of baseline noise (Figure 1). Although the QC requirements for array comparative genomic hybridisation (aCGH), which can be used to detect whole exon deletion and duplication mutations, are less stringent than those for sequencing, contamination or degradation of sample DNA can lead to suboptimal efficiency of labelling and hybridisation. Such difficulties arising in the practical procedure mean that the analysis of postmortem DNA can be time-consuming and challenging, and obtaining high quality data within a reasonable timeframe can be extremely difficult.

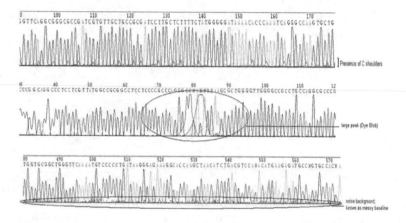

Figure 1. Electropherograms showing poor quality sequence data.

Long QT syndrome affects 1 in 2000 individuals [8] and contributes to 15-25% of sudden unexplained death in 1-40 year olds [9,10] and 10% of sudden unexplained deaths in infancy (SIDs) [11]. As a consequence, it is an important differential diagnosis to be considered in all cases of autopsy negative young sudden death. Molecular genetic testing is essential to make a postmortem diagnosis, given that screening for the electrocardiogram characteristics is no longer possible after death. Historically the turnaround time for diagnosis has been up to six months, due to the large number of genes to be analysed and the difficulties inherent in dealing with postmortem specimens (as detailed above). However, the demand by coroners for diagnostic laboratories to undertake more rapid analysis has been steadily increasing. A protocol tailored specifically to the treatment of postmortem specimens is necessary to meet this demand. Within our laboratory, we have successfully developed a robust process for sequence and dosage analysis of postmortem samples and have achieved an excellent turnaround time of 6-12 weeks. Here, we address the critical QC parameters that should be considered in order to obtain high quality data for rapid, accurate analysis. The discussion presented below concerns both sequence analysis and dosage analysis. The former uses conventional sequencing technology, while the latter involves the simultaneous high resolution screening of deletion and duplication mutations in multiple cardiac genes as opposed to the more conventional multiplex ligation dependent probe amplification (MLPA) technique, which many diagnostic laboratories still use [6].

2. Materials and methods

2.1. Sequencing

2.1.1. Primer design

We have used two approaches to design primers flanking each of the coding exons of the genes *KCNQ1* (LQT1), *KCNH2* (LQT2), *SCN5A* (LQT3), *KCNE1* (LQT5), *KCNE2* (LQT6), and *KCNJ2* (LQT7), including at least 50 base pairs of the flanking intronic regions. The first used the primer design program called PrimerQuest (Integrated DNA Technologies Inc; http://www.idtdna.com/Scitools/Applications/Primerquest/Advanced.aspx). This program allows the region in a sequence file to be specified, against which primers are designed to flank the targeted region. The designed primers for each exon are then checked *in silico* for annealing characteristics using the Macintosh-based program, Amplify. Finally, all primers were checked for single nucleotide polymorphisms (SNPs) using the software tool available from the National Genetic Reference Laboratory, Manchester (http://ngrl.man.ac.uk/SNPCheck/SNPCheck.html). This bioinformatics program uses the current National Center for Biotechnology Information (NCBI) build of the human genome and the current release of the Single Nucleotide Polymorphism database (dbSNP) to identify the position in the sequence where the primers bind and to detect any known SNPs at these sites

Following the above approach, we developed an alternate design protocol [12,13]. Each mRNA sequence of interest was identified through the public UCSC genome browser page http://genome.ucsc.edu. This website provides a direct link to ExonPrimer for the design of primers specific to the mRNA sequence. ExonPrimer uses exon position information provided by the UCSC genome browser in combination with the primer design tool Primer3 to create primer pairs according to set parameters, while avoiding pairing to homologous regions within the genome. Exon and amplicon size are provided and multiple alternative primer sets are given. Following primer design, all primers were checked for single nucleotide polymorphisms (SNPs), as described above. Following a negative SNP check the primer sequences were evaluated using the UCSC genome browser to confirm the identification of single amplicons. Each primer was then tailed with an M13 sequence and manufactured by Integrated DNA Technologies Inc or Life Technologies. In this way, primers are designed to allow amplification of all exons of interest and the corresponding splice sites using a single set of PCR conditions such that PCR (and subsequent sequencing) can be performed under identical conditions within a 96-well PCR plate.

2.1.2. DNA extraction

Genomic DNA (gDNA) was extracted from peripheral blood leucocytes (EDTA blood samples) using the Gentra Puregene DNA Extraction kit (Qiagen), according to the manufacturer's instructions.

A standard phenol/chloroform protease protocol was used to extract gDNA from postmortem tissue specimens. A small section (2mm x 2mm x 4mm) is usually cut from frozen tissue and diced as finely as possible using a scalpel blade. The tissue is placed into a 1.5ml microcentrifuge tube with 450µl of 1x TES Buffer (1M NaCl, 0.5M Tris-HCl, 10mM EDTA), 60µl of 20µg/µl Proteinase K (Roche) and 10µl of 10% SDS, and incubated overnight with vigorous shaking. Following digestion, an equal volume of phenol is added and the sample is vortexed vigorously. Once homogenous, the sample is centrifuged to separate the layers and the top aqueous layer is removed and transferred to a fresh 1.5ml centrifuge tube. An equal volume of chloroform is then added to the aqueous layer. This is vortexed, centrifuged, and the aqueous (top) layer again transferred to a fresh tube. A 2x volume of 100% ethanol is added to the aqueous layer to precipitate the DNA, followed by centrifugation at 13,000rpm and the supernatant is removed. The pellet is then washed with 70% ethanol and re-centrifuged for 2 minutes at 13,000rpm. The supernatant is again removed, and the pellet air dried prior to re-suspension in TE buffer (10mM Tris-HCl, 1mM EDTA, pH 7.0-8.0).

The quality and quantity of extracted gDNA is measured using a NanoDrop ND-1000 Spectrophotometer.

2.1.3. PCR

PCR amplification is performed in a final 25µl reaction volume with the following reagents: Faststart buffer (Roche Applied Science), 2mM $MgCl_2$ (Roche Applied Science), M13-tailed forward and reverse primers at 0.8µM each (synthesised by Integrated DNA Technologies Inc), 0.4mM dNTPs (GE Healthcare Ltd), 1 unit Faststart Taq DNA polymerase (Roche Applied Science) and 5µl GC-rich solution (Roche Applied Science). 50ng of gDNA is included in each reaction. PCR amplification is carried out with the following conditions: denaturation at 95°C for 5 minutes, followed by 35 cycles of 94°C for 45 seconds, 60°C for 30 seconds and 72°C for 30 seconds, with a final extension of 72°C for 10 minutes.

2.1.4. Sequencing (Figure 2)

5µL of each PCR is cleaned with ExoSAP-IT (Affymetrix, USB) prior to bidirectional DNA sequencing using M13 forward and reverse primers and Big-Dye Terminator v3.0 (Applied Biosystems Ltd). 20µl of each sequenced product is manually purified using the CleanSEQ Sequencing Purification System (Agencourt Bioscience). Four different drying times prior to elution (20 minutes, 24 hours, four days and seven days) were assessed to establish an optimal drying time for generating high quality sequencing data. 15µL of purified product was then subjected to capillary electrophoresis using the Applied Biosystems model 3130xl Genetic Analyzer.

The analysis of sequence traces is performed using Variant Reporter v1.0 (Applied Biosystems). Variant Reporter uses advanced algorithms and quality metrics to automate the detection of variants and to streamline the analysis process.

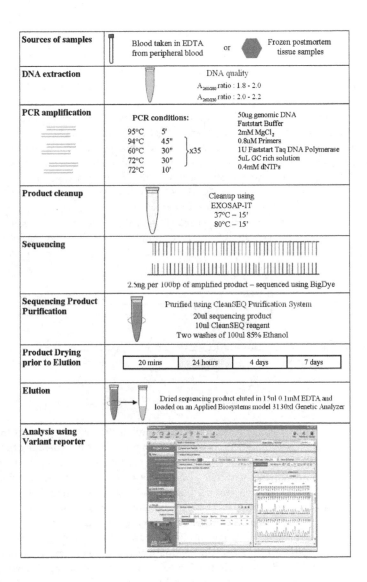

Figure 2. Flowchart of the sequencing method used in our laboratory.

2.2. Array comparative genomic hybridization (aCGH)

A Roche NimbleGen 12x135K Custom CGH Array was used for dosage analysis. This bespoke CGH array has been designed to screen for dosage changes within the genes responsible for LQT1-12 (*KCNQ1, KCNH2, SCN5A, ANK2, KCNE1, KCNE2, KCNJ2, CACNA1C, CAV3, SCN4B, AKAP9,* and *SNTA1*), the LQT-associated genes *GPD1L, KCNE3, SCN1B, SCN3B, CACNB2,* and the CPVT1 (*RYR2*) and CPVT2 (*CASQ2*) genes.

Two hundred and fifty nanograms of gDNA are processed according to the manufacturer's instructions (NimbleGen Array User's Guide: CGH and CNV Arrays v8.0; http://www.nimblegen.com). In brief, extracted gDNA from samples and Promega controls are denatured in the presence of a Cy3- (test) or Cy5- (control) labelled random primers and incubated with the Klenow fragment of DNA polymerase, together with dNTPs (5mM of each dNTP), at 37°C for 2 hours. The reaction is terminated by the addition of 21.5μL of 0.5M ED-TA, prior to isopropanol precipitation and ethanol washing. Following quantification, the test and sex-matched control samples are combined in equimolar amounts and applied to one of the twelve arrays on a microarray slide. Hybridisation is carried out in a Roche NimbleGen Hybridisation Chamber for a period of 48 hours. Slides are washed and scanned using a NimbleGen MS 200 Microarray Scanner. Array image files (.tif) produced by the MS 200 Data Collection Software are imported into DEVA v1.2.1 (Roche NimbleGen Inc) for analysis. Each genomic region exhibiting a copy number change within one of the LQT genes of interest were examined using the UCSC genome browser (http://genome.ucsc.edu/) to determine the location and significance of the change.

3. Results

In order to overcome the historical difficulties faced when performing Long QT syndrome testing using postmortem specimens and meet the demand by coroners for rapid results, we addressed the following parameters:

3.1. DNA purity

Since poor quality gDNA leads to suboptimal PCR amplification affecting downstream applications, the purity of gDNA is an important criterion for success in generating high quality sequencing data [14,15]. A NanoDrop ND-1000 spectrophotometer was used to measure the quality and quantity of the extracted gDNA. The ratio of absorbance at 260nm and 280nm (A260/280 ratio) is used to assess the purity of gDNA, which should be in the range of 1.8 to 2.0 to be accepted as pure gDNA. The ratio of absorbance at 260nm and 230nm (A260/230 ratio) is used as a secondary measure of nucleic acid purity, and for pure gDNA should be in the range of 2.0-2.2 [16]. Postmortem gDNA isolated using a standard phenol/chloroform protease protocol may contain residual phenol, chloroform or ethanol. These contaminants inhibit the activity of DNA polymerase in downstream applications (Figures 3-5) [14], so the purity of the gDNA must be strictly monitored. If a suboptimal A260/280 or A260/230 ratio indicates that the gDNA is of low quality, a secondary cleanup process should be considered. In our laboratory, we perform this cleanup using another phenol extraction and ethanol precipitation to further purify the gDNA sample [17].

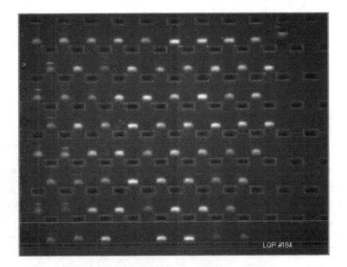

Figure 3. Agarose gel image of PCR amplification from an impure DNA with an acceptable $A_{260/280}$ ratio (1.88) but an acceptable $A_{260/230}$ ratio (2.5). NOTE: very few exons amplified effectively and strong primer dimers are visible.

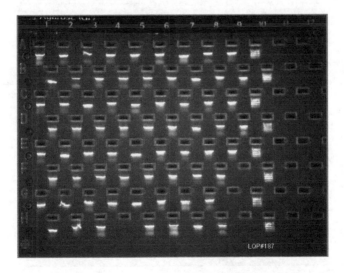

Figure 4. Agarose gel image of PCR products amplified from the same DNA sample after purification. NOTE: successful amplification and significantly reduced primer dimers.

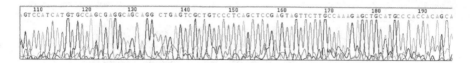

Figure 5. Electropherogram generated from an impure DNA sample with an acceptable $A_{260/280}$ ratio (1.95) but an unacceptable $A_{260/230}$ ratio (0.95). NOTE: significant baseline noise and data unable to be analysed.

3.2. Amount of DNA template used in a sequencing reaction

The extent of dilution of the cleaned PCR product prior to sequencing determines the amount of DNA template used in the sequencing reaction, which can affect the data quality for analysis [15]. The presence of excessive DNA template in a sequencing reaction will lead to rapidly progressive signal loss on the electropherogram (Figure 6), while using insufficient DNA template in a sequencing reaction will result in weak signal strength and a loss of peak shape (Figure 7), causing difficulties in basecalling and accurate analysis [15]. In order to obtain high quality data with good signal strength, the amplified product should be diluted in ddH_2O to as close as possible to 2.5ng per 100bp.

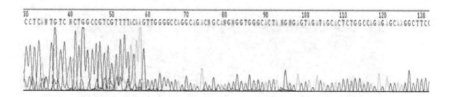

Figure 6. Electropherogram begins with strong high peaks, which fade rapidly.

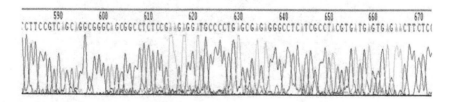

Figure 7. Electropherogram with increased background noise and loss of sharp peak shape.

3.3. CleanSEQ treatment of sequencing reactions

The sequenced product is purified using an Agencourt CleanSEQ system, which uses SPRI (Solid Phase Reversible Immobilization) magnetic bead-based technology. According to the manufacturer's recommendation, the sequencing product should be cleaned using undiluted CleanSEQ reagent, but in our experience, postmortem DNA samples should be cleaned using CleanSEQ reagent diluted 1:2 in ddH$_2$0 (figures 8,9).

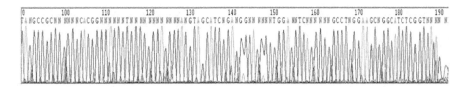

Figure 8. Electropherogram obtained from sequencing product cleaned with 10µl of undiluted CleanSEQ reagent: serious baseline noise and incorrect basecalling.

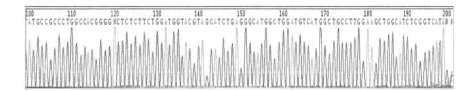

Figure 9. Electropherogram obtained from sequencing product cleaned using diluted CleanSEQ reagent: good quality trace.

3.4. Drying of DNA-bound beads prior to elution

The length of drying time following ethanol washing and prior to elution of the sequencing product from the CleanSEQ beads is one of the critical parameters for obtaining high quality sequence data. We assessed 4 different drying periods: 20 minutes, 24 hours, four days and seven days.

A drying time of 20 minutes, as recommended by the manufacturer, is frequently associated with the presence of large 'dye blobs', most probably as a result of residual ethanol in the eluted product (Figure 10); this problem resolves if drying time is extended to 24 hours (Figure 11). However, variable baseline noise on the electropherogram will be evident if the drying time exceeds four days (Figure 12); further increased background noise and loss of resolution occur when the drying time exceeds seven days (Figure 13).

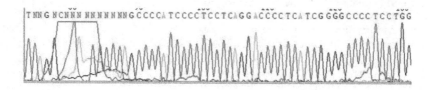

Figure 10. Electropherogram of purified products dried for 20 minutes prior to elution; presence of large dye blob.

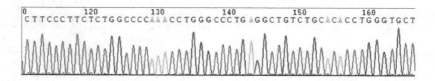

Figure 11. Electropherogram of purified products dried for 24 hours prior to elution; free of dye blobs, minimal baseline noise.

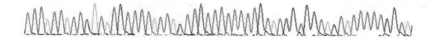

Figure 12. Electropherogram of purified products dried for 4 days prior to elution; presence of shoulders and messy baseline.

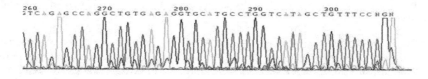

Figure 13. Electropherogram of purified products dried for 7 days prior to elution; extremely messy baseline and early loss of resolution.

4. Discussion

4.1. DNA quality

4.1.1. Sequence analysis

The gDNA used in a PCR should be as pure as possible in order to optimise the quality of the template that will be used in downstream applications. The purity of DNA is assessed in our laboratory using a NanoDrop ND-1000 spectrophotometer. It is important to consider both A260/280 and A260/230 as poor DNA quality will affect downstream applications [16,18]. An unacceptable A260/280 or A260/230 ratio indicates the presence of contaminants in the DNA; an abnormal A260/230 indicates the presence of residual phenol or other chemical from the extraction process, while an abnormal A260/280 most frequently indicates the presence of protein [16,18]. If any of the ratios appear to be abnormal, DNA purification should be considered before processing any further.

4.1.2. Dosage analysis (aCGH)

The quality requirements for gDNA used in an aCGH assay are not as stringent as those for a sequencing assay. An awareness of the presence of significant degradation is important; however, partial compensation for this can be made by increasing the volume of gDNA used in the amplification and labelling step. In our laboratory, we have found that doubling the volume of gDNA when degradation is visible on the 'check gel' (present in lanes 5-8 of Figure 14) is an effective counter-measure. The adequacy of amplification is measured using a NanoDrop ND-1000 spectrophotometer in order to allow the hybridisation of equimolar amounts of test and control DNA to the array slide. A post-amplification concentration of greater than 2500ng/µl is ideal for further processing; a sample with a post-amplification concentration of less than 1500ng/µl is unlikely to produce good quality data for analysis. Therefore, if there is sufficient volume of gDNA available, a repeat amplification with an increased volume of template gDNA should be undertaken.

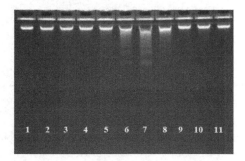

Figure 14. Agarose gel (2%) check of gDNA quality prior to aCGH.

4.2. Amount of DNA template used in a sequencing reaction

The DNA template should be diluted to 2.5ng per 100bp prior to sequencing. Incorrect quantification and dilution will alter the amount of input DNA template in a sequencing reaction, which can lead to problematic data for analysis. In our laboratory, we use Variant Reporter™ (Applied Biosystems Ltd) for automated analysis of sequence data. The signal strength of the sequence data is automatically assessed. Data with good signal strength is above the value of 200 in the Variant Reporter™ software. Sequence data with weak signal strength, a value below 100, indicates insufficient DNA template has been used in the sequencing reaction. Noisy background and a loss of sharp peak shape are also commonly evident. A repeat treatment with EXOSAP-IT and less extensive dilution of product is necessary to avoid inaccurate analysis using sequence data with unacceptable quality. In contrast, when excess DNA template is used in a sequencing reaction, a rapidly progressive signal loss is seen on the electropherogram. In this instance, trace quality can be improved by diluting the eluted product with water and reloading the sample on the capillary sequencing platform (we use an Applied Biosystems model 3130xl Genetic Analyzer).

4.3. CleanSEQ treatment of sequencing reactions

Agencourt CleanSEQ is routinely used to purify the sequenced products. According to the manufacturer's recommendation, 20µl of sequencing product should be cleaned with 10µl of CleanSEQ reagent. However, we found that this leads to an excess of CleanSEQ beads in relation to the amount of sequence product, therefore unwanted short fragments (e.g unincorporated dNTPs and excess primers) were able to bind to beads during purification, and the quality of sequence data generated was consequently reduced. We found that diluting the CleanSEQ beads 1:2 with ddH$_2$0 leads to much higher quality data.

4.4. Drying of DNA-bound beads prior to elution

This drying step is a critical QC consideration that significantly affects sequence quality. When the purified product is dried for 24 hours prior to elution, the subsequent electropherograms are free of dye blobs, C-shoulders and baseline noise, and consistently pass all QC metrics in Variant Reporter.

A drying time of 20 minutes, as suggested by manufacturer, was found to be problematic, causing the presence of dye blobs. Dye blobs are a common artefact due to either the presence of excess unincorporated dye or residual ethanol following product purification [15]. Previously, operators have focused on purifying sequenced products using an accurate final concentration of ethanol in an attempt to achieve consistency of evaporation/ drying between sequencing runs. Ethanol is highly volatile and it is therefore difficult to achieve consistency - even the short period of time in which the vessel containing the ethanol is open to allow access can result in a decrease in concentration. Here, we showed that the issue of dye blobs can be resolved by simply extending the drying time to 24 hours, allowing adequate time for all ethanol to evaporate completely, despite any minor differences in the concentration of ethanol used.

On the other hand, we found that the quality of sequence data is adversely affected if the drying time is extended to more than 4 days. This suggests that the stability of purified sequencing products is another factor that affects data quality. High quality sequence data was obtained with a drying time of 24 hours; however, the sequences were suboptimal when elution and electrophoresis were carried out at day 4 or day 7 of drying. This indicates that purified sequencing product is most stable for the first 24 hours and that consideration of the sample stability should be taken into account when aiming for high quality data.

4.5. Analysis parameters

4.5.1. Sequencing

All sequence traces are analysed in our laboratory using Variant Reporter Software v1.0 (Applied Biosystems). The current CMGS best practice guidelines for Sanger sequence analysis in diagnostic laboratories [19] recommend a PHRED score of at least 20 for bidirectional data (corresponding to 99% confidence that the base is called correctly), and a PHRED score of at least 30 for unidirectional data (99.9% confidence that each base is called correctly). The procedure we describe above produces bidirectional sequence data that meet our laboratory's even more stringent analysis criteria: a Variant Reporter trace score of 35, corresponding to a false base call rate of 0.031%.

4.5.2. Dosage analysis

In order to provide simultaneous dosage analysis of all the Long QT syndrome genes, we developed a custom designed Roche NimbleGen 12x135K CGH array. As part of the validation of this array we analysed twenty patients with known copy number abnormalities [20]. Analysis of the data from these individuals with known copy number changes allowed precise threshold criteria to be developed. It was determined that a $\log_2$ratio $\leq$-0.4 over 6 contiguous probes is indicative of a deletion, and a $\log_2$ratio of $\geq$0.4 over 15 contiguous probes indicative of a duplication.

4.6. Other parameters

It is important to monitor other QC parameters when it comes to sequence analysis of Long QT specimens: the freshness of the Polymer (POP-7) and the usage of the capillaries in the Applied Biosystems model 3130xl Genetic Analyzer.

Polymer (POP-7) is used to separate DNA fragments on genetic analyzers and the polymer remains stable for up to 7 days [15]. The capillary in the genetic analyzer should be replaced after 1000 injections. Within our laboratory, we perform a regular weekly maintenance of the analyzer, and the capillary is replaced when 600 injections are reached. From past experience, both the freshness of polymer and the usage of the capillary play a vital role in the data quality. Electropherograms with reduced resolution and peak shape are produced when either of these two parameters is suboptimal. In order to achieve high quality data, both freshness of polymer and usage of the capillary should be closely monitored.

5. Conclusions

We have successfully established a robust method for processing postmortem specimens for Long QT diagnostic testing in a timely manner. The electropherograms in Figure 15 are indicative of the high quality data routinely produced, despite the limitations inherent in the types of specimens that are referred. The blood sample used to extract gDNA for sequencing in this example was heavily haemolysed on arrival at the laboratory.

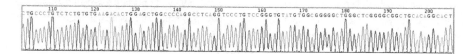

Figure 15. High quality sequence data generated from a haemolysed blood specimen; flat baseline along with distinct and evenly spaced peaks allow accurate basecalling.

The QC parameters described above should be monitored closely in order to consistently achieve optimal results (Figure 16). Although the basic procedure is essentially the same as that routinely used for sequence and aCGH analysis, the poor quality of postmortem specimens as a source of template DNA mean that particular attention needs to be paid to each step, in particular the critical initial assessment of DNA quality, the addition of the appropriate volume of template DNA to the sequencing reaction, and the drying time of the beads used in the purification procedure prior to elution.

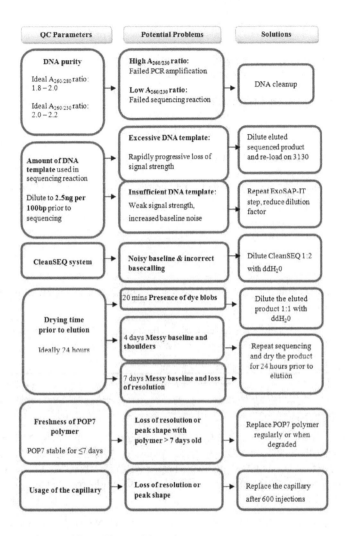

Figure 16. Flowchart of potential QC problems and their solutions.

Acknowledgements

We acknowledge the assistance of Dr Andrew Dodd in the initial design of primers against the coding regions of the LQT genes, and Mr Daniel Lai for his assistance in optimizing aspects of our amplicon clean-up.

Author details

Stella Lai[1], Renate Marquis-Nicholson[1,2*], Chuan-Ching Lan[1], Jennifer M. Love[1], Elaine Doherty[1], Jonathan R. Skinner[3] and Donald R. Love[1,2*]

*Address all correspondence to: donaldl@adhb.govt.nz

1 Diagnostic Genetics, Auckland City Hospital, New Zealand

2 School of Biological Sciences, The University of Auckland, New Zealand

3 Inherited Disease Group New Zealand, Paediatric Cardiac Services, Starship Childrens' Hospital, New Zealand

References

[1] Hunter, J. D., Sharma, P., & Rathi, S. (2008). Long QT syndrome. *Contin Educ Anaesth Crit Care Pain.*, 8, 67-70.

[2] Modell, S. M., & Lehmann, M. H. (2006). The long QT syndrome family of cardiac ion channelopathies: a HuGE review. *Genet Med.*, 8(3), 143-55.

[3] Alders, M., & Mannens, M. M. A. M. (2003). Romano-Ward Syndrome. Feb 20 [Updated 2012 May 31]., *In: Pagon RA, Bird TD, Dolan CR, et al., editors. GeneReviews™ [Internet]. Seattle (WA): University of Washington, Seattle;,* 1993Available from:, http://www.ncbi.nlm.nih.gov/books/NBK1129/.

[4] Yang, Y., Yang, Y., Liang, B., Liu, J., Li, J., Grunnet, M., Olesen, S. P., Rasmussen, H. B., Ellinor, P. T., Gao, L., Lin, X., Li, L., Wang, L., Junjie, J. X., Liu, Y. Y., Liu, Y. Y., Zhang, S. S., Lian, D. D., Peng, L. Y., Jespersen, T., & Chen, Y. H. (2010). Identification of a Kir3.4 mutation in congenital long QT syndrome. *Am. J. Hum. Genet.*, 86, 872-880.

[5] Dan, M., & Roden, M. D. (2008). Long-QT Syndrome. *N Engl J Med.*, 358, 169-176.

[6] Eddy, C. A., MacCormick, J. M., Chung, S. K., Crawford, J. R., Love, D. R., Rees, M. I., et al. (2008). Identification of large gene deletions and duplications in KCNQ1 and KCNH2 in patients with long QT syndrome. *Heart Rhythm*, 5(9), 1275-1281.

[7] Bonin, S., Petrera, F., Niccolini, B., & Stanta, G. (2003). PCR analysis in archival post mortem tissues. *Mol Pathol.*, 56, 184-186.

[8] Schwartz, P. J., Stramba-Badiale, M., Crotti, L., Pedrazzini, M., Besana, A., Bosi, G., et al. (2009). Prevalence of the congenital long-QT syndrome. *Circulation*, 120(18), 1761-1767.

[9] Skinner, J. R., Crawford, J., Smith, W., Aitken, A., Heaven, D., & Evans, CA. (2011). Prospective, population-based long QT molecular autopsy study of postmortem negative sudden death in 1 to 40 year olds. *Heart Rhythm*, 8(3), 412-419.

[10] Gladding, P. A., Evans, C. A., Crawford, J., Chung, S. K., Vaughan, A., Webster, D., et al. (2010). Posthumous diagnosis of long QT syndrome from neonatal screening cards. *Heart Rhythm*, 7(4), 481-486.

[11] Skinner, J. R. (2010). Sudden Unexplained Death in Infancy and Long QT syndrome. *Current Pediatric Reviews*, 6, 48-55.

[12] Doherty, E., Marquis-Nicholson, R., Love, J. M., Brookes, C., Prosser, D., & Love, D. R. (2011). Primer Design to Sequence Analysis- a Pipeline for a Molecular Genetic Diagnostic Laboratory, Applications and Experiences of Quality Control, Ognyan Ivanov (Ed.). 978-9-53307-236-4, InTech, Available from, http://www.intechopen.com/books/applications-and-experiences-of-quality-control/primer-design-to-sequence-analysis-a-pipeline-for-a-molecular-genetic-diagnostic-laboratory.

[13] Lai, D., & Love, D. R. (2012). Automation of a primer design and evaluation pipeline for subsequent sequencing of the coding regions of all human Refseq genes. *Bioinformation*, 8(8), 363-366.

[14] Verhagen, O. J., Wijkhuijs, A. J., van der Sluijs-Gelling, A. J., Szczepanski, T., van der Linden-Schrever, B. E., Pongers-Willemse van, M. J., Wering, E. R., van Dongen, J. J., & van der Schoot, C. E. (1999). Suitable DNA isolation method for the detection of minimal residual disease by PCR techniques. *Leukemia*, 13(8), 1298-1299.

[15] Applied Biosystems Chemistry Guide, second edition. (2009). DNA Sequencing by Capillary Electrophoresis. Available from:, http://www3.appliedbiosystems.com/cms/groups/mcb_support/documents/generaldocuments/cms_041003.pdf.

[16] T009 - Technical Support Bulletin and 260/230Ratios. (2008). Available from:, http://www.nanodrop.com/Library/T009-NanoDrop%201000-&-NanoDrop%208000-Nucleic-Acid-Purity-Ratios.pdf.

[17] Powell, R., & Gannon, F. (2002). Purification of DNA by phenol extraction and ethanol precipitation. *Oxford Practical Approach Series, Oxford University Press.*, Available from:, http://fds.oup.com/www.oup.co.uk/pdf/pas/9v1-7 -3.pdf.

[18] T042 - Technical Bulletin. (2011). Assessment of Nucleic Acid Purity. Available from:, http://www.nanodrop.com/Library/T042-NanoDrop-Spectrophotometers-Nucleic-Acid-Purity-Ratios.pdf.

[19] Ellard, S., Charlton, R., Yau, M., Gokhale, D., Taylor, G., Wallace, A., & Ramsden, S. C. (2009). Practice guidelines for Sanger Sequencing Analysis and Interpretation. Available from:, http://www.cmgs.org/BPGs/pdfs%20current%20bpgs/Sequencingv2.pdf.

[20] Marquis-Nicholson, R., Doherty, E., Thrush, A., Love, J. M., Lan-C, C., George, A. M., & Love, D. R. (2012). Array-based identification of copy number changes: simultaneous gene-focused and low resolution whole genome analysis. *Sultan Qaboos University Medical Journal*, submitted.

Chapter 9

Quality Control Considerations for Fluorescence *In Situ* Hybridisation of Paraffin-Embedded Pathology Specimens in a Diagnostic Laboratory Environment

Lisa Duffy, Liangtao Zhang, Donald R. Love and Alice M. George

Additional information is available at the end of the chapter

1. Introduction

Paraffin FISH testing is the application of the fluorescence *in situ* hybridisation (FISH) methodology to formalin fixed paraffin embedded sections (FFPE), and has proven a powerful tool for both histopathologists and cytogeneticists. Pathologists use the method to confirm or exclude a histological diagnosis, to differentiate between tumour subtypes, or as a confirmatory tool where the tissue morphology is poor or the immunohistochemistry (IHC) staining is uninformative [1]. Similarly, cytogeneticists find it useful when the tissue sample is insufficient or unsatisfactory for conventional culture methods, or when such methods fail to yield a result. The method can also be used to confirm abnormalities found in other tissue samples. Paraffin testing has a further advantage over conventional cytogenetic and molecular testing methods, as it can localize the anomaly within specific cells or tissue areas, and this provides the ability to study anomalies at a single cell level [2,3], unlike DNA techniques that pool DNA from hundreds of different cells [1,3].

Compared to FISH testing on conventional suspension samples (Figure 1), paraffin FISH can be labour intensive and highly variable due to differing fixation times between samples and referring histology labs, and the interpretation may be limited due to truncation of signal and overlapping cells [1,4].

Paraffin pretreatment steps

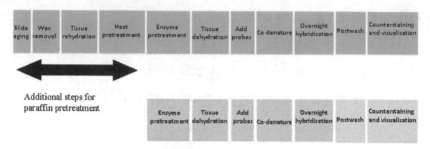

Additional steps for
paraffin pretreatment

Suspension pretreatment steps

Figure 1. A comparison of the paraffin pre-treatment process with the conventional FISH pre-treatment process on suspension semples.

For these reasons, it must be considered separately from the conventional suspension FISH method, and while it can be used as either a stand-alone technique, or an adjunct to conventional cytogenetics techniques [5], it must be noted that due to the use of interphase nuclei, a prior knowledge of the anomaly of interest is required.

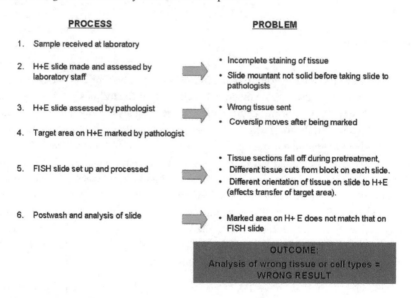

Figure 2. Errors that occur during the paraffin pre-treatment process.

The basic premise of the method involves establishing the area of interest for testing on the H+E stained pathology slide, and transferring this area to an unstained paraffin slide, which is then pretreated, probed and co-denatured using the traditional FISH methodology [6,7]. However, one of the most crucial factors for paraffin analysis is the assessment of the correct target area before beginning the procedure – without this, an erroneous result may occur (Figure 2), which may be costly to patients if it results in the appropriate treatment being with held [1].

For this reason, robust internal and external quality control procedures are required for diagnostic paraffin FISH testing and the exclusion of non-target tissue before analysis decreases the likelihood of an incorrect result due to an analysis error [1]. This protocol therefore aims to provide a guide to some of the considerations and troubleshooting that are necessary when using the method for diagnostic medical testing. It is adapted from the method used by the Diagnostic Genetics Department, LabPlus at Auckland City Hospital, New Zealand. There are a number of variations to the basic FISH method that can be used depending on the nature and number of samples being processed, and new technology has also been developed to automate the process (Xmatrix, Abbott Molecular). In this protocol however, we have suggested extra steps that are designed to help improve the quality of the testing procedure for diagnostic use. Probes used for diagnostic testing are commercially available and may be downloaded and gathered from the websites of companies such as Abbott Molecular, Cytocell, Zytovision or Kreatech Diagnostics.

2. Method

One slide (2-5 micron thickness usually) is needed per probe or probe set, and if a haematoxylin and eosin (H+E) slide is not provided by pathologists, an extra slide must also go through the deparaffinisation steps before staining with the Shandon Rapid-Chrome™ Frozen Section Staining kit (alternatively the individual stain kit components can be made from powder).

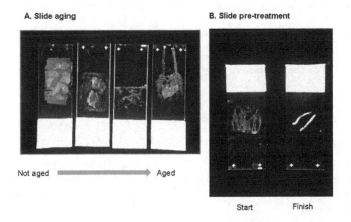

Figure 3. Slide pretreatment steps for paraffin FISH. (A) Appearance of unstain paraffin slides after aging in a 60ºC oven - note melted or "bubbled" appearance. (B) Unstained paraffin slides and after the pre-treatment steps.

1.   Deparaffinisation (approx. 60 minutes); see Figure 3

a.   Leave slide/s on the hotplate/in the oven at approximately 65°C for 30-60 minutes for aging (Figure 3).

b.   Perform deparaffinization by placing slide/s in xylene for at least 10 minutes in the fume hood, with intermittent shaking.

c.   Rehydrate slide/s by placing them for 2 minutes in each of 100%, 80%, and 70% ethanol solutions, followed by deionised water at room temperature.

2.   Haemotoxylin and Eosin (H+E) slides; see Figure 4

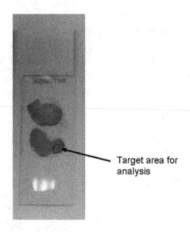

Target area for analysis

Figure 4. A haemotoxylin and eosin (H+E) stained slide with the target area for analysis marked by a pathologist.

a.   Take rehydrated slide/s and stain using the Shandon Rapid-Chrome™ Frozen Section Staining kit and mount the slide using Shandon Mount.

b.   Leave slides on the hotplate for at least 30 min to dry the mountant.

c.   Check slides for stain quality under a light microscope.

d.   Take slide/s to pathologist for marking (Figure 5).

3.   Heat Pre-treatment (approx. 30 minutes)

a.   Add 35µl of heat pre-treatment solution (Invitrogen Tissue Pre-treatment Kit) to the slide/s, cover with a 22x22mm (or bigger sized cover slip) glass cover slip and seal with rubber cement. Alternatively slides can be heat-pre-treated in coplin Jar at 95°C or pressure cooker.

b.   Heat slide/s on the thermal cycler for 15-60 minutes at 95°C (The time is dependent on the type of tissues and length of formalin fixation).

c. On completion, immerse slide/s with cover slip in deionised water to cool down and gently remove the cover slip.

d. Wash briefly in a coplin jar of deionised water at room temperature and drain off excessive water.

4. Enzyme Digestion (approx. 40 minutes).

a. Add an appropriate amount (~15μl) of enzyme reagent (Invitrogen Tissue Pre-treatment Kit) to the slide/s, depending on the size of hybridisation area, and cover with a square of parafilm.

b. Incubate slide/s for 15-45 minutes in a humidified chamber at 37°C (This time is dependent on the type of tumours and length of formalin fixation).

c. Remove cover slip/s and wash briefly in a coplin jar of deionised water at room temperature.

d. Dehydrate slide/s for 2 minutes each in each of 70%, 80% and 100% ethanol solutions and air dry at room temperature. Please note that a different ethanol series is used for the dehydration steps to avoid reagent contamination issues.

e. Check the tissue morphology of the pre-treated slide looks the same as that of the H+E.

f. The pre-treated paraffin slide/s should then be carefully matched against the marked H&E slide/s, and the area for testing transferred to the pre-treated slide/s using a marker pen initially, followed by the diamond-tipped engraver. This means that the area can still be visualised after the post-wash steps.

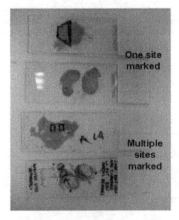 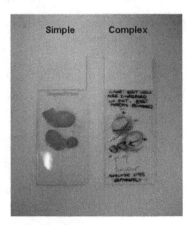

Figure 5. Haemotoxylin and eosin (H+E) stained slides marked with the target area for analysis. This reduces the volume of probe necessary and ensures that non-target tissue is excluded as much as possible before the FISH analysis procedure

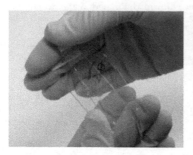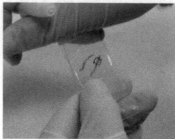

Figure 6. Transfer of target area for analysis from the H+E slide to the pre-treated FISH slide prior to the probing steps.

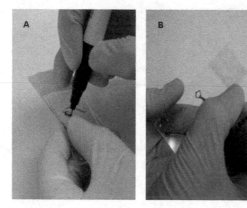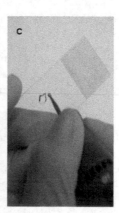

Figure 7. Engraving of target area on to the pre-treated paraffin FISH slide. (A) Draw target area onto bottom of slide with fix-resistant pen. (B & C) Engrave marked area onto bottom of slide using diamond-tipped engraver to keep area visible after post-wash steps.

5. Probe preparation (approx. 10 minutes)

   Use Ready-To-Use probes or refer to the probe preparation protocol outlined by the manufacturer.

6. Co-denaturation and hybridization (approx. 25 minutes)

a. Apply an appropriate amount (2-10μl) of probe mix to the hybridization site marked on each slide, depending on the size of cover slip being used, and seal with rubber cement. Leave the slide/s in the incubator or in a drawer at room temperature for a few minutes to allow the rubber cement to dry before placing them in the thermal cycler.

b. Denature slide/s together with probe mix for 10-20 min at 85°C or 5-10min at 95°C.

c. After co-denaturation, slide/s may be placed in a humidified box in the incubator at 37°C for at least 12-16 hours, usually no more than 72 hours.

7. Post Hybridization Wash (5 Minutes)

a. Briefly soak slide/s in 2xSSC and gently remove rubber cement.

b. Wash slide/s in 0.4xSSC/0.03% Tween 20 (or NP40) at 72°C for 2 min.

c. Place slide/s in 2xSSC/0.01% Tween 20 (or NP40) for 1 min.

d. Briefly drain slide/s, apply DAPI counter stain and put cover slip on.

e. Visualize FISHed-slide/s under fluorescence microscope.

When using indirectly labelled commercial probes that require antibody detection, signal detection must be done according to the manufacturer's instructions.

8. Analysis and interpretation; see Figure 8.

a. With a pathologist's consultation, check the H+E slide on a transmitted light microscope to assess whether the sample contains a mixture of cell types, as this may affect the interpretation of the FISH signal pattern.

b. Check the paraffin FISH slide on a fluorescence microscope using the 10x objective to ensure the area marked on the slide approximately matches that on the H+E slide.

c. Using two observers, analyse a minimum of at least 8 representative sites within the marked region (a minimum of 4 different areas per observer), scoring only cells that show both the target and control loci. Analysis of areas of areas where the cells are not overlapped is preferable, and a third analyst is required where there is discordance between two observers.

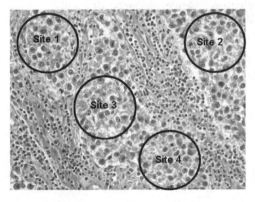

Each analyst must:

1. Check histology slide for mixed cell population

2. Check paraffin FISH slide to ensure that area matches

3. Score areas with minimal overlap

4. Observers score a minimum of 8 representative sites in marked area (different QAP programmes may use fewer number of sites.

Figure 8. Analysis principles for paraffin FISH slides.

3. Troubleshooting

Problem: Unclear whether slides have been aged before arrival, as repeating this step may decrease the hybridization efficiency of the probe.

[Step 1]

Solution: Although some waxes do not change in appearance, pre-aged slides generally have a bubbled or melted appearance of the wax compared to the smooth appearance of non-aged slides in general (N.B: some wax types do not change in appearance so this is a rule of thumb only).

Problem: The use of xylene to remove the wax from around the sample is not ideal as xylol is highly toxic.

[Step 1]

Solution: An alternative to xylene is HemoDe from Scientific Safety Solvents.

Problem: Finding that the wrong tissue was sent by the referring laboratory.

[Step 2]

Solution: Ask for a copy of the pathology report to be sent with all samples, and get pathologists to ring the referring laboratory to request the appropriate sample for testing.

Problem: Incomplete staining of the H+E slide causing correct target area to be missed by pathologist.

[Step 2]

Solution: Slides should be quality checked before taking them to a pathologist. Check the stain by eye to see if there are obvious colour differences across the slide – if one of the stains has been missed in an area it will appear either a dull purple (eosin missed) or a dull pink (haematoxylin missed or there is a problem with the pH of the bluing reagent) compared to the rest of slide. If there are any doubts, ask a histopathology technologist for assistance.

Problem: Cover slip moves after the slide has been marked because mountant is not completely hardened. This causes the target area to move.

[Step 2]

Solution: Leave the slides on the hotplate for a longer period of time, or change mountant to a faster drying version such as Entellan (Note: it is not possible to remove the Entellan with methanol after it has been cover slipped, hence why DPX is the preferred mountant).

The Rapid-Chrome™ Frozen Section Staining kit uses Shandon Mount; however alternatives such as Entellan are available.

Problem: Disappearance of tissue on slide during dehydration steps.

[Steps 3 and 4]

Solution: The ethanol series (in step 1) is necessary to rehydrate the tissue for the enzyme solution to act on, and may cause the tissue to become translucent, however it will become white again once the slide is dehydrated.

Problem: Scratching or loss of tissue during washing steps. Small tissue samples (e.g. core biopsies) may become fragile during the pretreatment steps and fall off the slide.

[Steps 3 and 4]

Solution: As the tissue becomes soft during pre-treatment it may easily fall off or get scratched; coplin jars of deionised water can be used to dip slides into rather than the more aggressive use of squirter bottles or running tap water (do not leave the pre treated slide in water for a long time, especially for a core biopsy or a tiny sample). The size of the tissue gives a good indication as to the fragility of the tissue, so this should be taken into account before beginning the pre treatment steps. Increasing the ageing step may also help to fix the tissue to the slide better, although it may also decrease the hybridization efficiency of the probe to the sample. Alternatively, skipping the heat pretreatment step and doing a reduced enzyme treatment on the sample may combat this.

Problem: The tissue does not look the same as the H+E slide after dehydration steps.

[Step 4]

Solution: This can either be due to loss of tissue during pretreatment or different cuts through the tissue block. Untreated slides should be closely examined to find one that appears to match the pretreated slide and a new H+E slide created using this slide. See also steps for reducing the loss of tissue during pretreatment.

Problem: Transfer of area is difficult due to a slight difference in the morphology of the tissue in different layers of the tissue section, or different orientation of tissue on pre-treated slide to that of the H+E slide.

[Step 4]

Solution: If the morphology of tissue on the pre-treated slide looks different to that of the H +E slide, check it against the remaining untreated slides to see if it looks like tissue has been lost during the pre-treatment procedure. If tissue has been lost, simply start the procedure over again with a new slide. If the morphology of the tissue appears different between the untreated slides, ask a pathologist for help selecting an appropriate slide to pre-treat, and try to find two similar untreated slides. Pre-treat one and make the other into an H+E slide to allow for more accurate marking.

Problem: There is more than one target area marked on slide – is more probe required?

[Step 4 and 5]

Solution: Assess the size of the areas – if there are several small areas, the total volume of probe does not need to be increased, simply aliquot the volume of probe equally over the different areas and place a small cover slip over each. More than one aliquot of probe is only required if the areas are greater than can be covered by a 13mm diameter cover slip.

Problem: The hybridisation buffer for a probe runs out.

[Step 5]

Solution: As hybridisation buffers are all fairly similar, it is fine to use the buffer of similar probe as a substitution. Alternatively, hybridization mix can be made up:

Hybridization mix

(10% dextran sulphate, 50% formamide in 2xSSC, 0.1% SDS, pH 7.0)

1. Mix 12.5ml formamide, 2.5ml 20xSSC pH7.0 and 10ml MilliQ water. Adjust pH to 7.0 with HCl then transfer to a 50ml Falcon tube.

2. Add 2.5mg dextran sulphate and place on a roller mixer at room temperature for 1-2 hours.

3. Add 25μl Tween 20 and invert to mix.

4. Aliquot 500μl into sterile eppendorf tubes. Store at -20°C and use a fresh aliquot each time.

Problem: A thermal cycler is not available for use.

[Step 6]

Solution: Denaturation of the slide(s) can be done separately using 70% formamide/2xSSC, as it gives better quality denaturation although the downside is that it is highly toxic. The hybridisation steps can also be done adequately in a programmable system (e.g. Thermobyte).

Problem: The cover slip is hard to remove before the post wash steps.

[Step 7]

Solution: Place slide in 2xSSC solution and agitate gently after removing the rubber cement, and then remove cover slip. If the cover slip is still stuck to slide, slide the blade of a scalpel under one corner of the slide and lift gently before immersing the slide in a 2xSSC solution and agitating it gently. This may need to be repeated several times if the cover slip remains stuck.

Problem: Weak or patchy signal quality.

[Step 8]

Solution: This can be difficult to fix, as it primarily occurs as a result of poor handling and fixation of tissue prior to receiving the sample for FISH testing [8,9]. Different tissue samples may require the pretreatment times to be varied [10]. The heat pretreatment buffer prepares the tissue for the enzyme to act on and the enzyme degrades the cellular material away from the DNA, in order to allow the probe to anneal to the chromatin. Variation of either or both these times is effective, and the steps may be repeated on the probed slide to reduce the need for lengthy pretreatment times on a new slide. Bone samples such as trephines may show poor hybridization efficiency of the probe, and require hydrogen chloride treatment, unless the sample has already been decalcified prior to arrival.

Poor signal quality may also be a result of incorrect post wash stringency. There is an alternative wash technique that uses 50% formamide/2xSSC to increase the stringency of the wash. However, this is not always ideal, as it significantly increases the length of the post wash, and also uses formamide which is extremely toxic [11].

Problem: High levels of cross hybridization due to non-specific binding of probes.

[Step 8]

Solution: This is due to incorrect stringency of the post wash [1]. For a quick fix, slides can be rewashed using the quick wash procedure reported here, or alternatively washing at a higher temperature or use of a different post wash procedure can be tried [11].

Problem: Cells only show one signal colour.

[Step 8]

Solution: Only cells showing both the control and target loci should be scored (e.g. 2R2G), so if both the control probe and the probe for the region of interest are on the same chromosome, it is most likely to be due to poor hybridisation of one of the probes. First check to see using single colour filters whether the signal colour is present but weak – if it is, repeat the pre-treatment and hybridisation steps again on the same slide (for a shorter time e.g. 15/15 buffer: enzyme treatment).

Problem: Using an indirectly labeled probe and can't get a good signal quality.

[Step 8]

Solution: In most cases, amplification with only a primary antibody is necessary, and further amplification can also increase the level of background on the slide(s). However if the signal is not bright enough, carefully remove the cover slip, rinse slide in 1xPBS (or SSC) and perform further amplification steps with secondary or tertiary antibodies as many times as necessary. After adding each antibody, slides should be covered with parafilm and incubated in a humidified chamber at 37°C for 5 minutes before being washed in 4xSSC/0.05% Tween20 for 2 minutes. Then mount with 8µl Vectashield antifade solution with DAPI.

Problem: Distinguishing between real signal and background or 'rubbish' on slide.

[Step 8]

Solution: Look at the signal intensity on single colour filters – rubbish generally appears to be brighter and shinier compared to real signals, and background will appear fuzzy and indistinct compared to real signal. High background may be due to the slides not being properly sealed with rubber cement during the pretreatment steps, as this allows the solution to evaporate and the tissue to dry out.

Problem: High background on the slides when analyzing.

[Step 8]

Solution: High background may be due to insufficient removal of material during the pretreatment steps. With high case numbers, solutions can become contaminated, therefore the solutions in the pretreatment steps need to be changed regularly, and it pays to have an additional coplin jar of 100% ethanol to dip the slides into after the xylol step in order to reduce contamination from the xylol solution. Alternatively, background may be due to the cover slip not being sealed properly during the pretreatment and co-denaturation steps, causing the tissue to dry out. By placing the slide in the incubator to allow the rubber cement to dry before these steps, this effect can be reduced. The use of a glass coverslip rather than a plastic coverslip also helps, as plastic acts as an insulator, and therefore will hold the temperature and increase the drying of the tissue.

The use of detergents in the post wash steps also helps to solubilize proteins, and if Tween20 is not effective, then NP-40 can also be used.

Problem: There is a mixed cell population in the marked target area (e.g. Tumour cells with non-target lymphocytes also present); see Figure 9.

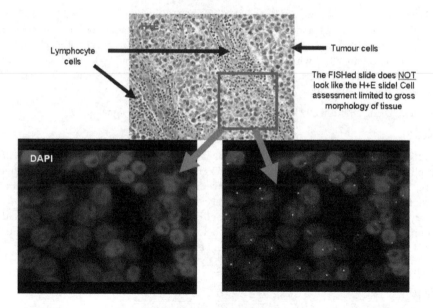

Figure 9. The analysis of slides with mixed tissue populations.

[Step 8]

Solution: Check the H+E slide first before analysing the FISH slide to see whether there is clustering of cell types, or differences in morphology between the different cell types. Then scan the marked target area on the FISH slide using the 10x objective to find areas which appear to be targeted cells and switch to a higher objective for confirmation and then analyse using appropriate filter. Consideration of accidental analysis of non-target cells must also be taken into account when interpreting such cases, therefore increasing the number of cells or sites analysed will increase the accuracy of the analysis. Alternatively, it may be possible to get a pathologist to mark several smaller sites containing only target cells, as this reduces the risk of error before beginning the analysis.

Problem: Target area marked is very small, so it is difficult to test a variety of areas.

[Step 8]

Solution: While this makes analysis difficult, switching to the 10x objective and moving the stage to a different position will reduce the likelihood of reanalyzing the same cells. Numerical scoring is also preferable in such a case, as it provides a reliable basis for interpretation.

Problem: The cells are highly dispersed or highly clustered, making analysis difficult.

[Step 8]

Solution: Select good areas where the cells are not overlapping using the DAPI filter and use numerical scoring of individual cell signal patterns (this may mean increasing the number of sites examined if the cells are widely dispersed). If a gene rearrangement probe is being used, it may be sufficient just to report the presence or absence of a rearrangement without doing individual cell analysis.

Problem: Distinguishing between real loss and gain of signal compared to artefact.

[Step 8]

Solution: If the target abnormality is either a gain (trisomy/tetrasomy) or loss (deletion) of a signal, it pays to establish thresholds using normal control slides to estimate the level of artefactual gain or loss of signal, and to check the manufacturer's product information to see if splitting of the probe or non-target binding/polymorphisms are common with the probe. The variance in the signal patterns can also be checked – if the percentage of cells showing a 1R2G signal pattern is roughly equivalent to those showing a 2R1G signal, then it is reasonable to assume that it is due to artefactual truncation of signal.

Problem: There is discordance between analysts.

[Step 8]

Solution: Get a third analyst to score the sample. If two analysts have similar results, discard the third analysis, or if all three give different results, take an average of all three results to allow robust interpretation. If the three results differ hugely, it is preferable to confirm the result with a secondary probe where possible, or request a repeat sample from another block. Where the interpretation is still not clear, the case can be reported as inconclusive or failed.

Problem: A low level abnormality, multiple clones or mosaicism is suspected.

[Step 8]

Solution: Where the result is not straightforward use quantitative scoring and use appropriate thresholds for interpretation. Paraffin FISH is not the most suitable method of detection for these cases, although methods that involve taking thicker slices of the section have been developed [12].

4. Conclusion

The role of pathologists is crucial to the analysis of paraffin FISH sections from the beginning of the process. They can help to eliminate very basic laboratory errors, such as identifying whether incorrect tissue has been sent prior to processing the slides, and can also help to identify the appropriate target tissue within the paraffin section prior to analysing the sample, so that inappropriate tissues can be reduced or eliminated. When analysing products of conception, the fetal component can be very small compared to the maternal component, and without guidance of pathologists, an erroneous result may occur. Similarly, in breast cancer samples, it is important to eliminate areas of contained carcinoma (*in situ* components such as DCIS and LCIS) and lymphocytes, as these may result in false positive or negative results, which can be deleterious if treatments such as Herceptin are then withheld from the patient. Some samples such as lymphomas or graft versus host disease may require extensive guidance from pathologists as knowledge of the disease characteristics will allow for highly targeted analysis. In follicular lymphoma, the follicles need to be identified so that centrocytes and centroblasts are targeted for analysis, and normal lymphocytes and reactive cells are avoided when analysing the sample (Swerdlow et al. 2008). For this reason, it is best to include a variety of areas to get a representative result. It should be noted that external quality assurance programmes may differ in the number of sites required for analysis. Generally speaking, fewer sites are required, if initially the non-target tissue is eliminated.

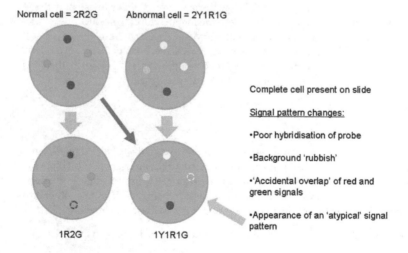

Figure 10. Artefactual signal changes on suspension FISH slides.

Despite such assistance however, care must also be taken during the analysis of paraffin samples, as in many cases it is impossible to completely remove the non-target tissue from the area of interest. It is therefore important to check the H+E slide before beginning the analysis, as this will give an indication as to whether the sample is made up solely of target tissue, or whether it contains a mixture of target and non-target tissue that must be taken into account when making the final interpretation.

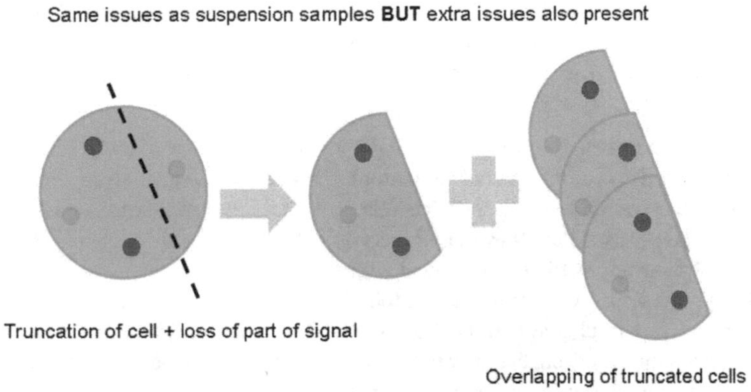

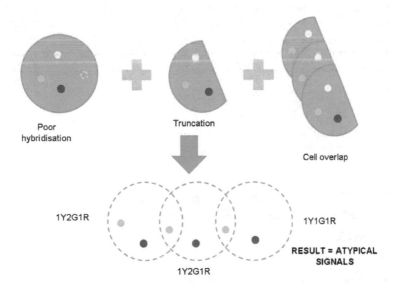

Same issues as suspension samples **BUT** extra issues also present

Truncation of cell + loss of part of signal

Overlapping of truncated cells

Figure 11. Artefactual considerations for paraffin FISH samples - truncation and overlapping of cells in specimen.

Poor
hybridisation

Truncation

Cell overlap

1Y2G1R

1Y1G1R

1Y2G1R

**RESULT = ATYPICAL
SIGNALS**

Figure 12. The need for thresholds for paraffin FISH analysis.

Due to both the potential for analysis of the incorrect target cells as outlined, and the artefactual variation that can arise when using the FISH technique [13], it is necessary to establish robust thresholds to guide the interpretation of results. Signal pattern changes can occur due to poor hybridization of probe, background 'rubbish-autofluorescence' or 'accidental overlap' of red and green signals (Figure 10).

These can lead to the appearance of false or atypical signal patterns; therefore thresholds need to be established to distinguish between false positives and negatives. Paraffin analysis requires higher thresholds than those for suspension cultures, as there is the additional complication of overlap and truncation of cells [1,12], causing artefactual gain or loss of signals (Figures 11 and 12).

Thresholds are of particular importance when dealing with cases that show atypical, non-target (e.g. unexpected loss or increase of copy number instead of a gene rearrangement) or low level abnormalities, or those where mosaicism or multiple clones appear to be present, as it is unclear in most cases as to how they may impact on patient treatment. While paraffin FISH is usually not the most appropriate way to deal with such cases, but when tissue is scarce or has already been processed, it can sometimes be the only option for testing. Numerical scoring of the tissue in such cases will give an indication of the major signal pattern(s) and the level of variation inherent in the tissue, particularly in tumours where there can be concurrent increase in the ploidy level, together with loss or gain of the target loci. This will allow a judgment to be made about whether the variation is likely to be artefactual or not, as false aneuploidies will show almost equivalent levels of loss between target and control loci.

Due to the potential complexities of paraffin analysis, the use of both cytogenetic and pathology external quality control programs such as the College of American Pathologists (CAP) and Australasian Society of Cytogeneticists (ASoC) is recommended, as it allows quality issues to be addressed from both the cytogenetic and pathology perspectives. This provides a balanced perspective on the degree of analytical stringency that is required prior to releasing result.

Appendices

Materials

Reagents

Biotin and Digoxygenin

Bovine serum albumin (BSA) Deionised water

Enzyme reagent (Invitrogen cat #00-8401)

Ethanol (70%, 80% and 100%)

Heat pre-treatment solution pH7.0 (Invitrogen cat #00-8401)

Hybridisation buffer

Non ionic detergent: NP40 (Vysis 30-80482). Store in -20°C.

Phosphate Buffered Saline (PBS)

0.01% pepsin/HCl solution

Purified H_2O

DNA probes

Shandon Rapid-Chrome™ Frozen Section Staining kit

2X SSC/0.1% Tween20

0.4xSSC/0.3%Tween20 solution

2xSSC/0.01% Tween20 solution

Vectashield antifade mounting solution with 1.5µg/ml DAPI (Vector laboratories Cat # H-1200). Store in the dark at 4°C.

Xylol

Equipment

Atlas cooler box

Blotting paper

Centrifuge –Heraeus Biofuge Pico

Coverslips (13mm diameter round, 22x22mm and 24 x 50mm)

Diamond pen or diamond-tipped engraver –Easy Marker Engraver (Taiwan)

Eppendorf tubes

Fix-resistant marker pen

Fluorescence microscope - Zeiss Axio Imager.M1 microscope, Zeiss Axioplan microscope, Olympus BX60 fluorescence microscope

Glass coplin jars

H&E slide

Hotplate

Humidified box

Incubator – Contherm Scientific NZ

Parafilm

Pipettes (2 ul and 100ul)

Pipette tips

Poly-lysine slides (with tissue sections of 2-5µm thickness)

Rubber cement – Weldtite Vulcanising Rubber Solution

Safety goggles

Scalpel

Scissors

Slide drying racks

Thermal cycler – MJC Research PTC- 100 and PTC-200 Peltier Thermal Cyclers

Transmitted light microscope (Zeiss)

Fine tweezers (2 pairs)

Water bath – Grant Instruments (Cambridge)

Recipes

Biotin- and Avidin-conjugated antibodies

Store antibodies as 20µl aliquots at 4°C in sterile eppendorf tubes. Do not freeze.

Texas Red Avidin DCS (Biotek/Vector Laboratories Cat #A-2016).

Add 0.5ml of MilliQ water to 1mg lyophilised antibody for a final concentration of 2mg/ml.

Fluorescein Avidin DCS (Cell sorter grade), (Biotek/Vector Laboratories Cat #A-2011).

2mg/ml stock solution aliquotted at 20µl and stored in the dark at 4°C. Dilute 1:400 in 4xSSC/1% BSA immediately prior to use.

Biotinylated goat anti-avidin D (Biotek/Vector Laboratories Cat #BA0300).

Add 1ml of MilliQ water to 0.5mg lyophilised antibody for a final concentration of 0.5mg/ml.

Bovine Serum albumin (BSA)

1% BSA in 4xSSC. Dissolve 0.25g of BSA (Sigma A-7030) in 25ml 4xSSC pH 7.0. Store at 4°C for up to 1 month.

FITC– conjugated anti-digoxygenin antibodies

Store antibodies as 50µl aliquots at 4°C in sterile eppendorf tubes. Do not freeze.

Anti-digoxigenin-fluorescein, FAB fragments (Boehringer Mannheim Cat #1207741).

Add 1ml of MilliQ water to 200µg lyophilised antibody for a final concentration of 0.2mg/ml.

Rabbit fluorescein anti-sheep IgG(H+L) (Biotek/Vector Laboratories Cat #FI-6000).

Add 1ml of MilliQ water to 1.5mg lyophilised antibody for a final concentration of 1.5mg/ml.

Goat fluorescein anti-rabbit IgG(H+L) (Biotek/Vector Laboratories Cat #FI-1000).

Add 1ml of MilliQ water to 1.5mg lyophilised antibody for a final concentration of 1.5mg/ml.

Ethanol 100% Molecular biology grade.

Ethanol 80% Mix ethanol absolute (molecular biology grade) and distilled water in a 4:1 ratio (v/v).

Ethanol 70% Mix ethanol absolute (molecular biology grade) and distilled water in a 7:3 ratio (v/v).

Hydrochloric acid (HCl)

0.2M HCl. Add 2.4ml of 5N HCl to 60mls of MilliQ water.

0.01N HCl. Add 1mL of 5N HCl to 499mLs of distilled water. Store at room temperature for up to 1 year.

Phosphate buffered saline (PBS)

1xPBS. Ca^{++} and Mg^{++} free. Dissolve 8.0g sodium chloride, 0.2g potassium chloride, 2.89g $Na_2HPO_4.12H_2O$ and 0.2g KH_2PO_4 in order in 750ml of MilliQ water. Adjust the volume to 1 litre and autoclave. Store at room temperature.

Pre-treatment reagents for paraffin embedded tissue – Zymed (Invitrogen) Spot-light™HER2 CISH kit (84-0146)

Reagent A. 1 litre of heat pretreatment solution, pH 7.0 (Ready-To-Use).

Reagent B. 5 ml of enzyme pretreatment reagent (Ready-To-Use).

Saline sodium citrate (SSC)

20xSSC (7.0). Dissolve 175.3g sodium chloride and 88.2g trisodium citrate in 800ml MilliQ water. (or use SSC that comes with the Vysis kits; add 4 bottles to make 1L), pH to 7.0 and adjust the final volume to 1 litre. Autoclave and store at room temperature.

4xSSC (pH7.0). Add 200ml of 20xSSC to 700ml MilliQ water. pH to 7.0 and adjust the final volume to 1 litre. Autoclave and store at room temperature.

4XSSC/0.05% Tween20. Add 500µl Tween20 to 1 litre of 4xSSC. Mix well.

2XSSC/0.1% NP40. Add 1mL of NP40 to 1L of 2XSSC (pH7.0)

2xSSC (pH7.0). Add 100ml 20xSSC (pH 7.0) to 800ml MilliQ water. pH to 7.0 and adjust the final volume to 1 litre. Autoclave and store at room temperature.

1xSSC (pH 7.0). Add 50ml of 20xSSC (pH 7.0) to 950ml of milliQ water. Adjust the pH to 7.0, autoclave and store at room temperature.

0.4XSSC/0.3% NP40 (Quickwash buffer). Add 20ml of 20xSSC and 3ml of NP40 to 900ml MilliQ water. Adjust the pH to 7.0 and final volume to 1 litre. Store at room temperature.

Caution

All reagents are potentially hazardous. Appropriate safety procedures must be followed when handling these materials. Avoid contact with skin and mucous membranes, and heating of slides should be performed in a fume hood, as formalin fixed specimens may produce toxic fumes when heated during processing. For more information consult the Hazardous Substances Data Bank (HSDB) - http://toxnet.nlm.nih.gov/cgi-bin/sis/htmlgen?HSDB.

Formamide: perform steps involving formamide in hood to avoid inhalation of fumes

Xylene: perform steps involving xylene in hood to avoid inhalation of fumes

Commercial probes and hybridisation buffer solutions: Wear gloves at all times, and when co-denaturing probes use a fume hood, as formamide may be present in probe mixtures and give off toxic fumes.

Author details

Lisa Duffy[1], Liangtao Zhang[1], Donald R. Love[1,2] and Alice M. George[1*]

*Address all correspondence to: AliceG@adhb.govt.nz

1 LabPlus, Auckland City Hospital, Auckland, New Zealand

2 School of Biological Sciences, The University of Auckland, New Zealand

References

[1] Pfeifer, J. D. (2006). *Molecular Genetic Testing in Surgical Pathology,* Lippincott Williams and Wilkens, 474.

[2] Vorasanova, S. G., Yurov, Y. B., & Iourov, I. Y. (2010). Human interphase chromosomes: a review of available molecular cytogenetic technologies. *Molecular Cytogenetics,* 3(1), 1-15.

[3] Maierhofer, C., Gangnus, R., Diebold, J., & Speicher, M. R. (2003). Multicolour deconvolution microscopy of thick biological specimens. *Am. J. Path.,* 162(2), 373-379.

[4] Ventura, R. A., Martin-Subero, J. I., Jones, M., Mc Parland, J., Gesk, S., Mason, D. Y., & Siebert, R. (2006). FISH Analysis for the Detection of Lymphoma-Associated Chromosomal Abnormalities in Routine Paraffin-Embedded Tissue. *J. Med. Diagn.,* 8(2), 141-151.

[5] George, T. I., Wrede, J. E., Bangs, C. D., Cherry, A. M., Warnke, R. A., & Arber, D. A. (2005). Low-Grade B-Cell Lymphomas With Plasmacytic Differentiation Lack PAX5 Gene Rearrangements. *J. Med. Diag.,* 7(3), 346-351.

[6] Naeim, F., Rao, P. N., Song, S., & Grody, W. W. (2008). Principles of Molecular Techniques. *In: Naeim F, Rao PN, Song S, Grody WW, editors. Hematopathology: Morphology, Immunophenotype, Cytogenetics and Molecular Approaches*, Elsevier Inc., Chapter 4, 72-74.

[7] Solovei, I., Grasser, F., & Lanctôt, C. (2007). FISH on Histological Sections. *Cold Spring Harb. Protoc.*, doi:10.1101/pdb.prot4729.

[8] Varella-Garcia, M. (2006). Stratification of non-small cell lung cancer patients for therapy with epidermal growth factor receptor inhibitors: the EGFR fluorescence in situ hybridization assay. *Diagnostic Pathology*, 1, 19 .

[9] Kaeda, S. (2009). Molecular Pathology and Genetic Testing from the Perspective of a Commercial Laboratory. *Connection*, 7-11.

[10] Srinivasan, S., Sedmak, D., & Jewell, S. (2002). Effect of fixatives and tissue processing on the content and integrity of nucleic acids. *Am. J. Path.*, 161(6), 1961-1971.

[11] Barch, M. J., Knutsen, T., & Spurbeck, J. (1997). Molecular Cytogenetics: Definitions, Clinical Aspects, and Protocols. *In: The AGT Cytogenetics Laboratory Manual* (Third Edition), Lippincott-Raven, Chapter 13, 557-595.

[12] Thompson, C., Le Boit, P. E., Nederlof, P. M., & Gray, J. W. (1994). Thick-section fluorescence in situ hybridization on formalin-fixed, paraffin embedded archival tissue provides a histogenetic profile. *Am. J. Path.*, 144(2), 237-243.

[13] Iourov, I. Y., Soloviev, I. V., Vorsanova, S. G., Monakhov, V. V., & Yurov, Y. B. (2005). An approach for quantitative assessment of fluorescence in situ hybridization (FISH) signals for applied human molecular cytogenetics. *J. Histo. & Cyto.*, 53(3), 401-408.

[14] Swerdlow, S. H., Campo, E., Harris, N. L., Jaffe, E. S., Pileri, S. A., Stein, H., Thiele, J., & Vardiman, J. W. (2008). *WHO classification of tumours of Haematopoeitc and Lymphoid Tissues* (4th Edition), International Agency for Research on Cancer (IARC), 220-226.

Chapter 10

Quality Control of Biomarkers: From the Samples to Data Interpretation

F. G. Ravagnani, D. M. Saidemberg, A. L. C. Faria,
S. B. Sartor, D. N. Oliveira and R. R. Catharino

Additional information is available at the end of the chapter

1. Introduction

The recent advances in biotechnology and the improved understanding of disease's mechanisms and pathophsyology have strongly shifted the treatment paradigm of empiric knowledge to targeted therapy. Science has enhanced its ability to guide application of new and existing treatments with development, assay verification, biological validation and application of biomarkers; however, in order to be successful, it is needed a thorough understanding of the relationship between the choice of a biomarker and its influence on the treatment effects. [1]

Current biochemical and molecular biological knowledge states that genetic information flows from genomic DNA to mRNA transcripts, which are then translated to proteins; this class of molecules, which also include enzymes, directly influence the concentrations of their substrates and products, which are integrating parts in several tightly-controlled metabolic pathways. Finally, the existence and multiple interactions of these low-molecular weight metabolites within a cell, tissue, or organism, generates a phenotype. [2]

Metabolome, the link between phenotype and genotype, is the last comprehensive grouping for downstream products of the genome and contemplates the total complement of all the low-molecular weight molecules (metabolites) in a cell, tissue, or organism, required for growth, maintenance, or basal function in any given specific physiological state. [3] The potential size of the metabolome is arguable, as studies suggest more and more that an important role is played by residing microflora and its metabolic products. [2]

The monitoring of metabolite changes has been the primary indicator of disease, and has made it possible to diagnose it in individuals. For that reason, the measurement of metabolites has become an essential part of clinical practice. Employing a wide range of biological fluids, such as blood (including both plasma and serum), saliva, cerebrospinal fluid (CSF), synovial fluid, urine, semen, and tissue homogenates have ensured the widespread use of metabolites as a very powerful diagnostic tool. [4]

Despite significant advances in analytical technologies the past few years, the discovery of metabolomic biomarkers in biological fluids still remains a challenge. As discussed, metabolome plays an important role in biological systems, hence, are attractive candidates to understand disease phenotypes. [5-6] It represents a diverse group of low-molecular weight structures including lipids, amino acids, peptides, nucleic acids, organic acids, vitamins, thiols, carbohydrates and a few others. [7]

Biomarkers are defined as "characteristics that are objectively measured and evaluated as indicators of normal biological processes, pathogenic processes or pharmacological responses to therapeutic intervention". They can be categorized as biomarkers of exposure, biomarkers of effect and biomarkers of susceptibility. [8] Those characteristics are informative for clinical outcome and can be broadly understood as prognostic or predictive biomarkers. [9-10]

Along the variety of chemical classes and physical properties that constitute metabolites, as well as the dynamic range of metabolite concentrations across large orders of magnitude, it becomes clear why it is necessary to employ an extensive array of analytical techniques in metabolomic research, for it represents a comprehensive method for metabolite assessment. [11-12]

Enabling the parallel assessment of the levels of a broad number of endogenous and exogenous metabolites, it has been demonstrated to have great impact on investigation of physiological status, diseases diagnosis, biomarker discovery and identification of disrupted pathways due to disease or treatment. [13-14]

2. Mass Spectrometry and Biomarkers

2.1. Mass spectrometry in metabolomics

Nowadays, mass spectrometry is one of the most promising approaches for quantifying and qualifying known and unknown specific molecules within a very complex sample, and for elucidating the structure and chemical properties of different compounds. A mass spectrometer consists of three major components: (1) Ion Source: For producing gaseous ions from the substance being studied, some examples are electron impact (EI), chemical ionization (CI), electrospray ionization (ESI), atmospheric pressure chemical ionization (APCI), atmospheric pressure photon ionization (APPI), thermospray ionization (TSI), among others; (2) Analyzer: For resolving or separating ions according to their mass-to-charge ratios, some analyzer examples are: quadrupole, time of flight, ion traps, Fourier transform ion cyclotron resonance, orbitrap, among others; (3) Detector system: For detecting the ions and recording the relative abundance of each of the resolved ionic species, for example: electron multiplier, microchannel plate detector, Daly detector, Faraday cup, among others. The mass spectrometry technique relies on the capacity of converting neutral molecules into gaseous ions, with or without fragmentation, which are then characterized by their mass to charge ratios (m/z) and relative abundances. The introduction of a sample into the system, which can be a gas chromatography or liquid chromatography system is necessary to allow the study of different structures and ionic forms.

Historically, most studies with metabolites have been performed with a combination of high resolution capillary gas chromatography, combined with electron impact ionization mass spectrometry (GC-MS). This configuration allowed, for decades, the separation and identification of key micromolecules from complex mixtures, including fatty acids, amino acids, and organic acids in biofluids, generating diagnostic information for several metabolic disorders in qualitative and quantitative pathways [15-16].

Despite its age, GC is still a very useful and informative technique that seems to be far away from retirement; however, there are some limitations in relation to the size and metabolite types that can be analyzed by this technique, and the extensive sample preparation for this purpose. This resulted in the use of nuclear magnetic resonance (NMR) as a tool for metabolite profiling; however, besides the richness of information about molecular structures obtained by this approach, NMR has low sensitivity, allowing just the most abundant compounds to be identified. In contraposition of GC-MS and NMR, the mass spectrometry with a high performance liquid chromatographic system (LC-MS), and the possibility of tandem mass spectrometry (LC-MS) as post-source fragmentation, especially after soft ionization techniques, offers the possibility of analyzing a wide range of polar and medium polarity compounds with good quantification, sensibility and reproducibility [16].

According to Birkemeier et al. (2005) [17], the metabolomic approaches are in dynamic development and a diversity of synonyms have been suggested, such as metabonomics, metabolite profiling (fingerprinting), among others. Several analytical platforms have been introduced, including spectroscopies using diverse electromagnetic wavelengths, like metabolite profiling with the use of infrared spectroscopy (IR), near infrared (NIR), or ultraviolet (UV), besides gas chromatography coupled to mass spectrometry (GC-MS), liquid chromatography with electrospray ionization mass spectrometry (LC-ESIMS), capillary electrophoresis with mass spectrometry (CE-MS) or liquid chromatography with nuclear magnetic resonance (LC-NMR), and these are only a few examples of the technologies involved with metabolomic studies. There is not a single approach to analyze the wide range of chemically different biomolecules, but it is important to choose the technology that fits better to your target molecules [17].

Hollywood et al. (2006) [18] have summarized the main metabolomic strategies:

1. Metabolomic target analysis, which is a more restrict approach. For example, the metabolites originated from a particular enzymatic system after any kind of biotic or abiotic disturbance.

2. Metabolite profiling, which is focused in a group of specific metabolites, for example, lipids associated to a determined metabolic pathway; or related with clinical and pharmaceutical analyses, to map drug metabolism in an organism. This strategy can be also applied with

other approaches, e.g.: *a.* "Metabolite fingerprinting", this approach is used in order to classify samples based both in their biological relevance to the organism, and in their origin. The fingerprinting technology is fast, but not necessarily gives specific information about metabolites. *b.* "Metabolite footprinting", exometabolome or secretome, this is similar approach to the fingerprinting, however the target now is a non-invasive analysis, in order to identify the extracellular metabolites. This technique is generally employed to the study of culture cells, with the advantage of not needing to extract the metabolites, and not having to interrupt the metabolism in a given moment before the analysis. Otherwise, this technique can be used for analysing the secretion of any organism, including the secretome of human embryos before *in vitro* fertilization, with the purpose of finding viable embryos and general disease biomarkers.

3. Metabolomics itself, which is the comprehensible analysis of the whole metabolome (all the mensurable metabolites), under a specific analysis condition. This term is frequently mistaken with metabonomics, a technique that focus in a wider profile of metabolites involved with different metabolic pathways interacting under the effect of some external stimuli, including diseases, drugs, toxins, among other.

2.2. MALDI AND MALDI-Imaging

Matrix-assisted laser desorption/ionization (MALDI) is an ionization method with common applications to high mass biomolecules, being a key technique in mass spectrometry (MS), and more traditionally to the proteomics field. MALDI-MS is extremely sensitive, easy-to-apply, and relatively tolerant to contaminants [19]. Its high-speed data acquisition and large-scale, off-line sample preparation has made it once again the focus for high-throughput proteomic analyses. These and other unique properties of MALDI offer new possibilities in applications such as rapid molecular profiling and imaging by MS [19].

More recently, there is a growing focus on the use of MALDI ionization system to the analysis of small molecules, however it is important to take into consideration that the coupling of LC-MALDI is a more delicate issue than the coupling of HPLC with other ionization sources such as ESI, because MALDI, based on desorption of molecules from a solid surface layer, is a priori not compatible with LC or CE [20]. A simple alternative to this limitation is the automatic deposition of fractions from a chromatographic separation on a MALDI-TOF target. More advanced techniques have been developed recently: electrospray deposition, electrically mediated deposition, rotating ball inlet, continuous vacuum deposition, and continuous off-line atmospheric-pressure deposition. The current interfacing improvements will surely expand the use of LC-MALDI in the metabolomic area [20,21].

Another good advantage of MALDI ionization is the possibility of obtaining tissue imaging. This is a new technology that allows the simultaneous investigation of the content and temporal/spatial distribution of molecules within a tissue section, enabling to find the exact localization of any biomarker of interest for the prediction of pathologies and for the discovery of future secondary complications originated from different metabolic disease [22].

One of the most common applications for this new approach besides the well described proteomics application is the identification of membrane lipids, which have been successfully analyzed by different authors for several biological tissues. MS imaging of cryosections of mature cotton embryos revealed a distinct, heterogeneous distribution of molecular species of triacylglycerols and phosphatidylcholines, the major storage and membrane lipid classes in cotton embryos. Other lipids were imaged, including phosphatidylethanolamines, phosphatidic acids, sterols, and gossypol, indicating the broad range of metabolites and applications for this chemical visualization approach [23].

There are several possibilities for MALDI imaging technology; however applications to the study of small molecule biomarkers are becoming an interesting novel possibility for this ionization method, mainly when considering the development of new matrices which generate low noise levels in the low m/z range of the spectra. Bnabdellah et al. (2009) [24] have described the detection and identification of 13 primary metabolites (AMP, ADP, ATP, UDP-GlcNAc, among others), directly from rat brain sections by chemical mass spectrometry imaging. Matrix-assisted laser desorption/ionization tandem mass spectrometry (MALDI-MS/MS) was combined with 9-aminoacridine as a powerful matrix in this study.

Metabolite distribution via imaging mass spectrometry (IMS) is an increasingly utilized tool in the field of neurochemistry. As most previous IMS studies analyzed the relative abundances of larger metabolite species, it is important to expand its application to smaller molecules, such as neurotransmitters [25]. However, it has been pointed out two technical problems that must be resolved to achieve neurotransmitter imaging, the lower concentrations of bioactive molecules, compared with those of membrane lipids, require higher sensitivity and/or signal-to-noise (S/N) ratios in signal detection, and the rapid molecular turnover of the neurotransmitters; thus, tissue preparation procedures should be performed carefully to minimize *postmortem* changes [25].

Furthermore, matrix-assisted laser desorption/ionization (MALDI) imaging mass spectrometry has attracted great interest for monitoring drug delivery and metabolism. Since this emerging technique enables simultaneous imaging of many types of metabolite molecules, MALDI-IMS can visualize and distinguish the parent drug and its metabolites. As another important advantage, changes in endogenous metabolites in response to drug administration can be mapped and evaluated in tissue sections [26].

Another applications of MALDI and MALDI imaging to the study of small molecule biomarkers are the use of the method for detecting drug-related degradation products [27] analysis of drugs from intact biological samples and crude extracts, a method that can be applied to rapid drug screening and precise identification of toxic substances in poisoning cases and *postmortem* examinations [28], the application of MALDI imaging mass spectrometry to the study of elevated nigral levels of dynorphin neuropeptides in L-DOPA-induced dyskinesia in rat model of Parkinson's disease [29], it is also possible to point out the recent advances in the field of lipidomics and oxidative lipidomics based on the applications of mass spectrometry and imaging mass spectrometry as they relate to studies of phospholipids in traumatic brain injury [30] and the using of proteomic or lipidomic signatures for discovery and spatial mapping of molecular disturbances within the microenvironment of chronic wounds using MALDI imaging technology [31].

2.3. Orbitrap

The orbitrap mass analyzer is a powerful and relatively new technology, which operates in the absence of any magnetic or rf fields. In this analyzer, ion stability is achieved only due to ions orbiting around an axial electrode. Orbiting ions also perform harmonic oscillations along the electrode with frequency proportional to (m/z)-1/2. These oscillations are detected using image current detection and are transformed into mass spectra using fast FT, similarly to FT-ICR [32]. In an orbitrap, ions are injected tangentially into the electric field between the electrodes and trapped because their electrostatic attraction to the inner electrode is balanced by centrifugal forces. Thus, ions cycle around the central electrode in rings. In addition, the ions also move back and forth along the axis of the central electrode. Therefore, ions of a specific mass-to-charge ratio move in rings which oscillate along the central spindle. The frequency of these harmonic oscillations is independent of the ion velocity and is inversely proportional to the square root of the mass-to-charge ratio (m/z). The entire instrument operates in LC/MS mode (1 spectrum/s) with nominal mass resolving power of 60 000 and uses automatic gain control to provide high-accuracy mass measurements, within 2 ppm using internal standards and within 5 ppm with external calibration. The maximum resolving power exceeds 100 000 (Full Width at Half-Maximum – FWHM). Rapid, automated data-dependent capabilities enable real-time acquisition of up to three high-mass accuracy MS/MS spectra per second [32,33].

Some recent applications of this mass analyzer in the search of biomarkers include the on-tissue digestion of proteins followed by detection of the resulting peptides, taking advantage of the high resolution obtained. Trypsin was applied by a spraying device for MALDI imaging experiments in a LTQ-Orbitrap mass spectrometer. The mass accuracy under imaging conditions was better than 3 ppm RMS. This allowed for confident identification of tryptic peptides by comparison with liquid chromatography/electrospray ionization tandem mass spectrometry (LC/ESI-MS/MS) measurements of an adjacent mouse brain section [34].

Another possible application for this mass analyzer is the monitoring of metabolites in human urine, approximately 970 metabolite signals with repeatable peak areas could be putatively identified in human urine, by elemental composition assignment within a 3 ppm mass error. The ability of the methodology for the verification of non-molecular ions, which arise from adduct formation, and the possibility of distinguishing isomers could also be demonstrated. Careful examination of the raw data and the use of masses for predicted metabolites produced an extension of the metabolite list [35].

Orbitrap mass analyzer has been also successfully applied to the monitoring of environmental contamination. The use of pharmaceuticals in livestock production is a potential source of surface water, groundwater and soil contamination. A rapid, versatile and selective multi-method was developed and validated for screening pharmaceuticals and fungicides compounds, in surface and groundwater, in one single full-scan MS method, using benchtop U-HPLC-Exactive Orbitrap MS at 50,000 (FWHM) resolution. It demonstrates that the ultra-high resolution and reliable mass accuracy of Exactive Orbitrap MS permits the detection of pharmaceutical residues in a concentration range of 10-100 ng.L^{-1}, applying a post-target screening approach, in the multi-method conditions [36].

Other recent applications of orbitrap mass analyzer in the search of biomarkers include: the analysis of serotonin and related compounds in urine and the identification of a potential biomarker for attention deficit hyperactivity/hyperkinetic disorder [37,38]; the quantitative profiling of phosphatidylethanol molecular species, which are a group of aberrant phospholipids formed in cell membranes in the presence of ethanol by the catalytic action of the enzyme phospholipase D on phosphatidylcholine in human blood, by liquid chromatography high resolution mass spectrometry performed on an LTQ-Orbitrap XL hybrid mass spectrometer equipped with an electrospray ionization source operated in negative ion mode [39]; frozen sections (12 μm thick) of an *ex vivo* tissue sample set comprising primary colorectal adenocarcinoma samples and colorectal adenocarcinoma liver metastasis samples were analyzed by negative ion desorption electrospray ionization (DESI), with spatial resolution of 100 μm using a computer-controlled DESI imaging stage mounted on a high resolution orbitrap mass spectrometer. DESI-IMS data were found to predominantly feature complex lipids, including phosphatidyl-inositols, phophatidyl-ethanolamines, phosphatidyl-serines, phosphatidyl-ethanolamine plasmalogens, phosphatidic acids, phosphatidyl-glycerols, ceramides, sphingolipids, and sulfatides among others, were identified based on their exact mass and MS/MS fragmentation spectra [40]; among several other applications of this promising technology to the discovery of important biomarkers in different biological systems, taking advantage of the high resolution and speed for LC-MS of this new analytical system.

2.4. Gas Chromatography

Gas chromatography (GC) can be understood as the chromatographic technique in which a gas is the mobile phase and, since 1952, when the first paper in this field was published, GC has always been considered simple, fast and applicable to the separation of many volatile materials, especially petrochemicals, for which distillation was the preferred method of separation at that time. Now, GC is a very important technique, and global market for instruments is estimated around to US$ 1 billion or over 30,000 instruments annually [41].

Chromatography is the separation process of a mixture into individual components; through the separation process, each component in the sample can be identified (qualitatively) and measured (quantitatively). There are several kinds of chromatographic techniques with theirs corresponding instruments, and gas chromatography is one of those techniques. GC is used for compounds that are thermally stable and volatile - or that can become volatilizable. Because of its simplicity, sensitivity and effectiveness in separating components, GC is one of the most important tools in chemistry. The principle of basic operation of this instrument involves the evaporation of the sample in a heated inlet port (injector), separation of the components in a mixture employing a prepared column specially and detection of each component by a specific detector. At the end of the process, the amplified detector signals are often recorded and evaluated by integrator software, calculating the analytical results. The sample is introduced into a stream of inert gas, the carrier gas, and transported through the column by its flow. The column can be a packed column or a capillary column, depending on the properties of the sample. As the gas flow passes through the column, the components of the sample move in velocities that are influenced by the degree of interaction of each component with the stationary phase in the column. Consequently, the different components are separated. Since the processes are temperature-dependent, the column is usually contained in a thermostat-controlled oven. Once that the components are eluted from the column, they can be quantified by a suitable detector and/or be collected for further analysis. There are some types of detectors and the choice of the ones depends on the type of components that will be detected and measured. The most common detectors are: flame ionization detectors (FIDs), thermal conductivity detectors (TCDs), electron capture detectors (ECDs), alkali flame ionization detectors – also called nitrogen/phosphorous detectors (NPDs), flame photometric detectors (FPDs) and photo ionization detectors (PIDs). Several of these are further described in separate leaflets [41,42].

GC is a widely used method for separating and analyzing organic compounds. There are a variety of applications for gas chromatography in every laboratory and in different processes within several industries. In chemical, petrochemical and pharmaceutical industries we can have measurements of any kind of organic compounds, such as process control as well as product control. Also for environmental measurements: aromatic pollutants in air and water, detection and measurement of pesticides, etc. Beside the wide application of GC, there are a few examples of applications on which this analysis technique plays an important role [43,44,45,46].

The detection of reliable biomarkers is a major research activity within the field of proteomics and a growing trend on metabolomics. A biomarker can be a single molecule or set of molecules that can be used to differentiate between normal and diseased states and can be separated and detected by Gas Chromatography - Mass Spectrometry (GC/MS). This combined technique is used to identify the presence of different substances in a given sample.

Kuhara et al. (2011) [47] has used a GC/MS-based approach to investigate the metabolome in urine of patients whom had been previously diagnosed with citrin deficiency. In this noninvasive technique, urine metabolic profiling provided should assist in the rapid and more reliable differential chemical diagnosis of citrin deficiency from other hyperammonemic syndromes.

Another application of GC/MS in biomarker analysis is its application on the studies of volatile organic compounds (VOCs). These compounds are exhaled in breath and provide valuable information about the human health status. The composition of the breath is variable and depends on the disease's characteristics; for example, a sweetened smell indicates diabetes, while the odor of rotten eggs, which are caused by sulfur-containing compounds, suggests liver problems [48,49]. Rudnicka (2011) [50] employed solid phase micro-extraction technique and gas chromatography coupled to time of flight in mass spectrometry (GC–TOF/MS) for the analysis of VOCs on exhaled air from patients with lung cancer and healthy persons. The total number of identified compounds in breathing samples equal 55 and the compound that enables as an indication of lung cancer was isopropyl alcohol.

These studies show how highly important and relevant are the studies on the use of chromatographic techniques for biomarker analysis and identification. It shows a wide range of applications in a field not yet fully developed, which still may be a very suitable area for new ideas and uses for the next couple decades.

3. Statistical and chemometrical analysis of biomarkers

In metabolomics, as well as in other branches of science and technology, there is a steady trend towards the use of more variables (properties) to characterize observations (e.g., samples, experiments, time points). Often, these measurements can be arranged into a data table, where each row constitutes an observation and the columns represent the variables or factors we have measured (e.g., wavelength, mass number, chemical shift, etc). This development generates huge and complex data tables, which are hard to summarize and overview without appropriate tools. Recently, with development of "omics" technologies (metabolomics, proteomics, foodomics, genomics, etc), the adoption of chemometric methods has been playing a very important role in planning and analyzing the obtained results. That includes efficient and robust methods for modeling and analysis of complex chemical or biological data tables that produce interpretable and reliable models capable of handling incomplete, noisy, and collinear data structures. These methods include principal component analysis (PCA) and partial least squares (PLS). It is also completely important to emphasize that chemometrics also provides a straightforward way to collect relevant information through statistical experimental design (SED) [51,52,53].

Multivariate statistical analysis such as Principal Components Analysis (PCA) is probably the most widely used technique for analyzing metabolomics. PCA technique is robust and objective and it is an appropriate way to reduce data sets containing high numbers of variables. By reducing the number of original variables to a smaller number of independent variables, this approach highlights fundamental differences between groups of variables. PCA has been extensively used in metabonomics literature. Despite apparent satisfying published results, the known large sensitivity of PCA to noise can suggest that improvements are expected with more robust methods to identify biomarkers in noisy data. Moreover, the traditional use of PCA remains highly questionable: biomarkers are identified from the loadings of the two first principal components, while the two first components do not necessarily contain the most relevant variations between altered and normal spectra. Sometimes, the results of the initial unsupervised analysis are confirmed by a second supervised analysis. This one employs classification methods as Partial Least Squares (PLS), SIMCA and neural networks, allowing firstly to separate normal and altered spectra, and secondly to identify more robust biomarkers [54,55].

Other data analysis methods frequently employed for disease diagnosis and biomarker identification in metabolomics are Univariate Testing, Soft independent modeling of class analogy (SIMCA), Linear discriminant analysis (LDA), Partial least squares discriminant analysis (PLS-DA), Orthogonal projection to latent structures discriminant analysis, (OPLS-DA), Neural networks (NN), Self organizing maps (SOM) and Support vector machines (SVM). Regardless of the chosen method, both statistical and biological validations are critical. Multivariate methods are of special importance to metabolomics since one biomarker often will not be sufficiently specific for a given condition by itself. There is a wide range of methods and it is natural that this can seem confusing to the non-specialist. The literature has already shown in previous works that it is more important that the chosen method is used correctly than the methodology itself. The reason for this is that all methods are data-driven, and since the parameter definition is through pre-processing, the contained features are static. Many statistical methods will highlight the same metabolites with similar classification ability. It is clear, however, that pre-processing and scaling of the data can lead to dramatically different results, both with regard to chosen biomarkers and classification ability of the model [53].

4. Bibliography

Aitio A, Apostoli P. Quality assurance in biomarker measurement. Toxicol Lett. 1995 May; 77(1-3):195-204.

Aitio A, Bernard A, Fowler BA, Nordberg G. Biological Monitoring and Biomerkers. Handbook on the Toxicology of Metals. Third Edition. 2007; Chapter 4: 65-78.

Christians U, Klepacki J, Shokati T, Klawitter J, Klawitter J. Mass spectrometry-based multiplexing for the analysis of biomarkers in drug development and clinical diagnostics – How much is too much ? Microchem. J. 2012, *doi:10.1016/j.microc.2012.02.001*

Hendriks MMWB, Eeuwijk FA, Jellema RH, Westerhuis JA, Reijmers TH, Hoefsloot HCJ, Smilde AK. Data-processing strategies for metabolomics studies. Trends in Analytical Chemistry. 2011; 30 (10): 1685-98.

Holland NT, Smith MT, Eskenazi B, Bastaki M. Biological sample collection and processing for molecular epidemiological studies. Mutat Res. 2003 Jun;543(3):217-34.

Lampe JW, Rock CL. Biomarkers and biological indicators of chance. Nutrition in the Prevention and Treatment of Disease. 2001; Chapter 10:139-153.

Lee JW, Hall M. Method validation of protein biomarkers in support of drug development or clinical diagnosis/prognosis. J Chromatogr B Analyt Technol Biomed Life Sci. 2009 May 1;877(13):1259-71.

Roux A, Lison D, Junot C, Heilier JF. Applications of liquid chromatography coupled to mass spectrometry-based metabolomics in clinical chemistry and toxicology: A review. Clin Biochem. Jan;44(1):119-35.

Author details

F. G. Ravagnani[1,2], D. M. Saidemberg[1], A. L. C. Faria[1], S. B. Sartor[1], D. N. Oliveira[1] and R. R. Catharino[1*]

*Address all correspondence to: rrc@fcm.unicamp.br

1INNOVARE Biomarkers Laboratory, Department of Clinical Pathology, School of Medical Sciences, University of Campinas, Brazil

2 Laboratory of Bioenergetics, Department of Clinical Pathology, School of Medical Sciences, University of Campinas, Brazil

References

[1] Lee, J., et al. (2011). Proteomics and biomarkers in clinical trials for drug development. 74(12), 2632-264.

[2] Roberts, L. D., Souza, A. L., Gerszten, R. E., & Clish, C. B. (2012). Targeted Metabolomics. *Current Protocols in Molecular Biology*, Unit 30.2.

[3] Goodacre, R. (2003). Metabolic Profiling: Its Role in Biomarker Discovery and Gene Function Analysis. Kluwer Academic Publishers, London.

[4] Ryan, D., Robards, K., Prenzler, P. D., & Kendall, M. (2011). Recent and potential developments in the analysis of urine: a review. *Anal Chim Acta*, 684, 8-20.

[5] Koulman, A., Lane, G. A., Harrison, S. J., & Volmer, D. A. (2009). From differentiating metabolites to biomarkers. *Anal Bioanal Chem*, 394, 663-70.

[6] de la Luz-Hernández, K. R., Rojas-del Calvo, L., Rabasa-Legón, Y., Lage-Castellanos, A., Castillo-Vitlloch, A., Díaz, J., et al. (2008). Metabolic and proteomic study of NS0 myeloma cell line following the adaptation to protein-free medium. *J Proteomics*, 71, 133-47.

[7] Ryan, D., Robards, K., Prenzler, P. D., & Kendall, M. (2011). Recent and potential developments in the analysis of urine: a review. *Anal Chim Acta*, 684, 8-20.

[8] Atkinson, A. J. C. W., De Gruttola, V., De Mets, D. L., Downing, G. J., Hoth, D. F., Oates, J. A., et al. (2001). Biomarkers and Surrogate Endpoints: Preferred Definitions and Conceptual Framework. *Clin Pharmacol Ther*, 69, 89-95.

[9] Simon, R., & Altman, D. G. (1994). Statistical aspects of prognostic factor studies in oncology. *Br J Cancer*, 69, 979-85.

[10] Sargent, D. J., Conley, B. A., Allegra, C., & Collette, L. (2005). Clinical Trial designs for predictive marker validation in cancer treatment trials. *J Clin Oncol*, 23, 2020-7.

[11] Nicholson, J. K., & Lindon, J. C. (2008). Systems biology: metabonomics. *Nature*, 455, 1054-1056.

[12] Arakaki, A. K., Skolnick, J., & McDonald, J. F. (2008). Marker metabolites can be therapeutic targets as well. *Nature*, 456, 443.

[13] de la Luz-Hernández, K. R., Rojas-del Calvo, L., Rabasa-Legón, Y., Lage-Castellanos, A., Castillo-Vitlloch, A., Díaz, J., et al. (2008). Metabolic and proteomic study of NS0 myeloma cell line following the adaptation to protein-freemedium. *J Proteomics*, 71, 133-47.

[14] Schauer, N., Steinhauser, D., Strelkov, S., Schomburg, D., Allison, G., Moritz, T., Lundgren, K., Roessner-Tunali, U., Forbes, M. G., Willmitzer, L., Fernie, Ar., & Kopka, J. (2005). GC-MS libraries for the rapid identification of metabolites in complex biological samples. *FEBS Letters*, 579, 1332-1337.

[15] Want, E. J., O'maille, G., Smith, Brandon. T. R., Uritboonthai, W., Qin, C., Trauger, S. A., & Siuzdak, G. (2006). Solvent-Dependent Metabolite Distribution, Clustering, and Protein Extraction for Serum Profiling with Mass Spectrometry. *Anal Chem*, 78, 743-752.

[16] Birkemeyer, C., et al. (2005). Metabolome analysis: the potential of in vivo labeling with stable isotopes for metabolite profiling. *Trends Biotechnol*, 23, 28-33.

[17] Hollywood, K., Brison, D., & Goodacre, R. (2006). Metabolomic: current technologies and future trends. *Proteomics*, 6, 4716-4723.

[18] Cramer, R. (2009). MALDI MS. *Methods Mol Biol*, 564, 85-103.

[19] Villas-Bôas, S. G., Mas, S., Akesson, M., Smedsgaard, J., & Nielsen, J. (2005). Mass spectrometry in metabolome analysis. *Mass spectrometry reviews*, 24(5), 613-646.

[20] Wehr, T. (2003). Coupling liquid-phase separations and MALDI-MS. *LCGC North America*, 10, 974-982.

[21] Seeley, E. H., & Caprioli, R. M. (2011). MALDI imaging mass spectrometry of human tissue: method challenges and clinical perspectives Trends. *Biotechnol*, 29(3), 136-146.

[22] Horn, P. J., Korte, A. R., Neogi, P. B., Love, E., Fuchs, J., Strupat, K., Borisjuk, I., Shulaev, V., Lee, Y. J., & Chapman, K. D. (2012). Spatial mapping of lipids at cellular resolution in embryos of cotton. *Plant Cell*, 24(2), 622-36.

[23] Benabdellah, F., Touboul, D., Brunelle, A., & Laprévote, O. (2009). In situ primary metabolites localization on a rat brain section by chemical mass spectrometry imaging. *Anal Chem*, 81(13), 5557-60.

[24] Sugiura, Y., Zaima, N., Setou, M., Ito, S., & Yao, I. (2012). Visualization of acetylcholine distribution in central nervous system tissue sections by tandem imaging mass spectrometry. *Anal Bioanal Chem*, In press.

[25] Sugiura, Y., & Setou, M. (2010). Imaging mass spectrometry for visualization of drug and endogenous metabolite distribution: toward in situ pharmacometabolomes. *J Neuroimmune Pharmacol*, 5(1), 31-43.

[26] Huang, J. T., Hannah-Qiuhua, L., Szyszka, R., Veselov, V., Reed, G., Wang, X., Price, S., Alquier, L., & Vas, G. (2012). Molecular imaging of drug-eluting coronary stents: method development, optimization and selected applications. *J Mass Spectrom*, 47(2), 155-62.

[27] Kuwayama, K., Tsujikawa, K., Miyaguchi, H., Kanamori, T., Iwata, Y. T., & Inoue, H. (2012). Rapid, simple, and highly sensitive analysis of drugs in biological samples using thin-layer chromatography coupled with matrix-assisted laser desorption/ionization mass spectrometry. *Anal Bioanal Chem.*, 402(3), 1257-67.

[28] Ljungdahl, A., Hanrieder, J., Fälth, M., Bergquist, J., & Andersson, M. (2011). Imaging mass spectrometry reveals elevated nigral levels of dynorphin neuropeptides in L-DOPA-induced dyskinesia in rat model of Parkinson's disease. *PLoS One*, 6(9):e25653.

[29] Sparvero, L. J., Amoscato, A. A., Kochanek, P. M., Pitt, B. R., Kagan, V. E., & Bayir, H. (2010). Mass-spectrometry based oxidative lipidomics and lipid imaging: applications in traumatic brain injury. *J Neurochem.*, 115(6), 1322-36.

[30] Taverna, D., Nanney, L. B., Pollins, A. C., Sindona, G., & Caprioli, R. (2011). Multiplexed molecular descriptors of pressure ulcers defined by imaging mass spectrometry. *Wound Repair Regen.*, 19(6), 734-44.

[31] Makarov, A. (2000). Electrostatic Axially Harmonic Orbital Trapping: A High-Performance Technique of Mass Analysis. *Anal. Chem.*, 72 (6), 1156-1162.

[32] Makarov, A., Denisov, E., Kholomeev, A., Balschun, W., Lange, O., Strupat, K., & Horning, S. (2006). Performance Evaluation of a Hybrid Linear Ion Trap/Orbitrap Mass Spectrometer. *Anal. Chem.*, 78 (7), 2113-2120.

[33] Schober, Y., Guenther, S., Spengler, B., & Römpp, A. (2012). High-resolution matrix-assisted laser desorption/ionization imaging of tryptic peptides from tissue. *Rapid Commun Mass Spectrom.*, 26(9), 1141-6.

[34] Zhang, T., Creek, D. J., Barrett, M. P., Blackburn, G., & Watson, D. G. (2012). Evaluation of coupling reversed phase, aqueous normal phase, and hydrophilic interaction liquid chromatography with Orbitrap mass spectrometry for metabolomic studies of human urine. *Anal Chem.*, 84(4), 1994-2001.

[35] Chitescu, C. L., Oosterink, E., de Jong, J., & Stolker, L. A. A. (2012). Accurate mass screening of pharmaceuticals and fungicides in water by U-HPLC-Exactive Orbitrap MS. *Anal Bioanal Chem*, In press.

[36] Moriarty, M., Lee, A., O'Connell, B., Kelleher, A., Keeley, H., & Furey, A. (2011). Development of an LC-MS/MS method for the analysis of serotonin and related compounds in urine and the identification of a potential biomarker for attention deficit hyperactivity/hyperkinetic disorder. *Anal Bioanal Chem.*, 401(8), 2481-93.

[37] Moriarty, M., Lehane, M., O'Connell, B., Keeley, H., & Furey, A. (2012). Development of a nano-electrospray MSn method for the analysis of serotonin and related compounds in urine using a LTQ-orbitrap mass spectrometer. *Talanta*, 90, 1-11.

[38] Nalesso, A., Viel, G., Cecchetto, G., Mioni, D., Pessa, G., Favretto, D., & Ferrara, S. D. (2011). Quantitative profiling of phosphatidylethanol molecular species in human blood by liquid chromatography high resolution mass spectrometry. *J Chromatogr A.*, 1218(46), 8423-31.

[39] Gerbig, S., Golf, O., Balog, J., Denes, J., Baranyai, Z., Zarand, A., Raso, E., Timar, J., & Takats, Z. (2012). Analysis of colorectal adenocarcinoma tissue by desorption electrospray ionization mass spectrometric imaging. *Anal Bioanal Chem*, In press.

[40] McNair, H. M., & Miller, J. M. (2009). Basic gas chromatography. Hoboken, N.J., John Wiley & Sons.

[41] Barry, R. L. G. E. F. (2004). Modern Practice of Gas Chromatography. Hoboken, NJ, Wiley and Sons.

[42] Fenoll, J., Hellin, P., et al. (2007). Multiresidue method for analysis of pesticides in pepper and tomato by gas chromatography with nitrogen, Äìphosphorus detection. Food Chemistry, 105(2), 711-719.

[43] Shahdousti, P., Mohammadi, A., et al. (2007). Determination of valproic acid in human serum and pharmaceutical preparations by headspace liquid-phase microextraction gas chromatography-flame ionization detection without prior derivatization. Journal of Chromatography B-Analytical Technologies in the Biomedical and Life Sciences, 850(1-2), 128-133.

[44] Botalova, O., Schwarzbauer, J., et al. (2009). Identification and chemical characterization of specific organic constituents of petrochemical effluents. Water Res, 43(15), 3797-3812.

[45] Tran, K., Eide, D., et al. (2012). Finding of pesticides in fashionable fruit juices by LC,ÄìMS/MS and GC,ÄìMS/MS. Food Chemistry, 134(4), 2398-2405.

[46] Kuhara, T., Ohse, M., et al. (2011). A GC/MS-based metabolomic approach for diagnosing citrin deficiency. Analytical and Bioanalytical Chemistry, 400(7), 1881-1894.

[47] Deng, C., Zhang, J., et al. (2004). Determination of acetone in human breath by gas chromatography, Mass spectrometry and solid-phase microextraction with on-fiber derivatization. Journal of Chromatography B, 810(2), 269-275.

[48] Buszewski, B., Kesy, M., et al. (2007). Human exhaled air analytics: biomarkers of diseases. Biomed Chromatogr, 21(6), 553-566.

[49] Rudnicka, J., et al. (2011). Determination of volatile organic compounds as biomarkers of lung cancer by SPME-GC-TOF/MS and chemometrics. Journal of Chromatography B-Analytical Technologies in the Biomedical and Life Sciences, 879(30), 3360-3366.

[50] Lindon, J. C., Nicholson, J. K., et al. (2007). The handbook of metabonomics and metabolomics. Amsterdam; Oxford, Elsevier.

[51] Trygg, J., Holmes, E., et al. (2007). Chemometrics in metabonomics. Journal of Proteome Research, 6(2), 469-479.

[52] Madsen, R., Lundstedt, T., et al. (2010). Chemometrics in metabolomics--a review in human disease diagnosis. Anal Chim Acta, 659(1-2), 23-33.

[53] Holmes, E., & Antti, H. (2002). Chemometric contributions to the evolution of metabonomics: mathematical solutions to characterising and interpreting complex biological NMR spectra. Analyst., 127(12), 1549-1557.

[54] Rousseau, R., Govaerts, B., et al. (2008). Comparison of some chemometric tools for metabonomics biomarker identification. Chemometrics and Intelligent Laboratory Systems, 91(1), 54-66.

Chapter 11

The Investigation of Gene Regulation and Variation in Human Cancers and Other Diseases

Shihori Tanabe and Sun Ha Jee

Additional information is available at the end of the chapter

1. Introduction

Dynamic regulation of genes is an important part of the cell life cycle in health and disease. The regulation includes the variety and alteration of genome and gene expression, and the concept such as quality of genome will be useful to predict and assess the developmental stages of the cells, disease status and drug sensitivity. Recent technologies and worldwide sequencing projects have revealed 26,383 annotated genes in the 2.91-Gigabase human genome [1,2]. The main molecular functions of the annotated genes, as categorized by Gene Ontology (GO), are enzyme, signal transduction, nucleic acid binding, cell adhesion, chaperone, cytoskeletal structural protein, extracellular matrix, immunoglobulin, ion channel, motor, structural protein of muscle, protooncogene, select calcium binding protein, intracellular transporter, and transporter [1,3]. Despite a wealth of knowledge, the function of 42% of the annotated genes remains unknown [1]. When the human genome sequence was published in 2001 [1], there were a predicted 39,114 genes, of which 59% were of unknown function. According to the International Human Genome Sequencing Consortium, the number of identified genes is approximately 32,000, of which 51% show a match within InterPro, a database that integrates diverse information about protein families, domains, and functional sites [2-5]. In 2001, InterPro combined sequence and pattern information from four databases (PRINTS, PROSITE, Pfam, Prosite Profile); however, it now includes information from an additional eight databases (SMART, ProDom, PIRSF, SUPERFAMILY, PANTHER, CATH-Gene3D, TIGRFAM, and HAMAP) [2,4-16]. In [2], the InterPro entries are collapsed into 12 broad categories: cellular processes, metabolism, DNA replication/modification, transcription/translation, intracellular signaling, cell–cell communication, protein folding and degradation, transport, multifunctional proteins, cytoskeletal/structural, defense and immunity, and miscellaneous function. The rate of single nucleotide polymorphism (SNP) variation has been reported as 1 in 1250 base pairs [1] and more than 1.4 million SNPs have been identified [2] (Table 1).

Size of the genome	2.91 Gbp	[1]
Number of annotated genes	26,383	[1]
Main molecular functions of annotated genes	enzyme, signal transduction, nucleic acid binding, cell adhesion, chaperone, cytoskeletal structural protein, extracellular matrix, immunoglobulin, ion channel, motor, structural protein of muscle, protooncogene, select calcium binding protein, intracellular transporter, transporter	[1]
Percentage of annotated genes with unknown function	42%	[1]
Number of hypothetical and annotated genes	39,114	[1]
Percentage of hypothetical and annotated genes with unknown function	59%	[1]
Number of identified genes	approx. 32,000	[2]
Percentage of matches with InterPro	51%	[2]
Rate of SNP variation	1/1250 bp	[1]
SNPs identified	more than 1.4 million	[2]

Table 1. Genomic and gene characteristics revealed by the Human Genome Project.

Among the databases combined in InterPro (Table 2), PRINTS, PROSITE, and Pfam contain protein families in which the homology between each protein is predicted by the degree of sequence similarity [8]. The others—SMART, ProDom, PIRSF, SUPERFAMILY, PANTHER, CATH-Gene3D, TIGRFAM, and HAMAP [4-16]—have unique characteristics and URLs, and have been developed sharing information among each other and incorporating information from GO. In detail, PRINTS is a collection of diagnostic protein family "fingerprints", which are groups of conserved motifs, evident in multiple sequence alignments [6]; PRO-SITE is a protein domain database for functional characterization and annotation that consists of documentation entries describing protein domains, families, and functional sites as well as associated patterns and profiles to identify them [7]; Pfam contains collections of protein families, each represented by multiple sequence alignments and hidden Markov models, available via servers in the UK, the USA, and Sweden [8]; SMART (Simple Modular Architecture Research Tool) is an online resource for the identification and annotation of protein domains and the analysis of protein domain architectures [9]; ProDom is a comprehensive set of protein domain families generated automatically from the UniProt database [10]; PIRSF is a classification system that reflects evolutionary relationships among full-length proteins and domains [11]; SUPERFAMILY is a database of structural and functional annotation for all proteins and genomes [12]; PANTHER is a classification system that classifies genes by their functions using published experimental evidence and evolutionary relationships to predict function even in the absence of direct experimental evidence [13]; CATH-Gene3D is a comprehensive database of protein domain assignments for sequences from the major sequence databases [14]; TIGRFAM is a collection of protein family definitions built to aid high-throughput annotation of specific protein functions [15]; and HAMAP is composed of two databases: the proteome database and the family database, and of an automatic annotation pipeline mainly focused on microbial proteomes [16]. Hidden Markov models are usually used for the database algorithm.

Database Name	Context	URL	Reference
InterPro	integrative predictive models of protein families, domain and functional sites of multiple databases such as PRINTS, PROSITE, Pfam, SMART, ProDom, PIRSF, SUPERFAMILY, PANTHER, CATH-Gene3D, TIGRFAM, and HAMAP	http://www.ebi.ac.uk/interpro/	[4], [5]
PRINTS	a collection of diagnostic protein family "fingerprints" which are groups of conserved motifs, evident in multiple sequence alignments	http://www.bioinf.manchester.ac.uk/dbbrowser/PRINTS/index.php	[6]
PROSITE	a protein domain database for functional characterization and annotation which consists of documentation entries describing protein domains, families and functional sites as well as associated patterns and profiles to identify them	http://prosite.expasy.org/	[7]
Pfam	a database of collection of protein families, each represented by multiple sequence alignments and hidden Markov models, available via servers in the UK, the USA and Sweden	http://pfam.sanger.ac.uk/http://pfam.janelia.org/http://pfam.sbc.su.se/	[8]
SMART	an online resource for the identification and annotation of protein domains and the analysis of protein domain architectures, of which abbreviation is Simple Modular Architecture Research Tool	http://smart.embl.de/	[9]
ProDom	a comprehensive set of protein domain families automatically generated from the uniProt knowledge Database	http://prodom.prabi.fr/prodom/current/html/home.php	[10]
PIRSF	the classification system which reflects evolutionary relationships of full-length proteins and domains	http://pir.georgetown.edu/pirsf/	[11]
SUPERFAMILY	a database of structural and functional annotation for all proteins and genomes	http://supfam.org/SUPERFAMILY/	[12]
PANTHER	the classification system which classifies genes by their functions using published scientific experimental evidence and evolutionary relationships to predict function even in the absence of direct experimental evidence	http://www.pantherdb.org/	[13]
CATH-Gene3D	a comprehensive database of protein domain assignments for sequences from the major sequence databases	http://gene3d.biochem.ucl.ac.uk/	[14]

Database Name	Context	URL	Reference
TIGRFAM	a collection of protein family definitions built to aid in high-throughput annotation of specific protein functions	http://www.jcvi.org/cgi-bin/tigrfams/index.cgi	[15]
HAMAP	a system which composed of two databases, the proteome database and the family database, and of an automatic annotation pipeline	http://hamap.expasy.org/	[16]

Table 2. Database information.

2. Gene regulation

2.1. Gene markers for cancer and cancer stem cells

Several molecular markers of cancer have been identified [17]. Metastatic cancer cells can transfer into bodily fluids through the cellular epithelia, which enables the detection of cancer markers in bodily fluids such as blood plasma, urine, or saliva [17]. The different types of cancer markers include genomic DNA point mutations, microsatellite alterations, promoter hypermethylation, viral sequences, aberrant chromosomal copy number, chromosomal translocations, deletions, or loss of heterozygosity, telomere extension, alterations in RNA or protein expression, and mitochondrial DNA mutations [17].

Molecular markers of cancer include *TP53* (encoding p53), which has been shown to be mutated in head and neck, lung, colon, pancreatic, and bladder cancer [17,18]; colon, lung, esophagus, breast, liver, brain, reticuloendothelial tissue, and hematopoietic tissue cancers [19]; and bladder cancer [20]. Mutation of the epidermal growth factor receptor (*EGFR*) gene is an important predictive/prognostic factor for EGFR-tyrosine kinase inhibitor therapy in non-small cell lung cancer [21]. *RAS* oncogene mutations have been identified in colorectal tumors [22]. Microsatellites, which are tandem iterations of simple di-, tri-, or tetranucleotide repeats, have been reported to be unstable in some inherited diseases and in some types of cancer [23], including head and neck, lung, breast, and bladder cancer [17,23].

The expression levels of the cell cycle-related proteins p21 (*CDKN1A*), p53 (*TP53*), cyclin D1 (*CCND1*), and aurora kinase A (*AURKA*) may be used as prognostic markers to predict recurrence in stage II and stage III colon cancer [24]. In addition, markers of the epithelial–mesenchymal transition (EMT)–such as reduced expression of keratins, a switch from E-Cadherin to N-Cadherin, and enhanced migration in D492M cells—might be a useful marker in breast cancer [25]. Furthermore, expression of the stem cell markers cytokeratins 15 and 19 was altered in squamous cell carcinoma: cytokeratin 15 levels were decreased and the localization of cytokeratin 19 was altered [26]. *KLK3*, which encodes prostate-specific antigen, a member of the kallikrein family of serine proteases, is a biomarker for prostate cancer detection and disease monitoring [27,28]. Mitochondrial DNA mutations have been associated with bladder, head and neck, lung, colorectal, and pancreatic cancer [29-32] (Table 3).

Highly parallel identification of cancer-related genes using small hairpin RNA screening has revealed that the expression of known and putative oncogenes, such as *EGFR, KRAS, MYC, BCR-ABL, MYB, CRKL,* and *CDK4* that are essential for cancer proliferation, is altered in cancer cells [33]. Other genes such as *PTPN1, NF1, SMARCB1,* and *SMARCE1* have been identified as essential for the imatinib response of leukemia cells, and *TOPOIIA* expression is involved in resistance to etoposide, an anti-topoisomerase II agent, in small cell lung cancer [33-36].

Marker	Cancer Type	Reference
	head and neck cancer	[18]
	bladder cancer	[20]
TP53 mutation		
	lung cancer (small cell lung cancer and non-small cell lung cancer); breast, colon, esophagus, liver, bladder, ovary, and brain cancers; sarcomas, lymphomas, and leukemias	[19]
EGFR mutation	non-small cell lung cancer	[21]
RAS mutation	colorectal tumors	[22]
DNA microsatellite alterations	bladder cancer	[23]
alteration in cell cycle mRNA expression	colon cancer	[24]
alteration in cytokeratin mRNA expression	squamous cell carcinoma	[26]
alteration in kallikrein mRNA expression	prostate cancer	[27]
	bladder cancer, head and neck cancer, lung cancer	[29]
mitochondrial DNA mutations	colorectal tumors	[30], [32]
	pancreatic cancer	[31]

Table 3. Genomic markers of cancer.

2.2. Genes related to cell proliferation

Cyclins, which regulate the cell cycle, play important roles in cell proliferation and the uncontrolled cell proliferation that is the most important factor in tumorigenesis [37]. Tumor cells accumulate mutations that result in constitutive mitogenic signaling and defective responses to anti-mitogenic signals that contribute to unscheduled proliferation [38]. In cancer, unscheduled proliferation, genomic instability, and chromosomal instability are the three major factors in cell cycle dysregulation [38]. Regulation of the cell cycle is mainly conducted by complexes of cyclins and cyclin-dependent kinases [38]. Cyclin D1 in cell migration and proliferation is temporo-spatially separated by its biphasic expression induced by thrombin, a G protein-coupled receptor agonist, which is mediated by nuclear factor of activated T cells c1 (*NFATC1*) and signal transducer and activator of transcription 3 (*STAT3*) [39]. Cyclin D1 regulates kinase activity and the G_1–S phase transition in the cell cycle; deregulated cyclin D1 expression is well documented in breast, colon, and prostate cancers [39,40]. The expression of cyclin D1 is regulated by several factors including cytokines such as interleukin 3 and interleukin 6 *via* STAT3 and STAT5, or extracellular matrix factors such as collagen, fibronectin, and vitronectin, which activate focal adhesion kinase upon integrin clustering, and hepatocyte nuclear factor 6 [41]. Cyclin D1 is a crucial regulator of Wnt- and Notch-regulated development [41,42]. The binding of Wnt to its receptor, Frizzled, causes release of β-catenin to translocate from the cytoplasm to the nucleus, where it forms a complex with the ternary complex factor and/or the lymphoid enhancer-binding factor [41,43]. Cyclin D1 is induced by overexpression of β-catenin, which is a major component of adherens junctions that link the actin cytoskeleton to members of the cadherin family of transmembrane cell–cell adhesion receptors. It plays an important role in linking the cytoplasmic side of cadherin-mediated cell–cell contacts to the actin cytoskeleton [43]. Beta-catenin is upregulated in colorectal cancer, which is considered to trigger cyclin D1 gene expression followed by uncontrolled progression of the cell cycle [43]. In addition, β-catenin plays another role in signaling that involves transactivation, in complex with transcription factors of the lymphoid enhancing factor family in the nucleus [43]. The pathway involving β-catenin/LEF1 and elevation of cyclin D1 might be crucial for tumorigenesis [43]. Inhibiting EglN2, a member of the EglN (also called PHD or HPH) family of prolyl hydroxylases that regulates the heterodimeric transcription factor hypoxia-inducible factor (HIF), causes a decrease in the expression of its interaction partner cyclin D1 in cancer cells and impairs the cells' ability to proliferate *in vivo* [44].

Progression of the eukaryotic cell cycle is driven by cyclin-dependent protein kinases (CDKs), which are binding partner of cyclins. The CDK oscillator acts as the primary organizer of the cell cycle [45]. Phosphorylation of cyclin-Cdk complexes is one of the primary mechanisms of cell cycle regulation [46]. Cyclins are degraded by ubiquitin-mediated proteolysis [46]. The ubiquitylation and degradation of cyclin 1 and cyclin 2 are mediated by the SCF complex, a multi-subunit ubiquitin ligase that contains Skp1, a member of the cullin family (Cdc53) and an F-box protein, as well as a RING-finger-containing protein [46]. CDKs including CDK1, CDK2, CDK4, CDK6, and CDK11 have various functions that have been investigated using loss-of-function, target validation, and gain-of-function mouse models [38]. CDK1 is a mitotic CDK, also known as cell division control protein 2 (CDC2). It is one of the master regulators of mitosis as it controls the centrosome cycle as well as mitotic onset; deficiency in CDK1 results in embryonic lethality in the first cell divisions [38,47]. CDK2, CDK4, and CDK6 are interphase CDKs that are not essential for the mammalian cell cycle; they are, however, required for the proliferation of specific cell types [38]. Deficiency in CDK2, CDK4, and CDK6 caused mid-gestation embryonic lethality because of hematopoietic defects [38,47].

2.3. Genes related to cell differentiation

Inhibitor of differentiation 1 (Id1) is associated with the induction of cell proliferation and invasion [48], as well as the invasive features of cancer and the EMT [48]. The *HOX* genes encode homeodomain-containing transcription factors involved in the regulation of cellular proliferation and differentiation during embryogenesis [49]. The expression of HOXA1, which plays an important role in proliferation, apoptosis, adhesion, invasion, the EMT, and anchorage-independent growth, was significantly increased in oral squamous cell carcinoma compared with in healthy oral mucosa [49], and it might be a useful prognostic marker for patients with this disease [49].

Wnt/β-catenin signaling controls skeletal development and differentiation [50]. The initiating step of skeletal development is mesenchymal condensation, during which mesenchymal progenitor cells are at least bipotentiate [50]. Osteochondral progenitor cells differentiate into osteoblasts instead of chondrocytes when Wnt/β-catenin signaling is activated [50]. *In vitro* models using human pluripotent stem cell-derived neural progenitor cells have been used to examine whether G11778A-mutated mitochondrial DNA, which is associated with Leber's hereditary optic neuropathy, might be involved in the differentiation of neural progenitor cells into neurons, oligodendrocytes, and astrocytes [51]. The differentiation of neural progenitor cells can be visualized by staining for the neuronal marker class III beta-tubulin [51]. Alternative splicing of exons play an important role in cellular differentiation and pathogenesis [52]. Alternative splicing in colorectal cancer and renal cell cancer samples has been analyzed by the Bioinformatics Exon Array Tool (BEAT, http://beat.ba.itb.cnr.it/) using an Affymetrix GeneChip Exon Array [52]. When the dataset was analyzed using GO terms, the cell differentiation (GO:0030154)-related gene delta-like 1 (Drosophila) (*DLL1*) was found to be involved in colorectal cancer [52].

2.4. Genes related to apoptosis

Cell proliferation and death are regulated by various molecules. Recently, microRNAs have been revealed to play important roles during death receptor-mediated apoptosis (programmed cell death) [53]. Transfection with miR-133b caused a proapoptotic effect on tumor necrosis factor alpha (TNFα)-stimulated HeLa cells [53]: the expression of apoptosis regulatory proteins such as transgelin 2 (TAGLN2), myosin, heavy chain 9, non-muscle (MYH9), cytoskeleton-associated protein 4 (CKAP4), polypyrimidine tract binding protein 1 (PTBP1), glutathione-S-transferase pi 1 (GSTP1), and copine III (CPNE3) were down-regulated compared with in control cells [53]. The BCL protein family plays a major role in regulation of the apoptotic cascade [54]. BCL2-associated protein (BAX) promotes apoptosis and delays disease progression, and has been associated with longer disease-free survival in patients with a number of gastrointestinal cancers, such as esophageal, stomach, small intestine, and colon cancer; moreover, high BCL6 expression is correlated with worse prognosis in patients with other gastrointestinal tumors, such as esophageal adenocarcinoma [54]. There are two major cell death pathways that transduce the effects of various death inducers: the extrinsic death pathway that is mediated through cell death receptors of the TNF receptor family, such as the Fas receptor; and the intrinsic death pathway that proceeds through mitochondria [55]. The expression of apoptosis signal-regulating kinase (ASK1), which plays an important role as a mitogen-activated protein kinase kinase kinase in apoptosis signaling, is increased in gastric cancer [56]. Furthermore, the levels of cyclin D1 and phosphorylated JNK were higher in gastric cancer than in non-tumor epithelium [56]. ASK1 may play a role in the development of gastric cancer [56].

2.5. Detection of cell proliferation or apoptosis

Several methods have been suggested for the diagnosis of cancer [57]. Protein markers for cancer include prostate-specific antigen for prostate cancer, CA125 for ovarian cancer, carcinoembryonic antigen for colon cancer, human chorionic gonadotropin for trophoblastic cancer, and a-fetoprotein for hepatocellular carcinoma and germ cell tumors [57]. Assays to detect telomerase activity in clinical samples include the TRAP (telomere repeat amplification protocol) assay, which involves protein extraction and subsequent primer-directed PCR amplification of telomere extensions [57].

Assays for the detection of kinases that regulate cell growth, proliferation, differentiation, and metabolism have been developed [58]. The assay technology includes fluorescence polarization to detect protein phosphorylation, scintillation proximity to detect protein dephosphorylation by phosphatases, fluorescence resonance energy transfer to detect protein cleavage or modification, immunosorbent assays to detect phosphorylation state, luciferase-based ATP detection to detect the kinase-dependent depletion of ATP, luminescent oxygen channeling to detect phosphorylation, time-resolved fluorescence resonance energy transfer to detect phosphopeptide formation, and enzyme fragment complementation to detect molecular interactions with kinases [58,59]. Cell proliferation can also be determined by the tetrazolium hydroxide (XTT) cell proliferation assay, in which absorbance is measured by an ELISA reader under 490-nm-wavelength light (Biological Industries) [60].

Cell proliferation assays and apoptosis assays have been used to examine the effects of inhibitors on cancer cells [61]. The cell proliferation of Neuro-2A cells, neuroblastoma cells, can be determined using the CellTiter 96 Aqueous Non-Radioactive Cell Proliferation Assay reagent (Promega) [61]. A colony formation assay using Neuro-2A cells was used to determine the effect of an inhibitor of GSK-3β [61]. In this experiment, colonies were allowed to form for 10 days, after which the cells were fixed with 70% ethanol and stained with 1% methylene blue. Apoptosis was then measured by flow cytometry using an Annexin V-allophycocyanin (APC) /propidium iodide (PI) detection kit (BD PharMingen) [61]. Apoptosis was also determined using 4'6-diamidino-2-phenylindole (DAPI) staining, observing apoptotic nuclear morphology, and immunoblotting with antibodies to β-catenin, X-linked inhibitor of apoptosis, and BCL2 [61]. Cell cycle analysis using PI to quantify the proportions of cells in the G_1/G_0 or G_2–M phases was used to examine cell cycle status [61].

Viable cells can be determined using MTT (3-(4,5-dimethylthiazol-2-yl)-2,5-diphenyltetrazolium bromide) colorimetric assays [62]. Absorbance at 570 nm is used to detect the incorporation of MTT. Apoptosis can also be determined by caspase activation using an anti-poly ADP-ribose polymerase (PARP) antibody [62]. Viable cells can also be determined using a 3-(4,5-dimethyl-thiazol-2yl)-5-(3-carboxymethoxyphenyl)-2-(4-sulfophenyl)-2H-tetrazolium (MTS) kit (Promega) [63]. The terminal transferase dUTP nick end labeling (TUNEL) assay is commonly used to detect apoptosis [63]. Harvested cells are resuspended in DNA labeling solution consisting of TdT reaction buffer, TdT enzyme, and BrdUTP, then stained with PI to detect a fluorescein isothiocyanate-labeled anti-BrdU antibody [63]. Cell viability and proliferation assays were used to validate internal tandem duplication mutations in *FLT3* as a therapeutic target for human acute myeloid leukemia [64]. Cell viability and proliferation can be determined using a Vi-cell XR automated cell viability analyzer (Beckman Coulter) [64].

3. Genomic variation in disease

3.1. Genome-wide association studies in cancer

Despite extensive research efforts for several decades, the genetic basis of common human diseases such as cancers remains largely unknown [65]. Genome-wide association studies (GWAS) have emerged as an important tool for the discovery of genomic regions that harbor genetic variants conferring risk for various cancers [66,67]. Family-based linkage studies and studies comprising tens of thousands of gene-based SNPs can also assay genetic variation across the genome [68], but the National Institutes of Health guidelines for GWAS require a sufficient density of genetic markers to capture a large proportion of the common variants in the study population, measured in enough individuals to provide sufficient power to detect variants of modest effect [67]. The recent success of GWAS can be attributed to the convergence of new technologies that can genotype hundreds of thousands of SNPs in hundreds or thousands of samples [66,69].

GWAS have been conducted in the five of the most common cancer types: breast, prostate, colorectal, lung, and melanoma (Table 4) and have identified more than 20 novel disease loci, confirming that susceptibility to these diseases is polygenic [70]. For many years, human genetics has been used to map rare mutations with large effect sizes in families or genetically homogeneous populations, such as *BRCA1/BRCA2* mutations in Ashkenazi women with breast cancer and ovarian cancer [71]. A number of SNPs have now been associated with breast cancer; for example, a SNP in intron 2 of the *FGFR2* gene, which encodes a receptor tyrosine kinase that is amplified and overexpressed in 5–10% of breast tumors [72,73], and SNPs on chromosomes 16q and 5q. The locus on 16q contains a gene *TNRC9* and a hypothetical gene *LOC643714*. The function of TNRC9 is unknown but the presence of an HMG box motif suggests that it might act as a transcription factor. The 5q locus includes *MAP3K1*, which encodes a protein involved in signal transduction (but not previously known to be involved in cancer) and two other genes: *MGC33648* and *MIER3*. In addition, several of the breast cancer loci appear to be associated with specific subtypes of the disease. In particular, the *FGFR2* association is strongly associated with estrogen receptor-positive breast cancer, while the *TNRC9* SNP is associated with both estrogen receptor-positive and -negative breast cancer [74,75]. It is surprising that none of the strongest associations map to regions harboring estrogen/progesterone genes in women of European background, particularly because a GWAS in Asian women reported a convincing association with markers near the estrogen receptor alpha (*ESR1*) gene [76]. In prostate cancer, the first and most important region to emerge was 8q24. This region was first associated with prostate cancer through linkage studies by the deCode group, was followed up by association analyses [77], and has been confirmed in subsequent GWAS [78-81]. Another signal, on chromosome 10q13, points to a variant in the promoter of the *MSMB* gene, which encodes the PSP94 protein; this is now under intense investigation as a biomarker for prostate cancer [80,81].

In general, the susceptibility alleles discovered thus far are common—that is, with a frequency in one or more population of >10%, and each allele confers a small contribution to the overall risk of the disease. For nearly all regions conclusively identified by GWAS, the effect sizes per allele are estimated at <1.3. It was not anticipated that GWAS in certain cancers would yield many novel regions when other cancers strongly associated with particular environmental exposures have yielded so few regions. For example, prostate cancer, breast cancer, and colon cancer have been associated with 29, 13, and 10 regions of the genome, respectively, while there are only three associated regions for lung cancer in smokers, and three for bladder cancer despite analysis of sufficiently large data sets [67]. Several GWAS for lung cancer have identified the same locus on 15q25, suggesting that this is an important susceptibility locus for this disease [82-87]. This locus contains the nicotinic acetylcholine receptor subunit genes *CHRNA3* and *CHRNA5*, suggesting that susceptibility may be mediated through smoking behavior [86,87].

GWAS represent an important advance in discovering genetic variants influencing disease but have important limitations. There is a high potential for false-positive results, they do not yield information on gene function, they are insensitive to rare and structural variants, they require large sample sizes, and incur possible biases because of case and control selection and genotyping errors [88]. Clinicians and scientists must understand the unique aspects of these studies and be able to assess and interpret GWAS results for themselves and their patients. However, at present these studies mainly represent a valuable discovery tool for examining genomic function and clarifying pathophysiological mechanisms. However, through GWAS, the identification of variants, genes, and pathways involved in multiple cancers offers a potential route to new therapies, improved diagnosis, and better disease prevention [65].

Cancer type	Reference	Year	Platform [SNP passing QC]	Ethnic group	Initial sample size		Replication sample size		
					Cases	Controls	Ethnic groups	Cases	Controls
Breast cancer	[89]	2012	Affymetrix [555,525]	Korean	2,273	2,052	Korean	4,049	3,845
	[90]	2012	Affymetrix [690,947]	Chinese	2,918	2,324	Chinese	6,838	6,888
							Han Chinese	1,297	1,585
							Taiwan Chinese	1,066	1,065
							Korean	5,038	6,869
							Japanese	1,934	1,875

Cancer type	Reference	Year	Platform [SNP passing QC]	Ethnic group	Initial sample size		Replication sample size		
					Cases	Controls	Ethnic groups	Cases	Controls
	[91]	2012	Affymetrix [613,031]	Chinese	1,950	-	Chinese	4,160	-
	[92]	2012	Illumina [470,796]	Japanese	240	-	Japanese	222	-
	[93]	2011	Affymetrix [684,457]	East Asian	2,062	2,066	East Asians	15,091	14,877
	[94]	2011	Affymetrix [782,838]	European	302	321	European	1,153	1,215
	[95]	2011	Illumina [~296,114]	British	1,694	2,365	British	7,317	8,124
							European	1,145	1,142
	[96]	2010	Illumina [285,984]	Swedish & Finnish	617	4,583	European	1,001	7,604
	[97]	2010	Affymetrix [592,163]	European	899	804	European	1,264	1,222
	[98]	2010	Illumina [285,984]	European	2,702	5,726	European	7,386	7,576
	[99]	2010	Illumina [582,886]	UK	3,659	4,897	European	12,576	12,223
	[100]	2010	Illumina [528,252]	British	1,145	-	British	4,335	-
	[101]	2009	Illumina [528,173]		1,145	1,142		8,625	9,657
	[102]	2009	Affymetrix [up to 607,728]	Chinese	1,505	1,522	Chinese	1,554	1,576
	[103]	2008	Affymetrix [200,220]		30	30	-	-	-
	[104]	2008	Affymetrix [492,900]	Ashkenazi Jewish	249	299	Ashkenazi Jewish	1,193	1,166
	[105]	2007	Affymetrix [70,897]	Framing-ham	1,345	-	-	-	-
	[106]	2007	Perlegen [205,586]		390	634		26,646	24,889
	[107]	2007	Illumina [528,173]		1,145	1,142		1,176	2,072

Cancer type	Reference	Year	Platform [SNP passing QC]	Ethnic group	Initial sample size		Replication sample size		
					Cases	Controls	Ethnic groups	Cases	Controls
Prostate cancer	[108]	2012	Illumina [509,916]	European	1,176	1,101	European	1,964	3,172
	[109]	2012	Affymetrix & Illumina [1,117,531] (imputed)		4,723	4,792	-	-	-
	[110]	2011	NR [2.6 million] (imputed)	European	6,621	6,939	European	22,957	23,234
							Japanese	285	798
							Chinese	135	135
							African American	112	298
								7,140	5,455
	[111]	2011	Illumina [571,243]	European	2,782	4,458	European	8,217	6,732
	[112]	2011	Illumina [1,047,198]	African American	3,425	3,290	African American	1,275	1,695
							Senegalese	86	414
							Ghanaian	271	960
							Barbadian	246	253
	[113]	2011	Affymetrix [387,384]	European	202	100	European	1,122	1,167
	[114]	2010	Affymetrix [419,613]	Caucasian	222	415	Caucasian	500	155
	[115]	2010	Illumina [510,687]	Japanese	1,583	3,386	Japanese	3,001	5,415
	[116]	2009	Illumina [541,129]	European	1,854	1,894	European, Chinese, Japanese, African American, Latino, and Hawaiian	19,879	18,761
	[117]	2009	Illumina [310,520]	Icelandic	1,968	35,382	European	11,806	12,387
	[118]	2008	Illumina [541,129]	European	1,854	1,894		3,268	3,366

Cancer type	Reference	Year	Platform [SNP passing QC]	Ethnic group	Initial sample size		Replication sample size		
					Cases	Controls	Ethnic groups	Cases	Controls
	[119]	2008	Illumina [527,069]		1,172	1,157		3,941	3,964
	[120]	2007	Affymetrix & Illumina [60,275]		1,235	1,599		1,242	917
	[121]	2007	Affymetrix [70,897]	Framingham	1,345		-	-	-
	[122]	2007	Illumina [316,515]		1,453	3,064	East Asia	1,210	2,445
	[123]	2007	Illumina [538,548]		1,172	1,157		3,124	3,142
Colorectal cancer	[124]	2011	Illumina [378,739]	European	2,906	3,416	European	8,161	9,101
	[125]	2010	Illumina [~550,000] (imputed)	European	3,334	4,628	European	14,851	15,569
	[126]	2010	Affymetrix [460,945]	German	371	1,263	German Czech	4,121 794	7,344 815
	[127]	2008	Illumina [~548,586]		1,902	1,929		4,878	4,914
	[128]	2008	Illumina [541,628]		981	1,002		16,476	15,351
	[129]	2008	Illumina [547,647]		922	927		17,872	17,526
	[130]	2007	Illumina [547,647]		940	965		7,473	5,984
	[131]	2007	Illumina [547,647]		930	960		7,334	5,246
	[132]	2007	Affymetrix & Illumina [99,632]		1,257	1,336		6,223	6,443
Lung cancer	[133]	2011	Affymetrix [906,703]	Chinese	2,331	3,077	Chinese	6,313	6,409
	[134]	2011	Illumina [307,260]	White	327		European	587	

Cancer type	Reference	Year	Platform [SNP passing QC]	Ethnic group	Initial sample size		Replication sample size		
					Cases	Controls	Ethnic groups	Cases	Controls
	[135]	2011	Illumina [620,901] (pooled)	Italian	600	-	Italian	317	-
	[136]	2010	Affymetrix [265,996]	Han Chinese	245	-	Han Chinese	305	-
	[137]	2010	Affymetrix [246,758]	Korean	621	1,541	Korean	804	1,470
	[138]	2010	Illumina [542,050]		377	377		511	1,007
	[139]	2009	Illumina [515,922]	European	5,739	5,848	European	7,561	13,818
	[140]	2009	Illumina [511,919]	European	1,952	1,438	European	5,608	6,767
	[141]	2008	Illumina [317,498]		1,154	1,138		2,724	3,694
	[142]	2008	Illumina [306,207]		10,995 smokers			4,848 smokers	
	[143]	2008	Illumina [310,023]		1,926	2,522		2,513	4,752
	[144]	2007	Affymetrix [~116,204] (pooled)	Italian	338	335	Norwegian	265	356
Melanoma	[145]	2011	Illumina [594,997]	European	2,804	7,618	European	5,551	7,449
	[146]	2011	Illumina [5,480,804 (imputed)]	European	2,168	4,387	European	5,193	15,144
	[147]	2011	Illumina [818,977]	European	1,804	1,026	European	6,483	23,324
	[148]	2011	Illumina [491,227]	European	156	2,150	NR	-	-
	[149]	2009	Illumina [~317,000]	European	1,539	3,917	European	2,312	1,867

Table 4. Summary of GWAS for the five of the most common types of cancer.

3.2. Genetic risk score in cancer and diabetes

Type 2 diabetes mellitus and cancers are major health problems worldwide [150,151]. The recent increase in the prevalence of these diseases is largely attributable to environmental factors. However, convincing evidence shows that genetic factors may play an important role in these diseases [152,153]. Recent GWAS have led to the identification of a series of SNPs that are robustly associated with either the risk of diabetes or cancers [151,154-159]. For type 2 diabetes mellitus, common SNPs have been identified in the *PPARG, KCNJ11,* and *TCF7L2* genes, and have been widely replicated in populations of various ethnicities [160-162]. Other potential new loci include *HHEX, CDKAL1, CDKN2A/B, IGF2BP2, SLC30A8,* and *WFS1* [65,155-159,163,164]. A number of SNPs have been identified as associated with breast cancer risk, including *FGFR2, CASP8, ERBB4, TAB2, BARX2, TMEM45B, ESR1, FGFR2, TNRC9, MAP3K1, MGC33648, MIER3,* and *RAD51L1* [74,75,151] (Table 5).

Combining multiple loci with modest effects into a global genetic risk score (GRS) might improve the identification of those at risk for common complex diseases such as type 2 diabetes and cancers [165-167]. Several studies have developed methods to predict the risk of certain diseases, such as coronary heart disease, type 2 diabetes, and breast cancer, aggregating information from multiple SNPs into a single GRS [151,168,169]. For example, in the Atherosclerosis Risk in Communities study, the aggregation of multiple SNPs into a single GRS was responsible for improving the prediction of coronary heart disease incidence [168]. In a study that used a GRS to determine the risk of type 2 diabetes in US men and women, individuals in the highest quintile of GRS had a significantly increased risk of type 2 diabetes compared with those in the lowest quintile; however, the addition of a GRS to the conventional model consisting of lifestyle risk factors only increased the area under the curve by only 1% (AUC=0.78). In this instance, the GRS was determined to be useful only when combined with the body mass index or a family history of diabetes [169]. For breast cancer, a GRS was created using 14 SNPs previously associated with breast cancer, and was substantially more predictive of estrogen receptor-positive breast cancer than of estrogen receptor-negative breast cancer, particularly for absolute risk [151]. Further studies are needed to confirm whether a GRS improves disease risk prediction.

The GRS is calculated on the basis of reproducible tagging of SNP-associated loci reaching genome-wide levels of significance. The GRS can be created by two methods: a simple count method (count GRS) and a weighted method (weighted GRS) [169,170]. Both methods anticipate each SNP to be independently associated with risk. An additive genetic model is used for each SNP, applying a linear weighting of 0, 1, or 2 to genotypes containing 0, 1, or 2 risk alleles, respectively. This model is known to perform well even when the true genetic model is unknown or wrongly specified [171]. The count model assumes that each SNP in the panel contributes equally to the disease risk and is calculated by summing the values for each of the SNPs. The weighted GRS is calculated by multiplying each B-coefficient, the estimates resulting from an analysis carried out on variables that have been standardized, by the number of corresponding risk alleles (0, 1, or 2).

Disease	Reference	Year	Ethnic group	Participants	No. of SNPs	Genes found from GWAS
Type 2 diabetes	[165]	2008	Framingham	2,377 diabetic patients	18	NOTCH2 (rs10923931),
						BCL11A (rs10490072),
						THADA (rs7578597),
						IGF2BP2 (rs1470579),
						PPARg (rs1801282),
						ADAMTS9 (rs4607103),
						CDKAL (rs7754840),
						VEGFA (rs9472138),
						JAZF1 (rs86475),
						SLC30A8 (rs13266634),
						CDKNA/2B (rs10811661),
						HHEX (rs1111875),
						CDC123, CAMK1D (rs12779790),
						TCF7L2 (rs7903146),
						KCNJ11 (rs5219), INS (rs689),
						DCD (rs1153188),
						TSPAN8, LGR5 (rs7961581)
	[169]	2009	European	2,809 diabetic patients & 3,501 health controls	10	WFS1 (rs10010131),
						HHEX (rs1111875),
						CDKAL1 (rs7756992),
						IGF2BP2 (rs4402960),
						SLC30A8 (rs13266634),
						CDKN2A/B (rs10811661),
						TCF7L2 (rs12255372),
						PPARG (rs1801282),
						KCNJ11 (rs5219)
Breast cancer	[151]	2010	UK	10,306 breast cancer patients & 10,393 controls	14	FGFR2 (rs2981582),
						TNRC9 (rs3803662),
						2q35 (rs13387042),
						MAP3K1 (rs889312),
						8q24 (rs13281615),
						2p (rs4666451),
						5pas (rs981782),
						CASP8 (rs104548),
						LSP1 (rs3817198),
						5p (rs30099),
						TGFB1 (rs198/2073),
						ATM (rs1800054),
						TNRC9 (rs8051542),
						TNRC9 (rs12443621)

Table 5. Studies using a genetic risk score for cancers and diabetes, comprising SNPs identified in GWAS.

3.3. Cancer Cell Line Encyclopedia

The Cancer Cell Line Encyclopedia (CCLE) has made predictive modeling of anticancer drug sensitivity a realistic proposition, by determining genomic markers of drug sensitivity in cancer cells [172,173]. The CCLE contains information from 947 human cancer cell lines including data on gene expression, chromosomal copy number, and massively parallel sequencing data. It has been used to identify genetic, lineage-specific, and gene expression-based predictors of drug sensitivity [172]. This has revealed, for example, that the plasma cell lineage is correlated with sensitivity to IGF1 receptor inhibitors, aryl hydrocarbon receptor (*AHR*) expression is associated with MEK inhibitor efficacy in *NRAS*-mutant lines, and *SLFN11* expression is associated with sensitivity to topoisomerase inhibitors [172]. Genomic markers of drug sensitivity in cancer cells have also been systematically identified using the Genomics of Drug Sensitivity in Cancer database (http://www.cancerRxgene.org) [173]. These databases will enable to overview genome quality.

4. Conclusion

There are dramatic changes in the genomes of cancer cells, which vary according to cancer subtype. Integrative and wide investigations of cancer cell genomes have revealed mutations and alterations in gene expression that are associated with the disease. Databases that include abundant data related to gene and protein conformation, gene expression, and genomic mutations enable the construction of dynamic cellular simulations and disease models. New sequencing tools such as next-generation sequencing will reveal new horizons in the prediction of disease and drug sensitivity, which play an important role in personalized medicine. Appropriate translation of the abundance of information to clinical practice is one of most important future challenges for medicine. The quality of genome would be one of the important factors for detecting the development of the disease.

Acknowledgements

The authors are grateful to all those who helped with preparation of the manuscript. In particular, we thank Jaeseong Jo for his great assistance.

Author details

Shihori Tanabe[1*] and Sun Ha Jee[2]

*Address all correspondence to: stanabe@nihs.go.jp

1 National Institute of Health Sciences, Tokyo, Japan

2 Institute for Health Promotion, Yonsei University, Seoul, Korea

References

[1] Venter, J. C., Adams, M. D., Myers, E. W., Li, P. W., Mural, R. J., Sutton, G. G., et al. (2001). The sequence of the human genome. *Science*, 291(5507), 1304-1351.

[2] Lander, E. S., Linton, L. M., Birren, B., Nusbaum, C., Zody, M. C., Baldwin, J., et al. (2001). Initial sequencing and analysis of the human genome. Paper presented at International Human Genome Sequencing Consortium. *Nature*, 409(6822), 860-921.

[3] Ashburner, M., Ball, C. A., Blake, J. A., Botstein, D., Butler, H., Cherry, J. M., et al. (2000). Gene ontology: tool for the unification of biology. The Gene Ontology Consortium. *Nat. Genet.*, 25(1), 25-29.

[4] Hunter, S., Apweiler, R., Attwood, T. K., Bairoch, A., Bateman, A., Binns, D., et al. (2009). InterPro: the integrative protein signature database. *Nucleic Acids Res.*, 37, D211-D215.

[5] Hunter, S., Jones, P., Mitchell, A., Apweiler, R., Attwood, T. K., Bateman, A., et al. (2012). InterPro in 2011: new developments in the family and domain prediction database. *Nucleic Acids Res.*, 40, D306-D312.

[6] Attwood, T. K., Coletta, A., Muirhead, G., Pavlopoulou, A., Philippou, P. B., Popov, I., et al. (2012). The PRINTS database: a fine-grained protein sequence annotation and analysis resource--its status in 2012. *Database*, Oxford, bas019.

[7] Sigrist, C. J. A., Cerutti, L., de Castro, E., Langendijk-Genevaux, P. S., Bulliard, V., Bairoch, A., et al. (2010). PROSITE, a protein domain database for functional characterization and annotation. *Nucleic Acids Res.*, 38, D161-D166.

[8] Punta, M., Coggill, P. C., Eberhardt, R. Y., Mistry, J., Tate, J., Boursnell, C., et al. (2012). The Pfam protein families database. *Nucleic Acids Res.*, 40, D290-D301.

[9] Letunic, I., Doerks, T., & Bork, P. (2012). SMART7: recent updates to the protein domain annotation resource. *Nucleic Acids Res.*, 40, D302-D305.

[10] Bru, C., Courcelle, E., Carrère, S., Beausse, Y., Dalmar, S., & Kahn, D. (2005). The ProDom database of protein domain families: more emphasis on 3D. *Nucleic Acids Res.*, 33, D212-D215.

[11] Nikolskaya, A. N., Arighi, C. N., Huang, H., Barker, W. C., & Wu, C. H. (2007). PIRSF family classification system for protein functional and evolutionary analysis. *Evol. Bioinform*, Online, 2, 197-209.

[12] de Lima, Morais. D. A., Fang, H., Rackham, O. J. L., Wilson, D., Pethica, R., Chothia, C., et al. (2011). SUPERFAMILY 1.75 including a domain-centric gene ontology method. *Nucleic Acids Res.*, 39, D427-D434.

[13] Mi, H., Dong, Q., Muruganujan, A., Gaudet, P., Lewis, S., & Thomas, P. D. (2010). PANTHER version 7: improved phylogenetic trees, orthologs and collaboration with the Gene Ontology Consortium. *Nucleic Acids Res.*, 38, D204-D210.

[14] Lees, J., Yeats, C., Perkins, J., Sillitoe, I., Rentzsch, R., Dessailly, B. H., et al. (2012). Gene3D: a domain-based resource for comparative genomics, functional annotation and protein network analysis. *Nucleic Acids Res.*, 40, D465-D471.

[15] Selengut, J. D., Haft, D. H., Davidsen, T., Ganapathy, A., Gwinn-Giglio, M., Nelson, W. C., et al. (2007). TIGRFAMs and Genome Properties: tools for the assignment of molecular function and biological process in prokaryotic genomes. *Nucleic Acids Res.*, 35, D260-D264.

[16] Lima, T., Auchincloss, A. H., Coudert, E., Keller, G., Michoud, K., Rivoire, C., et al. (2009). HAMAP: a database of completely sequenced microbial proteome sets and manually curated microbial protein families in UniProtKB/ Swiss-Prot. *Nucleic Acids Res.*, 37, D471-D478.

[17] Sidransky, D. (2002). Emerging molecular markers of cancer. *Nat. Rev. Cancer*, 2(3), 210-219.

[18] Brennan, J. A., Mao, L., Hruban, R. H., Boyle, J. O., Eby, Y. J., Koch, W. M., et al. (1995). Molecular assessment of histopathological staging in squamous-cell carcinoma of the head and neck. *N. Engl. J. Med.*, 332(7), 429-435.

[19] Hollstein, M., Sidransky, D., Vogelstein, M., & Harris, C. C. (1991). p53 mutations in human cancers. *Science*, 253(5015), 49-53.

[20] Sidransky, D., Von Eschenbach, A., Tsai, Y. C., Jones, P., Summerhayes, I., Marshall, F., et al. (1991). Identification of p53 gene mutations in bladder cancers and urine samples. *Science*, 252(5006), 706-709.

[21] Rossi, A., & Galetta, D. (2012). Biomarkers for the targeted therapies of non-small cell lung cancer. *Current Biomarker Findings*, 2, 7-17.

[22] Sidransky, D., Tokino, T., Hamilton, S. R., Kinzler, K. W., Levin, B., Frost, P., et al. (1992). Identification of ras oncogene mutations in the stool of patients with curable colorectal tumors. *Science*, 256(5053), 102-105.

[23] Gonzalez-Zulueta, M., Ruppert, J. M., Tokino, K., Tsai, Y. C., Spruck, I. I. I. C. H., Miyano, N., et al. (1993). Microsatellite instability in bladder cancer. *Cancer Res.*, 53(23), 5620-5623.

[24] Belt, E. J. T., Brosens, R. P. M., Delis-van Diemen, P. M., Bril, H., Tijssen, M., van Essen, D. F., et al. (2012). Cell cycle proteins predict recurrence in stage II and III colon cancer. *Ann. Surg. Oncol.*, DOI: 10.1245/s10434-012-2216-7, Published online: 04 Feb 2012.

[25] Sigurdsson, V., Hilmarsdottir, B., Sigmundsdottir, H., Fridriksdottir, A. J. R., Ringnér, M., Villadsen, R., et al. (2011). Endothelial induced EMT in breast epithelial cells with stem cell properties. *PLoS One*, 6(9), e23833.

[26] Abbas, O., Richards, J. E., Yaar, R., & Mahalingam, M. (2011). Stem cell markers (cytokeratin 15, cytokeratin 19 and p63) in in situ and invasive cutaneous epithelial lesions. *Mod. Pathol.*, 24(1), 90-97.

[27] Kote-Jarai, Z., Amin, Al., Olama, A., Leongamornlert, D., Tymrakiewicz, M., Saunders, E., et al. (2011). Identification of a novel prostate cancer susceptibility variant in the KLK3 gene transcript. *Human Genet.*, 129(6), 687-694.

[28] Schröder, F., Hugosson, J., Roobol, M. J., Tammela, T. L. J., Ciatto, S., Nelen, V., et al. (2012). ERSPC Investigators. Prostate-cancer mortality at 11 years of follow-up. *N. Engl. J. Med.*, 366(11), 981-990.

[29] Fliss, M. S., Usadel, H., Caballero, O. L., Wu, L., Buta, M. R., Eleff, S. M., et al. (2000). Facile detection of mitochondrial DNA mutations in tumors and bodily fluid. *Science*, 287(5460), 2017-2019.

[30] Polyak, K., Li, Y., Zhu, H., Lengauer, C., Willson, J. K. V., Markowitz, S. D., et al. (1998). Somatic mutations of the mitochondrial genome in human colorectal tumours. *Nat. Genet.*, 20(3), 291-293.

[31] Lam, E. T., Bracci, P. M., Holly, E. A., Chu, C., Poon, A., Wan, E., et al. (2012). Mitochondrial DNA sequence variation and risk of pancreatic cancer. *Cancer Res.*, 72(3), 686-695.

[32] Skonieczna, K., Malyarchuk, B. A., & Grzybowski, T. (2012). The landscape of mitochondrial DNA variation in human colorectal cancer on the background of phylogenetic knowledge. *Biochim. Biophys. Acta*, 1825(2), 153-159.

[33] Luo, B., Cheung, H. W., Subramanian, A., Sharifnia, T., Okamoto, M., Yang, X., et al. (2008). Highly parallel identification of essential genes in cancer cells. *Proc. Natl. Acad. Sci.*, USA, 105(51), 20380-20385.

[34] Nitiss, J. L., Liu, Y., & Hsiung, Y. (1993). A temperature sensitive topoisomerase II allele confers temperature dependent drug resistance on amsacrine and etoposide: a genetic system for determining the targets of topoisomerase II inhibitors. *Cancer Res.*, 53(1), 89-93.

[35] Osheroff, N. (1989). Effect of antineoplastic agents on the DNA cleavage/religation reaction of eukaryotic topoisomerase II: inhibition of DNA religation by etoposide. *Biochemistry*, 28(15), 6157-6160.

[36] Hande, K. R. (1998). Etoposide: four decades of development of a topoisomerase II inhibitor. *European J. Cancer*, 34, 1514-1521.

[37] Sherr, C. J. (1996). Cancer cell cycles. *Science*, 274(5293), 1672-1677.

[38] Malumbres, M., & Barbacid, M. (2009). Cell cycle, CDKs and cancer: a changing paradigm. *Nat. Rev. Cancer*, 9(3), 153-166.

[39] Kundumani-Sridharan, V., Quyen, D. V., Subramani, J., Singh, N. K., Chin, Y. E., & Rao, G. N. (2012). Novel interactions between NFATc1 (nuclear factor of activated T cells c1) and STAT-3 (signal transducer and activator of transcription-3) mediate G protein-coupled receptor agonist, thrombin-induced biphasic expression of cyclin D1, with first phase influencing cell migration and second phase directing cell proliferation. *J. Biol. Chem.*, 287(27), 22463-22482.

[40] Landis, M. W., Pawlyk, B. S., Li, T., Sicinski, P., & Hinds, P. W. (2006). Cyclin D1-dependent kinase activity in murine development and mammary tumorigenesis. *Cancer Cell*, 9(1), 13-22.

[41] Klein, E. A., & Assoian, R. K. (2008). Transcriptional regulation of the cyclin D1 gene at a glance. *J. Cell Sci.*, 121, Pt 23, 3853-3857.

[42] Hsu, W., Shakya, R., & Costantini, F. (2001). Impaired mammary gland and lymphoid development caused by inducible expression of Axin in transgenic mice. *J. Cell Biol.*, 155(6), 1055-1064.

[43] Shtutman, M., Zhurinsky, J., Simcha, I., Albanese, C., D'Amico, M., Pestell, R., et al. (1999). The cyclin D1 gene is a target of the beta-catenin/LEF-1 pathway. *Proc. Natl. Acad. Sci.*, USA, 96(10), 5522-5527.

[44] Zhang, Q., Gu, J., Li, L., Liu, J., Luo, B., Cheung, H., et al. (2009). Control of cyclin D1 and breast tumorigenesis by the EglN2 prolyl hydroxylase. *Cancer Cell*, 16(5), 413-424.

[45] Coudreuse, D., & Nurse, P. (2010). Driving the cell cycle with a minimal CDK control network. *Nature*, 468(7327), 1074-1079.

[46] Bloom, J., & Cross, F. R. (2007). Multiple levels of cyclin specificity in cell-cycle control. *Nat. Rev. Mol. Cell Biol.*, 8(2), 149-160.

[47] Santamaría, D., Barrière, C., Cerqueira, A., Hunt, S., Tardy, C., Newton, K., et al. (2007). Cdk1 is sufficient to drive the mammalian cell cycle. *Nature*, 448(7155), 811-815.

[48] Tobin, N. P., Sims, A. H., Lundgren, K. L., Lehn, S., & Landberg, G. (2011). Cyclin D1, Id1 and EMT in breast cancer. *BMC Cancer*, 11, 417.

[49] Bitu, C., Destro, M., Carrera, M., Silva, S., Graner, E., Kowalski, L. P., Soares, F., et al. (2012). HOXA1 is overexpressed in oral squamous cell

carcinomas and its expression is correlated with poor prognosis. *BMC Cancer*, 12, 146.

[50] Yang, Y. (2012). Wnt signaling in development and disease. *Cell & Bioscience*, 2, 14.

[51] Iyer, S., Xiao, E., Alsayegh, K., Eroshenko, N., Riggs, M. J., Bennett, J. P., et al. (2012). Mitochondrial gene replacement in human pluripotent stem cell-derived neural progenitors. *Gene Ther.*, 19(5), 469-475.

[52] Consiglio, A., Carella, M., De Caro, G., Delle, Foglie. G., Giovannelli, C., Grillo, G., et al. (2012). BEAT: Bioinformatics Exon Array Tool to store, analyze and visualize Affymetrix GeneChip Human Exon Array data from disease experiments. *BMC Bioinformatics*, 13(Suppl 4), S21.

[53] Patron, J. P., Fendler, A., Bild, M., Jung, U., Müller, H., Arntzen, M., et al. (2012). MiR-133b targets antiapoptotic genes and enhances death receptor-induced apoptosis. *PLoS One*, 7(4), e35345.

[54] Alevizos, L., Gomatos, I. P., Smparounis, S., Konstadoulakis, M. M., & Zografos, C. (2012). Review of the molecular prolife and modern prognostic markers for gastric lymphoma: how do they affect clinical practice? *Can. J. Surg.*, 55(2), 117-124.

[55] Aoudjit, F., & Vuori, K. (2012). Integrin signaling in cancer cell survival and chemoresistance. *Chemother. Res. Pract.*, 2012, 283181.

[56] Hayakawa, Y., Hirata, Y., Nakagawa, H., Sakamoto, K., Hikiba, Y., Kinoshita, H., et al. (2011). Apoptosis signal-regulating kinase 1 and cyclin D1 compose a positive feedback loop contributing to tumor growth in gastric cancer. *Proc. Natl. Acad. Sci.*, USA, 108(2), 780-785.

[57] Cairns, P., & Sidransky, D. (1999). Molecular methods for the diagnosis of cancer. *Biochim. Biophys. Acta*, 1423(2), C11-C18.

[58] Glickman, J. F., Mc Gee, J., & Napper, A. (2004). *Assay development for protein kinase enzyme. Assay Guidance Manual [Internet]. Sittampalam GS, Weidner J, Auld D, et al., editors*, Bethesda (MD): Eli Lilly & Company and the National Center for Advancing Translational Sciences, 2012.

[59] Eglen, R. M., & Singh, R. (2003). Beta galactosidase enzyme fragment complementation as a novel technology for high throughput screening. *Comb. Chem. High Throughput Screen.*, 6(4), 381-387.

[60] Baran, Y., Zencir, S., Cakir, Z., Ozturk, E., & Topcu, Z. (2011). Imatinib-induced apoptosis: a possible link to topoisomerase enzyme inhibition. *J. Clin. Pharm. Ther.*, 36(6), 673-679.

[61] Dickey, A., Schleicher, S., Leahy, K., Hu, R., & Hallahan, D. (2011). Thotala DK GSK-3β inhibition promotes cell death, apoptosis, and in vivo tumor

growth delay in neuroblastoma Neuro-2A cell line. *J. Neurooncol.*, 104(1), 145-153.

[62] Wang, L., Hurley, D. G., Watkins, W., Araki, H., Tamada, Y., Muthukaruppan, A., et al. (2012). Cell cycle gene networks are associated with melanoma prognosis. *PLoS One*, 7(4), e34247.

[63] Kim, J., Chae, M., Kim, W. K., Kim, Y., Kang, H. S., Kim, H. S., et al. (2011). Salinomycin sensitizes cancer cells to the effects of doxorubicin and etoposide treatment by increasing DNA damage and reducing p21protein. *Br. J. Pharmacol.*, 162(3), 773-784.

[64] Smith, C. C., Wang, Q., Chin, C., Salerno, S., Damon, L. E., Levis, M. J., et al. (2012). Validation of ITD mutations in FLT3 as a therapeutic target in human acute myeloid leukaemia. *Nature*, 485(7397), 260-263.

[65] Wellcome Trust Case Control Consortium. (2007). Genome-wide association study of 14,000 cases of seven common diseases and 3,000 shared controls. *Nature*, 447(7145), 661-668.

[66] National Institutes of Health. (2007). Policy for sharing of data obtained in NIH supported or conducted genome-wide association studies (GWAS). *Federal Regist.*, 72(166), 49290-49297, http://www.grants.nih.gov/grants/guide/notice-files/NOT-OD-07-088.html, accessed 3 July 2012.

[67] Chung, C. C., Magalhaes, W. C., Gonzalez-Bosquet, J., & Chanock, S. J. (2010). Genome-wide association studies in cancer--current and future directions. *Carcinogenesis*, 31(1), 111-120.

[68] Hampe, J., Franke, A., Rosenstiel, P., Till, A., Teuber, M., Huse, K., et al. (2007). A genome-wide association scan of nonsynonymous SNPs identifies a susceptibility variant for Crohn disease in ATG16L1. *Nat. Genet.*, 39(2), 207-211.

[69] Manolio, T. A. (2010). Genomewide association studies and assessment of the risk of disease. *N. Engl. J. Med.*, 363(2), 166-176.

[70] Easton, D. F., & Eeles, R. A. (2008). Genome-wide association studies in cancer. *Hum. Mol. Genet.*, 17(R2), R109-R115.

[71] Miki, Y., Swensen, J., Shattuck-Eidens, D., Futreal, P. A., Harshman, K., Tavtigian, S., et al. (1994). A strong candidate for the breast and ovarian cancer susceptibility gene BRCA1. *Science*, 266(5182), 66-71.

[72] Adnane, J., Gaudray, P., Dionne, C. A., Crumley, G., Jaye, M., Schlessinger, J., et al. (1991). BEK and FLG, two receptors to members of the FGF family, are amplified in subsets of human breast cancers. *Oncogene*, 6(4), 659-663.

[73] Greenman, C., Stephens, P., Smith, R., Dalgliesh, G. L., Hunter, C., Bignell, G., et al. (2007). Patterns of somatic mutation in human cancer genomes. *Nature*, 446(7132), 153-158.

[74] Garcia-Closas, M., Hall, P., Nevanlinna, H., Pooley, K., Morrison, J., Richesson, D., et al. (2008). Heterogeneity of breast cancer associations with five susceptibility loci by clinical and pathological characteristics. *PloS Genet.*, 4(4), e1000054.

[75] Antoniou, A. C., Spurdle, A. B., Sinilnikova, O. M., Healey, S., Pooley, K. A., Schmutzler, R. K., et al. (2008). CIMBA. Common breast cancer-predisposition alleles are associated with breast cancer risk in BRCA1 and BRCA2 mutation carriers. *Am. J. Hum. Genet.*, 82(4), 937-948.

[76] Zheng, W., Long, J., Gao, Y. T., Li, C., Zheng, Y., Xiang, Y. B., et al. (2009). Genome-wide association study identifies a new breast cancer susceptibility locus at 6q25.1. *Nat. Genet.*, 41(3), 324-328.

[77] Amundadottir, L. T., Sulem, P., Gudmundsson, J., Helgason, A., Baker, A., Agnarsson, B. A., et al. (2006). A common variant associated with prostate cancer in European and African populations. *Nat. Genet.*, 38(6), 652-658.

[78] Yeager, M., Orr, N., Hayes, R. B., Jacobs, K. B., Kraft, P., Wacholder, S., et al. (2007). Genome-wide association study of prostate cancer identifies a second risk locus at 8q24. *Nat. Genet.*, 39(5), 645-649.

[79] Gudmundsson, J., Sulem, P., Manolescu, A., Amundadottir, L. T., Gudbjartsson, D., Helgason, A., et al. (2007). Genome-wide association study identifies a second prostate cancer susceptibility variant at 8q24. *Nat. Genet.*, 39(5), 631-637.

[80] Eeles, R. A., Kote-Jarai, Z., Giles, G. G., Olama, A. A., Guy, M., Jugurnauth, S. K., et al. (2008). Multiple newly identified loci associated with prostate cancer susceptibility. *Nat. Genet.*, 40(30), 316-321.

[81] Thomas, G., Jacobs, K. B., Yeager, M., Kraft, P., Wacholder, S., Orr, N., et al. (2008). Multiple loci identified in a genome-wide association study of prostate cancer. *Nat. Genet.*, 40(3), 310-315.

[82] Chanock, S. J., & Hunter, D. J. (2008). Genomics: when the smoke clears. *Nature*, 452(7187), 537-538.

[83] Hung, R. J., Mc Kay, J. D., Gaborieau, V., Boffetta, P., Hashibe, M., Zaridze, D., et al. (2008). A susceptibility locus for lung cancer maps to nicotinic acetylcholine receptor subunit genes on 15q25. *Nature*, 452(7187), 633-637.

[84] Mc Kay, J. D., Hung, R. J., Gaborieau, V., Boffetta, P., Chabrier, A., Byrnes, G., et al. (2008). Lung cancer susceptibility locus at 5p15. *Nat. Genet.*, 40(12), 1404-1406.

[85] Wang, Y., Broderick, P., Webb, E., Wu, X., Vijayakrishnan, J., Matakidou, A., et al. (2008). Common 5p15and 6p21.33 variants influence lung cancer risk. *Nat. Genet.*, 40(12), 1407-1409.

[86] Bierut, L. J., Madden, P. A., Breslau, N., Johnson, E. O., Hatsukami, D., Pomerleau, O. F., et al. (2007). Novel genes identified in a high-density genome wide association study for nicotine dependence. *Hum. Mol. Genet.*, 16(1), 24-35.

[87] Caporaso, N., Gu, F., Chatterjee, N., Sheng-Chih, J., Yu, K., Yeager, M., et al. (2009). Genome-wide and candidate gene association study of cigarette smoking behaviors. *PloS One*, 4(2), e4653.

[88] Pearson, T. A., & Manolio, T. A. (2008). How to interpret a genome-wide association study. *JAMA*, 299(11), 1335-1344.

[89] Kim, H. C., Lee, J. Y., Sung, H., Choi, J. Y., Park, S. K., Lee, K. M., et al. (2012). A genome-wide association study identifies a breast cancer risk variant in ERBB4 at 2q34: results from the Seoul Breast Cancer Study. *Breast Cancer Res.*, 14, R56.

[90] Long, J., Cai, Q., Sung, H., Shi, J., Zhang, B., Choi, J. Y., et al. (2012). Genome-wide association study in east Asians identifies novel susceptibility loci for breast cancer. *PLoS Genet.*, 8(2), e1002532.

[91] Shu, X. O., Long, J., Lu, W., Li, C., Chen, W. Y., Delahanty, R., et al. (2012). Novel genetic markers of breast cancer survival identified by a genome-wide association study. *Cancer Res.*, 72(5), 1182-1189.

[92] Kiyotani, K., Mushiroda, T., Tsunoda, T., Morizono, T., Hosono, N., Kubo, M., et al. (2012). A genome-wide association study identifies locus at 10q22 associated with clinical outcomes of adjuvant tamoxifen therapy for breast cancer patients in Japanese. *Hum. mol. genet.*, 21(7), 1665-1672.

[93] Cai, Q., Long, J., Lu, W., Qu, S., Wen, W., Kang, D., et al. (2011). Genome-wide association study identifies breast cancer risk variant at 10q21.2: results from the Asia Breast Cancer Consortium. *Hum. Mol. Genet.*, 20(24), 4991-4999.

[94] Sehrawat, B., Sridharan, M., Ghosh, S., Robson, P., Cass, C. E., Mackey, J. R., et al. (2011). Potential novel candidate polymorphisms identified in genome-wide association study for breast cancer susceptibility. *Hum. Genet.*, 130(4), 529-537.

[95] Fletcher, O., Johnson, N., Orr, N., Hosking, F. J., Gibson, L. J., Walker, K., et al. (2011). Novel breast cancer susceptibility locus at 9q31.2: results of a genome-wide association study. *J. Natl. Cancer Inst.*, 103(5), 425-435.

[96] Li, J., Humphreys, K., Darabi, H., Rosin, G., Hannelius, U., Heikkinen, T., et al. (2010). A genome-wide association scan on estrogen receptor-negative breast cancer. *Breast Cancer Res.*, 12(6), R93.

[97] Gaudet, M. M. , Kirchhoff, T., Green, T., Vijai, J., Korn, J. M., Guiducci, C., et al. (2010). Common genetic variants and modification of penetrance of BRCA2-associated breast cancer. *PloS Genet.*, 6(10), e1001183.

[98] Li, J., Humphreys, K., Heikkinen, T., Aittomäki, K., Blomqvist, C., Pharoah, P. D., et al. (2011). A combined analysis of genome-wide association studies in breast cancer. *Breast Cancer Res Treat.*, 126(3), 717-727.

[99] Turnbull, C., Ahmed, S., Morrison, J., Pernet, D., Renwick, A., Maranian, M., et al. (2010). Genome-wide association study identifies five new breast cancer susceptibility loci. *Nat. Genet.*, 42(6), 504-507.

[100] Azzato, E. M., Pharoah, P. D., Harrington, P., Easton, D. F., Greenberg, D., Caporaso, N. E., et al. (2010). A genome-wide association study of prognosis in breast cancer. *Cancer Epidemiol. Biomarkers Prev.*, 19(4), 1140-1143.

[101] Thomas, G., Jacobs, K. B., Kraft, P., Yeager, M., Wacholder, S., Cox, D. G., et al. (2009). A multistage genome-wide association study in breast cancer identifies two new risk alleles at 1p11and 14q24.1 (RAD51L1). *Nat. Genet.*, 41(5), 579-584.

[102] Zheng, W., Long, J., Gao, Y. T., Li, C., Zheng, Y., Xiang, Y. B., et al. (2009). Genome-wide association study identifies a new breast cancer susceptibility locus at 6q25.1. *Nat. Genet.*, 41(3), 324-328.

[103] Kibriya, M. G., Jasmine, F., Argos, M., Andrulis, I. L., John, E. M., Chang-Claude, J., et al. (2009). A pilot genome-wide association study of early-onset breast cancer. *Breast Cancer Res. Treat.*, 114(3), 463-477.

[104] Gold, B., Kirchhoff, T., Stefanov, S., Lautenberger, J., Viale, A., Garber, J., et al. (2008). Genome-wide association study provides evidence for a breast cancer risk locus at 6q22.33. *Proc. Natl. Acad. Sci.*, USA, 105(11), 4340-4345.

[105] Murabito, J. M., Rosenberg, C. L., Finger, D., Kreger, B. E., Levy, D., Splansky, G. L., et al. (2007). A genome-wide association study of breast and prostate cancer in the NHLBI's Framingham Heart Study. *BMC Med. Genet.*, 8(Suppl 1), S6.

[106] Easton, D. F., Pooley, K. A., Dunning, A. M., Pharoah, P. D., Thompson, D., Ballinger, D. G., et al. (2007). Genome-wide association study identifies novel breast cancer susceptibility loci. *Nature*, 447(7148), 1087-1093.

[107] Hunter, D. J., Kraft, P., Jacobs, K. B., Cox, D. G., Yeager, M., Hankinson, S. E., et al. (2007). A genome-wide association study identifies alleles in FGFR2

associated with risk of sporadic postmenopausal breast cancer. *Nat. Genet.*, 39(7), 870-874.

[108] Tao, S., Feng, J., Webster, T., Jin, G., Hsu, F. C., Chen, S. H., et al. (2012). Genome-wide two-locus epistasis scans in prostate cancer using two European populations. *Hum. Genet.*, 131, 1225-1234.

[109] Tao, S., Wang, Z., Feng, J., Hsu, F. C., Jin, G., Kim, S. T., et al. (2012). A genome-wide search for loci interacting with known prostate cancer risk-associated genetic variants. *Carcinogenesis*, 33(3), 598-603.

[110] Kote-Jarai, Z., Olama, A. A., Giles, G. G., Severi, G., Schleutker, J., Weischer, M., et al. (2011). UK Genetic Prostate Cancer Study Collaborators/British Association of Urological Surgeons' Section of Oncology; UK ProtecT Study Collaborators, The Australian Prostate Cancer BioResource; PRACTICAL Consortium. Seven prostate cancer susceptibility loci identified by a multi-stage genome-wide association study. *Nat. Genet.*, 43(8), 785-791.

[111] Schumacher, F. R., Berndt, S. I., Siddiq, A., Jacobs, K. B., Wang, Z., Lindstrom, S., et al. (2011). Genome-wide association study identifies new prostate cancer susceptibility loci. *Hum. Mol. Genet.*, 20(19), 3867-3875.

[112] Haiman, C. A., Chen, G. K., Blot, W. J., Strom, S. S., Berndt, S. I., Kittles, R. A., et al. (2011). Genome-wide association study of prostate cancer in men of African ancestry identifies a susceptibility locus at 17q21. *Nat. Genet.*, 43(6), 570-573.

[113] Fitz, Gerald L. M., Kwon, E. M., Conomos, M. P., Kolb, S., Holt, S. K., Levine, D., et al. (2011). Genome-wide association study identifies a genetic variant associated with risk for more aggressive prostate cancer. *Cancer Epidemiol. Biomarkers Prev.*, 20(6), 1196-1203.

[114] Penney, K. L., Pyne, S., Schumacher, F. R., Sinnott, J. A., Mucci, L. A., Kraft, P. L., et al. (2010). Genome-wide association study of prostate cancer mortality. *Cancer Epidemiol. Biomarkers Prev.*, 19(11), 2869-2876.

[115] Takata, R., Akamatsu, S., Kubo, M., Takahashi, A., Hosono, N., Kawaguchi, T., et al. (2010). Genome-wide association study identifies five new susceptibility loci for prostate cancer in the Japanese population. *Nat. Genet.*, 42(9), 751-754.

[116] Eeles, R. A., Kote-Jarai, Z., Al Olama, A. A., Giles, G. G., Guy, M., Severi, G., et al. (2009). UK Genetic Prostate Cancer Study Collaborators/British Association of Urological Surgeons' Section of Oncology; UK ProtecT Study Collaborators; PRACTICAL Consortium, Easton DF Identification of seven new prostate cancer susceptibility loci through a genome-wide association study. *Nat. Genet.*, 41(10), 1116-1121.

[117] Gudmundsson, J., Sulem, P., Gudbjartsson, D. F., Blondal, T., Gylfason, A., Agnarsson, B. A., et al. (2009). Genome-wide association and replication studies identify four variants associated with prostate cancer susceptibility. *Nat. Genet.*, 41(10), 1122-1126.

[118] Eeles, R. A., Kote-Jarai, Z., Giles, G. G., Olama, Guy. M., Jugurnauth, S. K., et al. (2008). UK Genetic Prostate Cancer Study Collaborators; British Association of Urological Surgeons' Section of Oncology; UK ProtecT Study Collaborators. Multiple newly identified loci associated with prostate cancer susceptibility. *Nat. Genet.*, 40(3), 316-321.

[119] Thomas, G., Jacobs, K. B., Yeager, M., Kraft, P., Wacholder, S., Orr, N., et al. (2008). Multiple loci identified in a genome-wide association study of prostate cancer. *Nat. Genet.*, 40(3), 310-315.

[120] Duggan, D., Zheng, S. L., Knowlton, M., Benitez, D., Dimitrov, L., Wiklund, F., et al. (2007). Two genome-wide association studies of aggressive prostate cancer implicate putative prostate tumor suppressor gene DAB2IP. *J. Natl. Cancer Inst.*, 99(24), 1836-1844.

[121] Murabito, J. M., Rosenberg, C. L., Finger, D., Kreger, B. E., Levy, D., Splansky, G. L., et al. (2007). A genome-wide association study of breast and prostate cancer in the NHLBI's Framingham Heart Study. *BMC Med. Genet.*, 8(Suppl 1), S6.

[122] Gudmundsson, J., Sulem, P., Manolescu, A., Amundadottir, L. T., Gudbjartsson, D., Helgason, A., et al. (2007). Genome-wide association study identifies a second prostate cancer susceptibility variant at 8q24. *Nat. Genet.*, 39(5), 631-637.

[123] Yeager, M., Orr, N., Hayes, R. B., Jacobs, K. B., Kraft, P., Wacholder, S., et al. (2007). Genome-wide association study of prostate cancer identifies a second risk locus at 8q24. *Nat. Genet.*, 39(5), 645-649.

[124] Peters, U., Hutter, C. M., Hsu, L., Schumacher, F. R., Conti, D. V., Carlson, C. S., et al. (2012). Meta-analysis of new genome-wide association studies of colorectal cancer risk. *Hum. Genet.*, 131(2), 217-234.

[125] Houlston, R. S., Cheadle, J., Dobbins, S. E., Tenesa, A., Jones, A. M., Howarth, K., et al. (2010). Meta-analysis of three genome-wide association studies identifies susceptibility loci for colorectal cancer at 1q41, 3q26.2, 12q13.13 and 20q13.33. *Nat. Genet.*, 42(11), 973-977.

[126] Lascorz, J., Försti, A., Chen, B., Buch, S., Steinke, V., Rahner, N., et al. (2010). Genome-wide association study for colorectal cancer identifies risk polymorphisms in German familial cases and implicates MAPK signalling pathways in disease susceptibility. *Carcinogenesis*, 31(9), 1612-1619.

[127] Houlston, R. S., Webb, E., Broderick, P., Pittman, A. M., Di Bernardo, M. C., Lubbe, S., et al. (2008). Meta-analysis of genome-wide association data identifies four new susceptibility loci for colorectal cancer. Paper presented at International Colorectal Cancer Genetic Association Consortium. *Nat. Genet.*, 40(12), 1426-1435.

[128] Tenesa, A., Farrington, S. M., Prendergast, J. G., Porteous, M. E., Walker, M., Haq, N., et al. (2008). Genome-wide association scan identifies a colorectal cancer susceptibility locus on 11q23 and replicates risk loci at 8q24 and 18q21. *Nat. Genet.*, 40(5), 631-637.

[129] Tomlinson, I. P., Webb, E., Carvajal-Carmona, L., Broderick, P., Howarth, K., Pittman, A. M., et al. (2008). A genome-wide association study identifies colorectal cancer susceptibility loci on chromosomes 10p14and 8q23.3. *Nat. Genet.*, 40(5), 623, 630.

[130] Broderick, P., Carvajal-Carmona, L., Pittman, A. M., Webb, E., Howarth, K., Rowan, A., et al. (2007). CORGI Consortium. A genome-wide association study shows that common alleles of SMAD7 influence colorectal cancer risk. *Nat. Genet.*, 39(11), 1315-1317.

[131] Tomlinson, I., Webb, E., Carvajal-Carmona, L., Broderick, P., Kemp, Z., Spain, S., et al. (2007). A genome-wide association scan of tag SNPs identifies a susceptibility variant for colorectal cancer at 8q24.2. *Nat. Genet.*, 39(8), 984-988.

[132] Zanke, B. W., Greenwood, C. M., Rangrej, J., Kustra, R., Tenesa, A., Farrington, S. M., et al. (2007). Genome-wide association scan identifies a colorectal cancer susceptibility locus on chromosome 8q24. *Nat. Genet.*, 39(8), 989-994.

[133] Hu, Z., Wu, C., Shi, Y., Guo, H., Zhao, X., Yin, Z., et al. (2011). A genome-wide association study identifies two new lung cancer susceptibility loci at 13q12.12 and 22q12.2 in Han Chinese. *Nat. Genet.*, 43(8), 792-796.

[134] Wu, X., Ye, Y., Rosell, R., Amos, C. I., Stewart, D. J., Hildebrandt, et., & al, . (2011). Genome-wide association study of survival in non-small cell lung cancer patients receiving platinum-based chemotherapy. *J. Natl. Cancer Inst.*, 103(10), 817-825.

[135] Frullanti, E., Galvan, A., Falvella, F. S., Manenti, G., Colombo, F., Vannelli, A., et al. (2011). Multiple genetic loci modulate lung adenocarcinoma clinical staging. *Clin. Cancer Res.*, 17(8), 2410-2416.

[136] Wu, C., Xu, B., Yuan, P., Miao, X., Liu, Y., Guan, Y., et al. (2010). Genome-wide interrogation identifies YAP1 variants associated with survival of small-cell lung cancer patients. *Cancer Res.*, 70(23), 9721-9729.

[137] Yoon, K. A., Park, J. H., Han, J., Park, S., Lee, G. K., Han, J. Y., et al. (2010). A genome-wide association study reveals susceptibility variants for non-small cell lung cancer in the Korean population. *Hum. Mol. Genet.*, 19(24), 4948-4954.

[138] Li, Y., Sheu, C. C., Ye, Y., de Andrade, M., Wang, L., Chang, S. C., et al. (2010). Genetic variants and risk of lung cancer in never smokers: a genome-wide association study. *Lancet Oncol.*, 11(4), 321-330.

[139] Landi, M. T., Chatterjee, N., Yu, K., Goldin, L. R., Goldstein, A. M., Rotunno, M., et al. (2009). A genome-wide association study of lung cancer identifies a region of chromosome 5p15associated with risk for adenocarcinoma. *Am. J. Hum. Genet.*, 85(5), 679-691.

[140] Broderick, P., Wang, Y., Vijayakrishnan, J., Matakidou, A., Spitz, M. R., Eisen, T., et al. (2009). Deciphering the impact of common genetic variation on lung cancer risk: a genome-wide association study. *Cancer Res.*, 69(19), 6633-6641.

[141] Amos, C. I., Wu, X., Broderick, P., Gorlov, I. P., Gu, J., Eisen, T., et al. (2008). Genome-wide association scan of tag SNPs identifies a susceptibility locus for lung cancer at 15q25.1. *Nat. Genet.*, 40(5), 616-622.

[142] Thorgeirsson, T. E., Geller, F., Sulem, P., Rafnar, T., Wiste, A., Magnusson, K. P., et al. (2008). A variant associated with nicotine dependence, lung cancer and peripheral arterial disease. *Nature*, 452(7187), 638-642.

[143] Hung, R. J., Mc Kay, J. D., Gaborieau, V., Boffetta, P., Hashibe, M., Zaridze, D., et al. (2008). A susceptibility locus for lung cancer maps to nicotinic acetylcholine receptor subunit genes on 15q25. *Nature*, 452(7187), 633-637.

[144] Spinola, M., Leoni, V. P., Galvan, A., Korsching, E., Conti, B., Pastorino, U., et al. (2007). Genome-wide single nucleotide polymorphism analysis of lung cancer risk detects the KLF6 gene. *Cancer Lett.*, 251(2), 311-316.

[145] Barrett, J. H., Iles, M. M., Harland, M., Taylor, J. C., Aitken, J. F., Andresen, P. A., et al. (2011). GenoMEL Consortium. Genome-wide association study identifies three new melanoma susceptibility loci. *Nat. Genet.*, 43(11), 1108-1113.

[146] Mac Gregor, S., Montgomery, G. W., Liu, J. Z., Zhao, Z. Z., Henders, A. K., Stark, M., et al. (2011). Genome-wide association study identifies a new melanoma susceptibility locus at 1q21.3. *Nat. Genet.*, 43(11), 1114-1118.

[147] Amos, C. I., Wang, L. E., Lee, J. E., Gershenwald, J. E., Chen, W. V., Fang, S., et al. (2011). GenoMEL Investigators. Genome-wide association study identifies novel loci predisposing to cutaneous melanoma. *Hum. Mol. Genet.*, 20(24), 5012-5023.

[148] Teerlink, C., Farnham, J., Allen-Brady, K., Camp, N. J., Thomas, A., Leachman, S., et al. (2012). A unique genome-wide association analysis in extended Utah high-risk pedigrees identifies a novel melanoma risk variant on chromosome arm 10q. *Hum. Genet.*, 131(1), 77-85.

[149] Bishop, D. T., Demenais, F., Iles, M. M., Harland, M., Taylor, J. C., Corda, E., et al. (2009). Genome-wide association study identifies three loci associated with melanoma risk. *Nat. Genet.*, 41(8), 920-925.

[150] King, H., Aubert, R. E., & Herman, W. H. (1998). Global burden of diabetes, 1995-2025: prevalence, numerical estimates, and projections. *Diabetes Care*, 21(9), 1414-1431.

[151] Reeves, G. K., Travis, R. C., Green, J., Bull, D., Tipper, S., Baker, K., et al. (2010). Incidence of breast cancer and its subtypes in relation to individual and multiple low-penetrance genetic susceptibility loci. *JAMA*, 304(4), 426-434.

[152] Kaprio, J., Tuomilehto, J., Koskenvuo, M., Romanov, K., Reunanen, A., Eriksson, J., et al. (1992). Concordance for type 1 (insulin-dependent) and type 2 (non-insulin-dependent) diabetes mellitus in a population-based cohort of twins in Finland. *Diabetologia*, 35(11), 1060-1067.

[153] Risch, N. (1990). Linkage strategies for genetically complex traits. I. Multilocus models. *Am. J. Hum. Genet.*, 46(2), 222-228.

[154] Grant, S. F., Thorleifsson, G., Reynisdottir, I., Manolescu, A., Sainz, J., Helgason, A., et al. (2006). Variant of transcription factor 7-like 2 (TCF7L2) gene confers risk of type 2 diabetes. *Nat. Genet.*, 38(3), 320-323.

[155] Sladek, R., Rocheleau, G., Rung, J., Dina, C., Shen, L., Serre, D., et al. (2007). A genome-wide association study identifies novel risk loci for type 2 diabetes. *Nature*, 445(7130), 881-885.

[156] Saxena, R., Voight, B. F., Lyssenko, V., Burtt, N. P., de Bakker, P. I., Chen, H., et al. (2007). Genome-wide association analysis identifies loci for type 2 diabetes and triglyceride levels. *Science*, 316(5829), 1331-1336.

[157] Scott, L. J., Mohlke, K. L., Bonnycastle, L. L., Willer, C. J., Li, Y., Duren, W. L., et al. (2007). A genome-wide association study of type 2 diabetes in Finns detects multiple susceptibility variants. *Science*, 316(5829), 1341-1345.

[158] Zeggini, E., Weedon, M. N., Lindgren, C. M., Frayling, T. M., Elliott, K. S., Lango, H., et al. (2007). Wellcome Trust Case Control Consortium (WTCCC). Replication of genome-wide association signals in UK samples reveals risk loci for type 2 diabetes. *Science*, 316(5829), 1336-1341.

[159] Zeggini, E., Scott, L. J., Saxena, R., Voight, B. F., Marchini, J. L., Hu, T., et al. (2008). Meta-analysis of genome-wide association data and large-scale

replication identifies additional susceptibility loci for type 2 diabetes. *Nat. Genet.*, 40(5), 638-645.

[160] van Dam, R. M., Hoebee, B., Seidell, J. C., Schaap de, Bruin. T. W., & Feskens, E. J. (2005). Common variants in the ATP-sensitive K+ channel genes KCNJ11 (Kir6.2) and ABCC8 (SUR1) in relation to glucose intolerance: population-based studies and meta-analyses. *Diabet. Med.*, 22(5), 590-598.

[161] Ludovico, O., Pellegrini, F., Di Paola, R., Minenna, A., Mastroianno, S., Cardellini, M., et al. (2007). Heterogeneous effect of peroxisome proliferator-activated receptor gamma2 Ala12 variant on type 2 diabetes risk. *Obesity (Silver Spring)*, 15(5), 1076-1081.

[162] Cauchi, S., El Achhab, Y., Choquet, H., Dina, C., Krempler, F., Weitgasser, R., et al. (2007). TCF7L2 is reproducibly associated with type 2 diabetes in various ethnic groups: a global meta-analysis. *J. Mol. Med.*, 85(7), 777-782.

[163] Steinthorsdottir, V., Thorleifsson, G., Reynisdottir, I., Benediktsson, R., Jonsdottir, T., Walters, G. B., et al. (2007). A variant in CDKAL1 influences insulin response and risk of type 2 diabetes. *Nat. Genet.*, 39(6), 770-775.

[164] Sandhu, M. S., Weedon, M. N., Fawcett, K. A., Wasson, J., Debenham, S. L., Daly, A., et al. (2007). Common variants in WFS1 confer risk of type 2 diabetes. *Nat. Genet.*, 39(8), 951-953.

[165] Meigs, J. B., Shrader, P., Sullivan, L. M., Mc Ateer, J. B., Fox, C. S., Dupuis, J., et al. (2008). Genotype score in addition to common risk factors for prediction of type 2 diabetes. *N. Engl. J. Med.*, 359(21), 2208-2219.

[166] Weedon, M. N., Mc Carthy, M. I., Hitman, G., Walker, M., Groves, C. J., Zeggini, E., et al. (2006). Combining information from common type 2 diabetes risk polymorphisms improves disease prediction. *PloS. Med.*, 3(10), e374.

[167] Wray, N. R., Goddard, M. E., & Visscher, P. M. (2007). Prediction of individual genetic risk to disease from genome-wide association studies. *Genome Res.*, 17(10), 1520-1528.

[168] Morrison, A. C., Bare, L. A., Chambless, L. E., Ellis, S. G., Malloy, M., Kane, J. P., et al. (2007). Prediction of coronary heart disease risk using a genetic risk score: the Atherosclerosis Risk in Communities Study. *Am. J. Epidemiol.*, 166(1), 28-35.

[169] Cornelis, M. C., Qi, L., Zhang, C., Kraft, P., Manson, J., Cai, T., et al. (2009). Joint effects of common genetic variants on the risk for type 2 diabetes in U.S. men and women of European ancestry. *Ann. Intern. Med.*, 150(8), 541-550.

[170] Ripatti, S., Tikkanen, E., Orho-Melander, M., Havulinna, Silander. K., Sharma, A., et al. (2010). A multilocus genetic risk score for coronary heart disease: case-control and prospective cohort analyses. *Lancet*, 376(9750), 1393-1400.

[171] Balding, D. J. (2006). A tutorial on statistical methods for population association studies. *Nat. Rev. Genet.*, 7(10), 781-791.

[172] Barretina, J., Caponigro, G., Stransky, N., Venkatesan, K., Margolin, Kim. S., et al. (2012). The Cancer Cell Line Encyclopedia enables predictive modelling of anticancer drug sensitivity. *Nature*, 483(7391), 603-607.

[173] Garnett, N. J., Edelman, E. J., Heidorn, S. J., Greenman, C. D., Dastur, A., Lau, K. W., et al. (2012). Systematic identification of genomic markers of drug sensitivity in cancer cells. *Nature*, 483(7391), 570-575.

Permissions

The contributors of this book come from diverse backgrounds, making this book a truly international effort. This book will bring forth new frontiers with its revolutionizing research information and detailed analysis of the nascent developments around the world.

We would like to thank Dr. Isin Akyar, for lending her expertise to make the book truly unique. She has played a crucial role in the development of this book. Without her invaluable contribution this book wouldn't have been possible. She has made vital efforts to compile up to date information on the varied aspects of this subject to make this book a valuable addition to the collection of many professionals and students.

This book was conceptualized with the vision of imparting up-to-date information and advanced data in this field. To ensure the same, a matchless editorial board was set up. Every individual on the board went through rigorous rounds of assessment to prove their worth. After which they invested a large part of their time researching and compiling the most relevant data for our readers. Conferences and sessions were held from time to time between the editorial board and the contributing authors to present the data in the most comprehensible form. The editorial team has worked tirelessly to provide valuable and valid information to help people across the globe.

Every chapter published in this book has been scrutinized by our experts. Their significance has been extensively debated. The topics covered herein carry significant findings which will fuel the growth of the discipline. They may even be implemented as practical applications or may be referred to as a beginning point for another development. Chapters in this book were first published by InTech; hereby published with permission under the Creative Commons Attribution License or equivalent.

The editorial board has been involved in producing this book since its inception. They have spent rigorous hours researching and exploring the diverse topics which have resulted in the successful publishing of this book. They have passed on their knowledge of decades through this book. To expedite this challenging task, the publisher supported the team at every step. A small team of assistant editors was also appointed to further simplify the editing procedure and attain best results for the readers.

Our editorial team has been hand-picked from every corner of the world. Their multi-ethnicity adds dynamic inputs to the discussions which result in innovative outcomes. These outcomes are then further discussed with the researchers and contributors who give their valuable feedback and opinion regarding the same. The feedback is then collaborated with the researches and they are edited in a comprehensive manner to aid the understanding of the subject.

Apart from the editorial board, the designing team has also invested a significant amount of their time in understanding the subject and creating the most relevant covers. They scrutinized every image to scout for the most suitable representation of the subject and create an appropriate cover for the book.

The publishing team has been involved in this book since its early stages. They were actively engaged in every process, be it collecting the data, connecting with the contributors or procuring relevant information. The team has been an ardent support to the editorial, designing and production team. Their endless efforts to recruit the best for this project, has resulted in the accomplishment of this book. They are a veteran in the field of academics and their pool of knowledge is as vast as their experience in printing. Their expertise and guidance has proved useful at every step. Their uncompromising quality standards have made this book an exceptional effort. Their encouragement from time to time has been an inspiration for everyone.

The publisher and the editorial board hope that this book will prove to be a valuable piece of knowledge for researchers, students, practitioners and scholars across the globe.

List of Contributors

Kung-Tien Liu and Chien-Hsin Chen
Everlight Chemical Industrial Corporation, Taiwan

Jian-Hua Zhao and Lee-Chung Men
Chemistry Division, Institute of Nuclear Energy Research, Taiwan

Stephen Inkoom
Radiation Protection Institute, Ghana Atomic Energy Commission, Legon, Accra, Ghana

Barbara Testagrossa, Giuseppe Acri, Federica Causa, Maria Giulia Tripepi and Giuseppe Vermiglio
Environmental, Health, Social and Industrial Department - University of Messina, Italy

Raffaele Novario
Department of Biotechnologies and Life Sciences– University of Insubria, Italy

Xuemin Zhu and Sen Qian
The Institute of High Energy Physics, Chinese Academy of Sciences, China

Bruna Galdorfini Chiari, Maria Gabriela José de Almeida, Marcos Antonio Corrêa and Vera Lucia Borges Isaac
Faculdade de Ciências Farmacêuticas, UNESP - Univ Estadual Paulista, Departamento de Fármacos e Medicamentos, Laboratório de Cosmetologia – LaCos, Araraquara, Laboratório de Cosmetologia, São Paulo, Brazil

Isin Akyar
Acibadem University Faculty of Medicine Department of Microbiology, Turkey

Onur Karatuna
Acibadem University, Istanbul, Turkey

Stella Lai, Chuan-Ching Lan, Jennifer M. Love and Elaine Doherty
Diagnostic Genetics, Auckland City Hospital, New Zealand

Renate Marquis-Nicholson and Donald R. Love
School of Biological Sciences, The University of Auckland, New Zealand

Jonathan R. Skinner
Inherited Disease Group New Zealand, Paediatric Cardiac Services, Starship Children's Hospital, New Zealand

Lisa Duffy, Liangtao Zhang and Alice M. George
LabPlus, Auckland City Hospital, Auckland, New Zealand
School of Biological Sciences, The University of Auckland, New Zealand

Donald R. Love
LabPlus, Auckland City Hospital, Auckland, New Zealand

D. M. Saidemberg, A. L. C. Faria, S. B. Sartor, D. N. Oliveira and R. R. Catharino
INNOVARE Biomarkers Laboratory, Department of Clinical Pathology, School of Medical Sciences, University of Campinas, Brazil

F. G. Ravagnani
INNOVARE Biomarkers Laboratory, Department of Clinical Pathology, School of Medical Sciences, University of Campinas, Brazil
Laboratory of Bioenergetics, Department of Clinical Pathology, School of Medical Sciences, University of Campinas, Brazil

Shihori Tanabe
National Institute of Health Sciences, Tokyo, Japan

Sun Ha Jee
Institute for Health Promotion, Yonsei University, Seoul, Korea